Physiotherapy in Orthopaedics

A problem-solving approach

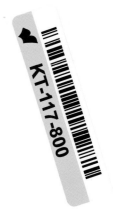

Karen Atkinson MSc GradDipPhys CertEd DipTP
Senior Lecturer, Department of Health Sciences,
University of East London, London

Fiona Coutts MSc MCSP
Principal Lecturer in Physiotherapy, Department of Health Sciences
University of East London, London

Anne-Marie Hassenkamp MSc MCSP MACP
Senior Lecturer, Department of Health Sciences,
University of East London, London

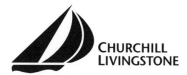

CHURCHILL
LIVINGSTONE

EDINBURGH LONDON NEW YORK PHILADELPHIA SYDNEY TORONTO 1999

CHURCHILL LIVINGSTONE
An Imprint of Harcourt Publishers Limited

Churchill Livingstone, Robert Stevenson House, 1–3 Baxter's Place,
Leith Walk, Edinburgh EH1 3AF, UK

First published 1999
  Reprinted 2000

ISBN 0 443 05074 0

British Library Cataloguing in Publication Data
A catalogue record for this book is available from the British Library.

Library of Congress Cataloging in Publication Data
A catalog record for this book is available from the Library of
Congress.

Medical knowledge is constantly changing. As new information
becomes available, changes in treatment, procedures, equipment
and the use of drugs become necessary. The authors and the
publishers have, as far as it is possible, taken care to ensure that the
information given in this text is accurate and up to date. However,
readers are strongly advised to confirm that information, especially
with regard to drug usage, complies with the latest legisation and
standards of practice.

The authors and publishers have made every effort to trace the
copyright holders for borrowed material. If they have inadvertently
over-looked any, they will be pleased to make the necessary
arrangements at the first opportunity.

The
publisher's
policy is to use
**paper manufactured
from sustainable forests**

Printed in China
NPCC/02

Contents

Preface

Orthopaedics is very wide-ranging and complex area of patient management. It encompasses conditions due to both trauma and disease which present within different client groups. Patients with orthopaedic problems are encountered throughout the physiotherapist's working life. They may present with a primary condition for the physiotherapist to treat specifically, or with problems requiring physiotherapy which have developed as a result of other pathologies. However, despite the importance of orthopaedic conditions to physiotherapy practice, it seems that orthopaedics is often preceived as a 'basic' subject which physiotherapy students should get to grips with early on in their programmes of study. Not surprisingly, given the wide variety of orthopaedic disorders which a physiotherapist may encounter, many students are daunted by the prospect of absorbing the knowledge and learning the skills necessary to work in this area.

As the authors of *Physiotherapy in Orthopaedics* we firmly believe that a good knowledge of orthopaedics is fundamental to sound physiotherapy practice. In preparing this text we have drawn on our many years of experience of clinical work in various orthopaedic settings and of teaching at both undergraduate and postgraduate levels. Its development was prompted after observing the difficulties that students (and some junior physiotherapists) have with their clinical reasoning when faced with apparently diverse patient problems. There is a tendency to rely on treatment 'recipes' so that when encountering patients with a particular injury or condition the student falls back on rote learning. We believe it is important that the therapist should learn to examine the person in front of them and then make decisions based on the information gathered. Although injuries and conditions vary, within the range of orthopaedics many of the signs and symptoms will be the same. Similarly, the physiotherapeutic interventions used in these situations are the same. The difficult part is being able to decompartmentalise them and this is where clinical reasoning and decision making are so important. It is for this reason that we have taken a problem-solving approach to the subject throughout the book.

The content of the book moves from normal to abnormal and from simple to complex. We have used case studies and self-assessment sections to encourage participation by the reader. The authors hope that this text will go some way towards helping undergraduate physiotherapy students to develop a reasoned and logical approach towards the management of their orthopaedic patients.

Introduction

How to use this book

Objectives

By the end of this section you should:

1. Be familiar with the format in which the book is presented, therefore making it easier for you to use.
2. Be aware of the aims and objectives of the book.
3. Understand the general framework within the text of moving from normal to abnormal, simple to complex and so on, and why this method is used.

OVERALL APPROACH TO ORTHOPAEDICS

This book is designed to look at orthopaedics somewhat differently from the way you may be used to. The overall approach is one of problem solving.

Usually in orthopaedics books, each condition is dealt with in turn, and the management described. Obviously the information given is extremely relevant, but can be quite repetitive with little stimulation or encouragement for you to apply your knowledge. If orthopaedic problems are looked at in a more global way, their management is often similar or at least may overlap in many areas, so perhaps each condition does not necessarily need to be considered as a totally separate unit. It would therefore seem reasonable to assume that the knowledge gained from dealing with one type of problem could be transferred to the management of others where appropriate.

In the light of this, the aim of the book is to tackle the subject from a different angle: groups of conditions with similar signs and symptoms are considered. For each group, problems are highlighted that patients with those conditions may experience. Then the interventions which may help to alleviate or remove those problems are presented.

You will be encouraged to take part in this process of problem solving, designing what you consider to be suitable strategies with regard to different scenarios. For ease of reference, the groups of conditions are considered in separate sections, but unnecessary repetition is avoided whenever possible. As well as physiotherapy aspects, the roles of other health care professionals, carers and of course the patients themselves are considered.

Issues regarding prevention and education related to patient management are also included whenever possible.

It is intended that by the time you have finished reading this book you will be able to consider a large range of orthopaedic patients and have a good idea of at least the types of treatment and advice that could benefit them. You will also be in a position to consider possible input from the rest of the health care team.

STRUCTURE OF THIS BOOK

General

Before you start to look at orthopaedics, it is a good idea for you to think about what 'problem solving' actually means, and what it involves. So first of all you will find a brief explanation of how the book is set out. Then Chapter 1 introduces you to the concepts of problem solving in the general sense; this will be put into the clinical perspective in Chapter 5.

The first five chapters are intended to be introductory, laying the foundations and giving the background necessary for you to be able to use the rest of the book successfully. They are also designed to make you think about different issues concerned with problem solving: the normal and abnormal changes occurring in the body throughout life, assessment and clinical practice.

Key words

Under each chapter heading you will find a list of key words. These highlight the major points that are covered in that section. All of the key words are defined in the glossary which you can find towards the back of the book.

Objectives and prerequisites

After the key words in each chapter there is a list of objectives which gives you an indication of what you can learn from reading and working through that section. Where appropriate, there are also some prerequisites so that you are aware of what you 'should know' before beginning that chapter.

Review points

At intervals within some chapters you will find sections headed 'Review points'. These indicate stages where you should review what has been covered before moving on to the next section. In this way you will keep a continual check on your progress.

Problem-solving exercises

As you work through the chapters of the book

you are presented with a number of problem-solving exercises. In the first chapter they deal with general problems, but later on they are related to clinical issues and case studies.

The exercises will be indicated as follows: **Problem-solving exercise 1.1** – the first number signifies the chapter you are in, and the second gives the sequence of the exercises (for example, in this case '1.1' denotes Chapter 1 and the first exercise within that chapter).

In connection with each problem-solving exercise there will usually be some questions. These are designed to direct you towards the areas you ought to be considering. They are indicated by capital letters **A**, **B**, etc.

Where the problem-solving exercises concern case studies, you are asked to consider each case in the light of the knowledge you have gained from earlier sections and to decide how you might manage it. It is envisaged that you will gradually develop some idea of clinical decision-making skills from this process. An example of this is prioritisation, which may involve the following types of question: 'Which of the patient's problems are the most important and need to be dealt with first?' or 'Will other members of the health care team be involved, and if so, which ones and when?' and so on.

The case studies are used to illustrate important points about the problem-solving approach and the management of particular client groups.

Suggested solutions to the problem-solving exercises may be given at the end of the appropriate chapter if they have not already been dealt with in the text.

Self-assessment questions

A number of self-assessment questions (SAQs) are included in each chapter. They are numbered, in Chapter 1 for example, as **SAQ 1.1**, **SAQ 1.2** etc., in Chapter 2 as **SAQ 2.1**, **SAQ 2.2** and so on. These questions will help you to determine how much you have understood from the preceding sections. As with the problem-solving exercises, where appropriate, solutions to the self-assessment questions are given at the end of the chapter. Sometimes, however, they are given immediately after the question and sometimes

solutions may be found from information given in the text.

The summary

Just before you reach the solutions for the exercises and questions in each chapter, you will find a summary. This, used in conjunction with the list of objectives at the beginning of the chapter, gives an overview of the areas you have covered. It also provides another indication of how much information you have absorbed.

AIMS AND RATIONALE

It is intended that, as you read, you will become an active participant in the process of problem-solving with a special emphasis on orthopaedics. You will gradually begin to understand, and feel ready to apply, the concepts presented in the text. This book has been designed with a pyramidal framework in mind (see Fig. I.1). It tackles issues by first addressing the simple and gradually expanding to encompass the more complex.

At the beginning, this takes the form of the

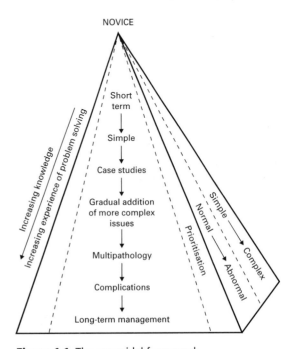

Figure 1.1 The pyramidal framework.

transition from the normal condition of the body through to abnormal; that is, when do normal changes in the tissues start to cause problems for the individual? An example of this is the natural ageing process: most older people will complain of some aches and pains, but at what point do these become severe enough to warrant intervention from health professionals? Following on from this, you are introduced to straightforward case studies which gradually progress by the addition of extra facets for you to consider, for example different age groups or possible complications. Later on, the actual case studies deal with more complex conditions, and the extra aspects and differences involved in short- and long-term management are brought in. So you start at the point of the pyramid and work your way down, gradually broadening your approach and considering more and more aspects in relation to the cases presented. This process will involve the transference of knowledge and the problem-solving skills you have obtained in the earlier sections.

Research has shown that people rely heavily on 'worked out' examples in solving exercise problems (Kahney 1993), especially in new areas. In accordance with this, you are initially provided with lots of information, help and guidance. But, as you work through the book, you are given less help and so do more of the problem solving independently. However, if you do run into problems, remember you can find the solutions at the ends of the chapters.

Summary

This section has introduced you to the general framework of the book, and the format of the chapters has been briefly explained. This includes Key words, Objectives, Prerequisites, Review points, Problem-solving exercises and Self-assessment questions. The aims and rationale of the book have also been briefly presented.

By working through the chapters and using the various methods described above to monitor and analyse your progress, you will become familiar with the problem-solving process and how this can be applied in the clinical orthopaedic setting.

REFERENCE

Kahney H 1993 Problem solving: current issues, 2nd edn. Open University Press, Buckingham

1

Introduction to problem solving

■ Problem solving ■ Decision making ■ Clinical reasoning

Objectives

By the end of this chapter you should:

1. Grasp the basic concepts of problem solving.
2. Begin to be able to appreciate the synthesis of the problem-solving approach with clinical orthopaedic practice.

Prerequisites

You should have read the introduction 'How to use this book' before starting this chapter.

PROBLEM SOLVING

Although a problem-solving approach has been heralded recently as a new and innovative way to deal with patient management in the clinical setting, it is in fact something that everyone is extremely familiar with. This process begins very early in life, although of course, those initial problems, such as 'How can I reach that lovely colourful toy?' seem very simple later on. But when a child is only just at the stage of starting to crawl, it must seem very complex. What may be problematic for a child may not be so for an adult. Reaching the toy will be a dilemma the first few times the situation is encountered, but it ceases to be a difficulty once the child learns how to do it.

For a physiotherapy student, discovering how to use an ultrasound machine could be a problem the first time, as it can seem rather complex and not easy to understand. It does not remain so for long however, whereas deciding on the physiotherapy needs of someone with rheumatoid arthritis will bring up new problems with each patient encountered as everyone is so different (May & Newman 1980). This type of problem is more difficult to cope with, and it is not possible to learn just one, straightforward solution.

Evidence from developmental studies demonstrates that a child's abilities to solve problems emerge spontaneously as more knowledge is acquired, and superficial concepts are replaced with deeper ones (Kahney 1993). These skills improve with maturity, as they are learned through experience. It is unlikely that anyone can get through a day without having to go through the problem-solving mechanism at some point. But even though this process begins from birth and continues throughout life, little thought is given to what is actually going on in the mind at the time.

People vary in their problem-solving styles, some being quite systematic, working through step by step, whereas others seem to find solutions by intuition. Or, there can be different approaches for different types of problem (May & Newman 1980). By the time you reach the stage of reading this book, you will have already developed your own approach to solving problems. If you are able to solve them with no difficulty, you probably never consider the process. However, now you are starting to think about problems in the clinical setting, where you have less, if any experience, you will need to develop different strategies to apply your knowledge in physiotherapy practice. But, in order to make the process a little simpler to start with, consider the more general problems in the list below:

- How can I pass my anatomy exam?
- What does 'systemic lupus erythematosus' mean?
- What is the best route to work tomorrow if there's a bus strike?
- If I have three different sized rings on pole one, how can I move them to pole two and not break the rules?
- How do I go about performing a literature search for my project?
- How do I go about writing a classic novel?
- Where did I put my keys?
- How am I going decide which of this patient's problems I need to concentrate on first?
- How can I make something of my life?
- How will I manage to live for the rest of the term/month when my grant/salary runs out?

Some of these problems may be things that you have to deal with regularly, or perhaps have dealt with in the past. The rest, you may never have to tackle yourself, but hopefully you can perceive that they could be problems for certain other people.

It is widely recognised that there is a need for problem solving in physiotherapy as well as in medical and other paramedical professions (Morris 1993). In fact, May & Newman (1980) state that 'problem solving is an integral part of effective physiotherapy practice'. If students or clinicians cannot recognise patients' problems then it will be difficult, if not impossible, to formulate goals and appropriate treatment plans. These of course are necessary in successful patient management.

Other concepts that you need to consider are decision making and clinical reasoning, which are intimately related to problem solving. You will explore these in more detail later. The 'reasoning' aspect is important as it refers to the thinking processes associated with clinical practice. According to Higgs (1992) this includes the ability to utilise thinking skills, reflection, review and evaluation. It also entails metacognition which involves an awareness of the thinking processes, and the ability to access data already stored in long-term memory.

Decision making is something that everyone does on a regular basis. Lindsay & Norman (1977) state that decision making is 'choice among complex issues involving combining psychological impressions of the issues and comparing these'. Psychological impressions are formed and then compared, the positive and negative factors being weighed to determine the final decisions made. But it is important to realise that the availability of data stored in memory will also play a large part in this, that is, what is already known also influences the decisions made. This relates directly to the reasoning skills mentioned previously. Perhaps the influence of the existing 'database' gives some clue to the individual differences found in problem solvers when faced with exactly the same issues and information. Even more fascinating is that one person may arrive at different decisions if the same things are compared, but considered in a different order (Lindsay & Norman 1977). Thus, it becomes obvious that there is a great deal of flexibility as well as variability in decision making.

So, what is problem solving?

Look back briefly at the list of general problems given earlier. According to Kahney (1993) all problems have two things in common:

1. a goal, e.g. something a person wants or wants to do/achieve, such as finding the keys or performing a literature search, and
2. something stopping them from immediately reaching that goal, that is, some kind of block which could be due, for example, to lack of resources or lack of knowledge.

This then gives the basis for the concept of problem solving: whenever a desired goal is blocked,

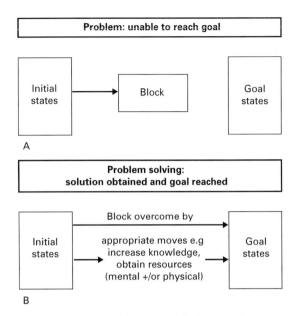

Figure 1.1 A. A problem: some block preventing solution. B. Problem solving: processes that allow goal achievement.

this amounts to a problem, and whatever is done to achieve the goal is problem solving. The block keeping the person from their goal has to be dealt with in some way, and this could involve mental or physical processes, or elements of both (Fig. 1.1).

Much of the work that has been carried out into problem solving has been in-depth study of what are known as transformational problems, i.e. where an initial state is transformed into a target state by certain moves. A simple example of this would be changing yellow into green by adding blue. If the resulting shade of green were too dark then it could be lightened by adding more yellow and so on until the desired shade was achieved.

So that you don't get too bored with reading for a long period, it's now time for you to have a go at problem solving. The intention of this is twofold:

— To show you a slightly more complex example of a transformational problem. (The exercise below is one commonly used by psychologists.)
— To let you 'have a go' at solving a problem

that should aid in your appreciation of the mental operations involved, which will be discussed later.

In order to get the most out of this exercise, you should observe yourself as you go through the stages of reaching a solution. Note what you do, the difficulties you have, the points of the problem that give you clues to move on. Quite a useful way of doing this is to jot down what you do as you go along – or even better, tape it. Say out loud everything you think as you work on the problem, and why you decide on certain moves. You can then look back on the stages you went through. This type of verbal record is known as a protocol.

Problem-solving exercise 1.1

THE TOWERS OF HANOI
There are three poles labelled 1, 2 and 3. On pole 1 there are three rings, a large, a medium and a small one. You must transfer all of the three rings from pole 1 to pole 2 (largest on the bottom,

then the medium and then the smallest on top). Both of these states, i.e. the initial state and the goal state are shown in Figure 1.2 below.

These are the rules: you can only move one ring at a time, you must not place the rings anywhere except on one of the other poles (e.g. not on floor or table) and lastly, you may not place a larger ring on top of a smaller one. If you have access to poles and rings, you can use these to help you; if not, three different sized coins can be used. As a last resort, do it on a piece of paper!

- **A.** How many moves did it take you to solve the problem? (It should take seven; see the end of the chapter.)

  Look back at your notes or listen to the tape you made whilst solving the problem of the Towers of Hanoi.

- **B.** Do you think you recorded everything that you thought?

- **C.** Do you think everything you did was accompanied by a specific thought?

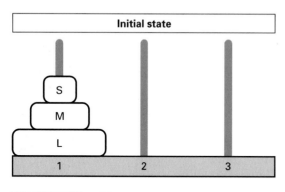

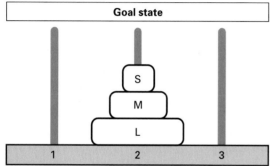

Figure 1.2 The Towers of Hanoi.

You will probably find that there are some gaps, and in fact, there may be episodes where you did not really know what you were thinking. According to Lindsay & Norman (1977) the reports that people give of their thoughts are not always accurate or complete. So this might give you an inkling of why working out problem-solving strategies is a problem in and of itself. Another point here is that you would probably tackle the same problem in a different way if it was presented to you a second time; this is because you would now have some experience of it. Even if quite a long period intervened between the first and second tries, you would probably remember the overall successful approach that you eventually came up with in the initial instance. Undoubtedly, experience changes the nature of the problem-solving task.

Review points
On studying the steps you went through when solving the Towers of Hanoi problem, you probably found that you broke the overall goal down into a number of smaller steps.

This is quite a usual technique where a person will try out a variety of simple strategies hoping each will yield some information. Some strategies work which gives more data; some do not and so backing up occurs followed by a different line of approach. But the questions are: How is the goal broken down? How are the strategies chosen? How is the strategy decided upon and how can it be decided whether it is leading to the goal or to a dead end (Lindsay & Norman 1977)?

The Towers of Hanoi is one type of problem used by psychologists to study the processes involved in problem solving, and a great deal of research has been carried out in this area. But why is there such a fascination with this subject? Well, the ideal situation would be to put all problems into groups or categories, and then to work out and understand the strategies used by successful problem solvers whilst reaching their solutions. If this could be done, then the next step, within the context of this book at least, would be to teach you the successful strategies used by expert clinicians in dealing with the management of their patients. You would then be good at problem solving in that situation yourselves – well at least you might be better at it!

Unfortunately, due to the extremely wide range of problems and differences in complexity and content, it would appear that this is very unlikely to happen. It is often difficult to see the common elements and similarities between two apparently simple problems, so this suggests that even the categorisation itself would be impossible.

This being said however, problems have been divided into broad categories or classes and these are:

- well defined
- ill defined.

Well defined problems

This category of problem is one where there is a clearly stated goal. It is well structured and all of the information necessary to solve the problem is provided. As you probably realise, you have just had experience of a well defined problem in the Towers of Hanoi example.

It is necessary to have a goal, and ways to tell whether the problem solving is proceeding as hoped. Kahney (1993) classes the information needed to solve a well defined problem into four sections:

1. Initial state of the problem.
2. Goal state.
3. Legal operators, that is, the things you are allowed to do to solve it.
4. Operator restrictions, that is, factors governing or constraining the use of legal operators. These could be seen as the 'rules' in some instances.

> ### Self-assessment questions
>
> ■ **SAQ 1.1.** Go back to the Towers of Hanoi problem and identify the four parts mentioned above, that is, initial state of the problem, goal state, legal operators and operator restrictions.
>
> ■ **SAQ 1.2.** Work out the initial states and goal states for the following problems:
> **A.** A game of Scrabble
> **B.** Solving a crossword clue.

A more general example of a well defined problem may be something like the earlier ones: 'What is the best route to work tomorrow if there is a bus strike?' or 'How do I go about performing a literature search for my project?' It is possible to work out the initial state, what the goal is and how you can achieve it. Also, if appropriate, what constraints or restrictions there might be.

Ill defined problems

Here, in comparison to the well defined problem, there is poor structure with little or no information regarding initial and goal states, or operators. If you try to analyse these problems, everything is rather vaguely defined. We had an example of this earlier in the problem: 'How can I pass my anatomy exam?' So how can this be analysed?

— *Initial state.* You are presented with an anatomy paper containing questions. You know how many to answer and how much time you've got.

— *Goal state*. This is the grade you want. So, if you want a good pass, your answers will have to be better than if you only want to scrape a pass. But how do you know whether your answers are worth a good pass? How do you know if your goal has been achieved? Presumably the only way you will know for certain is when you receive your results, by which time it could be a little late.

— *Operators*. Well there is really no information given here. You are not told about retrieving information from memory, making notes, doing essay plans, not including irrelevant material, division of time between questions, etc. In other words, all the things you are expected to know already about sitting an exam – but do you?

— *Operator restrictions*. Because you are in an exam situation, many of the ways you might normally use to obtain information are not available to you, such as asking your peers, looking at your notes, reading books, consulting a lecturer, etc. Even your time is restricted.

In this example, you have to take part in defining the problem. The extent to which the problem may be structured often depends on your prior knowledge and experience. If you have taken many exams before and are very familiar with the subject matter, you will augment the information given to you at the beginning with knowledge from long-term memory.

The boundary between well and ill defined problems becomes blurred when the solver's knowledge is taken into account. So this suggests that the amount of structure that a problem has initially, can be used to decide how it will be treated by the solver, rather than trying to put it into a particular category.

The most important thing for a problem solver to be able to recognise is when a solution arises. An example of this would be the couple who get into the car to go out for the day with a goal of 'having a good time'. There is no particular plan, but as they drive around they find a place to visit for the day, and later a good restaurant where they have an excellent meal to round things off. This all occurs while they are working on the problem of 'having a nice day out'; they know the sort of things they like and so they can recognise the situations that will satisfy their goal.

This approach of adding problems with indefinite goals widens the boundaries of well defined problems. But unfortunately for those people interested in analysing the 'solving process', it is the ill defined category of problem that comes up more frequently.

Most studies of problem solving concentrate on well defined problems. The goal of the work is to understand the processes people use in working through to the solution of problems. This involves the construction of internal models of the problem, the strategies used, the rules followed and the assessment of progress. Kahney (1993) gives some reasons for the use of the simpler, well defined problems in research work. 'Toy worlds' are set up and examined as models of reality to help in the understanding of how people behave in real world situations, because the real world is extremely complex and 'messy' and therefore difficult to study. These studies can be done in the laboratory setting, in easily observable stages with subjects needing no prior knowledge. Problems can be presented in different ways with different 'cover stories'. They can be scaled up, for example by repeating the Towers of Hanoi but increasing the number of rings to five. This may then show how the subjects use their previous experience with similar problems to help in solving the present one. These experiments take a relatively short time. This makes them manageable in comparison to the real world, where problems may take anywhere from a few minutes, to more than a lifetime to solve. This moves the question on from whether the problem is solved, to how it is solved.

Problem-solving exercise 1.2

THE CHINESE TEA CEREMONY
(*adapted from Kahney 1993*)

In a number of Himalayan villages, the innkeepers perform a very refined and civilised tea ceremony. It involves the innkeeper himself who is the host, and two guests, never more or less. One guest holds a more exalted position than the other. The guests arrive and are seated comfortably at the table. The host then performs three services for them.

1. Stoking the fire which is the least noble task.
2. Pouring the tea which is of medium nobility.
3. Reciting poetry which is the most noble of the three.

As the ceremony proceeds any person present may ask another 'Honoured Sir, may I perform this onerous task for you?' He may only ask to perform the least noble task that the other is performing. Then, if someone is already performing any tasks, he cannot ask to take on a task which is nobler than the least noble task he is already doing. According to custom, by the time the ceremony is completed, all tasks must be transferred from the host to the most senior guest.

■ **A.** How can this be done?

All of the information that you need to solve this problem is given to you.

Here's a clue: it is exactly the same in underlying structure as the Towers of Hanoi. This is an example of two problems that are identical in structure, but they have very different cover stories.

■ **B.** Did you have any idea of the similarity between the two problems before you were given the clue?

It is quite common for problems to appear different superficially but to have similar solutions. As you've probably found, this is not always easy to detect. It can be useful to find analogies between present problems and ones for which the solution is known, to recognise similarities and differences.

However, it is important not to waste time and effort looking for similarities when there may not be any, and what is really needed is a fresh approach (Lindsay & Norman 1977). Psychologists can draw up plans of the structure of problems called 'state space' diagrams. Some are quite difficult to work out as certain problems have the possibility of a lot of 'illegal moves'. But the path taken through a state space diagram can be used to analyse a person's problem-solving behaviour.

An example of a simple state space diagram can be seen in Figure 1.3 which shows the possible steps in making a cup of tea (after Kahney 1993).

Many well defined problems, for example those in mathematics, have direct and efficient solutions, that is, algorithms. Use the rules properly and you will always get the right answer. But when people are asked to solve these problems they often use rambling trial-and-error methods. Why is this? Well firstly, there could be difficulties in the person's understanding of the problem; not everyone will have perfect understanding of each one encountered. Secondly, algorithms and state space diagrams are very helpful if you can remember them, but each person will have a unique representation of the problem in his/her mind, and each will also have a different amount of data stored in memory which can be brought to bear on it. Some people will have more and some will have less.

A side issue, which nevertheless needs to be addressed briefly, is that of the quality of each step taken when solving a problem. If making a cup of tea is used as an example, it may not seem very complex to you, but it can still be difficult for someone who has never done it before. Any route taken through the state space diagram will result in a cup of tea being made – but will it be a good cup of tea?

Some people insist that a certain routine needs to be followed otherwise the result is poor, that is, the tea should never be put in before the milk, and then of course, how much milk should be added? This is a simple illustration. It is not just a matter of following a route through to a solution. In order to ensure a quality result, it is also extremely important to consider the fine detail, that is, the manner in which each step is performed.

THE ROLE OF MEMORY

Problem solving is limited by the constraints of

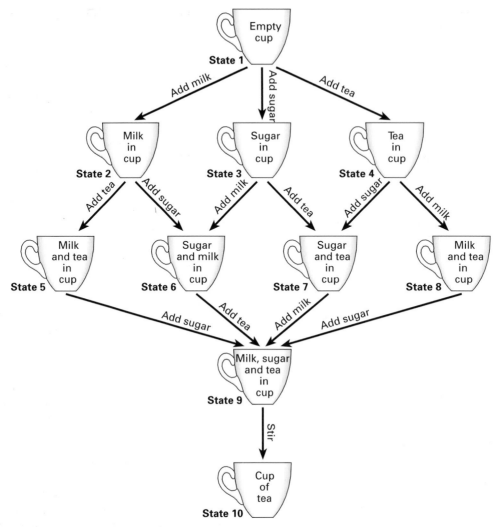

Figure 1.3 State space diagram for making a cup of tea. Any route taken through the plan will result in all the necessary constituents for a cup of tea being in the cup together.

short-term or working memory. It also depends on the information processing system, the time involved in storage, and retrieval in long-term memory. It is only possible to think ahead effectively when there is already some experience with the topic. According to Lindsay & Norman (1977), noughts and crosses is at the limit of human cognitive ability. For someone playing this game for the first time, there is no way that all of the possibilities can be kept in mind, due to the limits of working memory. If it were played by sheer reasoning alone, it would not be possible to do it. But it is played and in fact appears a very simple game, so why is this?

Well, because people have previous experience of playing the game they have learned certain structures which enable them to decide where to place the next symbol in the grid. If the first symbol is placed in the centre it will ensure a win, or at worst a draw. If the first player has already placed a symbol in the centre, then the second player must place his/hers in a corner, anything else guarantees a loss. Because it is possible to remember winning and losing configurations from previous games, it reduces the necessary amount of forward planning.

But is the human mind really so restricted as the noughts and crosses example suggests?

Yes and no.

Yes, because the limitations of working memory do restrict performance, it is not possible to plan very far ahead when solving problems, especially those encountered in everyday life. But then, no, because it is possible to augment the limited amount of working memory by the following methods:

1. We use external aids to thought such as writing, referral to notes, symbolic representation, etc.
2. We can use strategies to guide searches for solutions to problems. Algorithms have already been considered, which if followed, guarantee a solution. But they are not always helpful. The 'rule of thumb' problem-solving methods known as 'heuristics' can be useful. These methods often succeed but certainly do not guarantee success. For example, if you are lost in an unfamiliar city, your heuristic method of problem solving may be to ask someone the way. This usually works, but only if the person you ask knows the place you are wanting to get to.
3. We use the capacity and flexibility of long-term memory. This involves drawing on previous experience when confronted with a new problem. A person can become an 'expert' in a particular field because of thousands of hours of practice, acquiring large amounts of structured knowledge, which is stored in long-term memory. An example that is commonly used is that of expert chess players. They are often seen as having some sort of unique mental ability. However, this is not so. Everyone has the same capabilities. The expert chess players have a large amount of knowledge of the game obtained through experience. They have organised this into clusters of meaningful, well learned, structured information. These configurations can then be brought to bear on each new chess game. A novice however, needs to use working memory just to remember the rules and moves. The experts have all this already stored in long-term memory and so they can use the working memory to concentrate on the problem in

hand. It is possible for anyone to use this strategy and in fact many people do so much of the time without being conscious of it. The key factor is that the configurations stored in long-term memory are meaningful, making them easier to retain and to work with than those which make no sense.

Problem-solving exercise 1.3

How well can you remember a sequence of letters? The limit for most people is about 10. Look at the following letters once and then try to repeat them without looking at the page.

F T P G I B J Z M U

- **A.** Did you find them difficult to remember?
- **B.** If so, why do you think this is?

Each letter is a separate unit and must therefore be stored separately in memory.

Now consider what happens if letters are organised into some meaningful configuration; repeat the exercise with the following sequence of letters:

P R O C E S S I N G

Not only is it easy, but in fact you probably do not even think of them as separate at all, but as a contained unit, which is represented in memory as a single item. It is easy to remember even longer lists of letters in this way; try the one below:

> The book, *Physiotherapy in Orthopaedics: a problem-solving approach* introduces the reader to problem solving in the clinical setting.

Here, even though there are 112 letters, the exercise is relatively easy because the sequence of letters is meaningful to you.

The apparent skill of expert chess players deteriorates markedly when they asked to remember meaningless configurations of pieces on a chess board, just as yours does when asked to remember meaningless sequences of letters.

ANALOGICAL PROBLEM SOLVING

According to Kahney (1993), it has been shown that people actively use old knowledge in trying to understand new events or problems. This is known as analogical problem solving: analogies between old problems and new problems are identified. Most of the situations encountered in everyday life are fairly familiar and therefore analogous to previous experience. This means that each person already has a lot of the knowledge necessary to deal with each scenario. But it is not always easy to identify the analogy or to know how to apply the solution. Experiments have shown that subjects are good at using this method if they are given hints that this is what they should do; if the hints are not given, previous analogies are not so helpful.

This type of problem solving is useful in new situations, but again it does rely on retrieval of data from long-term memory. So, if the original problem can be remembered, this will help in solving the present one. There are, however, some difficulties with this. If long-term memory fails and the old problem cannot be retrieved, then the new problem has to be solved from the beginning. Also, it is possible that false analogies may be used which will lead to the wrong solution. For example, meeting one person with rheumatoid arthritis who copes very well with the long-term symptoms may lead you to assume that 'all people with rheumatoid arthritis cope well with the condition'. This in turn may lead to an incorrect reaction in a new situation.

But even with the disadvantages mentioned, there is no doubt that past experience does help in present problem solving. Clear differences can be seen between novices, those with intermediate amounts of experience, and experts. This is not to say that experts never have to problem solve or never come across unfamiliar situations. But because of the highly structured amounts of information they have in long-term memory, they have a marked advantage over novices in many tasks. They probably have memorised solutions to many types of problem they are likely to come across, whereas the novice has a much smaller store of answers to fall back on. Even if there is not a direct answer available to the experts, they will have evolved general strategies for dealing with particular types of problem within their own field, which novices will not yet have developed. Novices tend to concentrate on the objects mentioned in the problem rather than relating back to underlying principles. However, if experts are put into areas with which they are unfamiliar, their problem-solving skills will revert to those used by novices.

DECISION MAKING

This process is part of problem solving. As problems are present throughout life, specific choices between alternatives are regularly made. In the selection of these alternatives, relative merits are weighed and evaluated, even if this is done without any awareness of the steps gone through to come to a final decision.

If the choices are complex, there may be difficulties.

- It strains short-term memory to picture what may happen if a single alternative is chosen along with its implications, let alone a greater number to allow for comparison.
- Because there are usually many different factors involved in each alternative, there may be no clear way to compare them.
- Then, of course there are the unknown factors: who knows what will really happen? Sometimes the result of a decision depends very much on how someone else reacts to it (Lindsay & Norman 1977).

Because of this, it sometimes seems easier to give up, or to leave things as long as possible before making the decision, to not even try to consider alternatives and the implications of the choices. The decision is then only made when forced, and it is too late to change. This is often followed by a period of wondering what would have happened if a different choice had been selected. Would the outcome have been better?

There is a definite distinction between the rules that ought to be followed, and those that are. Someone may make a decision which appears illogical to you, but it may be perfectly sensible from their position, at least in terms of the information they had available at the time.

In general, the major principle of rational decision making is 'optimisation': everything else being equal, choose the alternative with the greatest value. However, this does not work very well in human decision making as each person will view gains and costs differently (Lindsay & Norman 1977).

The choices of a rational decision maker are determined by the expected values associated with possible decisions, that is the probabilities of events and the payoffs and penalties related to various outcomes. People do appear to operate according to the principles of optimisation, but this is not easy to predict because of other factors which are internal variables, such as fatigue or boredom. These need to be added to the equation in order to begin to understand individual differences in decision making.

Because of the limits of working memory, people are often forced into decisions which minimise 'cognitive strain', that is, they are unable to consider all of the important variables. They may use what appear to be logical strategies to come to their decisions, but they will probably not be the optimal ones. Inevitably they are unable to take into account everything that may impinge upon the situation.

Estimates of optimisation will also change, so a decision could be made at one time, and then a very different one made if the same information is considered at a later date. It is also true that different people have different judgements of the value of the same events.

This almost makes it sound as though it should be impossible to make decisions at all, but of course this is not the case. People are constantly choosing between alternatives and are often successful and happy with their choice.

In the clinical setting, your problem solving with patients is inseparable from the decision-making process. The decisions you make will influence whether or not you reach a satisfactory solution. This will be explored further in Chapter 5, but for now, two factors need to be kept in mind for successful problem solving and decision making:

1. When you are dealing with patients with a large variety of orthopaedic conditions, you will need to have an accessible, organised knowledge base from which to work, in order to reach effective solutions.
2. You must recognise patients' involvement in decision making and they should be encouraged to play a responsible role in their own health care (Higgs 1992).

Summary

This chapter has introduced you to the general issues surrounding problem solving and decision making. These are both processes which you use constantly on a day-to-day basis. You have been encouraged to start thinking about the mechanisms involved.

The synthesis of the problem-solving approach with clinical orthopaedic practice has been presented briefly, just to put it into context, and will be expanded upon later in the book.

On reading this summary, do you feel you have grasped the above points? If not, perhaps you should go back and re-read any appropriate parts of the chapter before moving on.

ANSWERS TO QUESTIONS AND EXERCISES

Problem-solving exercise 1.1 (page 8)

The Towers of Hanoi

■ **A.** How many moves should it take?

Answer: It should take seven moves as follows:
— *small ring to pole 2*
— *medium ring to pole 3*
— *small ring to pole 3*
— *large ring to pole 2*
— *small ring to pole 1*
— *medium ring to pole 2*
— *small ring to pole 2.*

Self-assessment questions (page 9)

■ **SAQ 1.1.** Go back to the Towers of Hanoi problem and identify the initial state of the problem, goal state, legal operators and operator restrictions.

Answer:
— *Initial state: three poles, number 1 on the left with three rings on it (small on top of medium on top of large), then two empty poles, number 2 in the middle and number 3 on the right.*
— *Goal state: the three rings on pole 2 in the same order as above.*
— *Legal operators: move rings from one pole to another.*
— *Operator restrictions:*
   a. *move one ring at a time*
   b. *do not place rings anywhere except on another pole*
   c. *do not place larger rings on top of smaller ones.*

■ **SAQ 1.2.** Work out the initial states and goal states for the following problems:

A. A game of Scrabble

Answer:
— *Initial state: an empty Scrabble board;*

every player has seven tiles each with a letter on; spare tiles in bag.
— *Goal state: the highest number of points (gained by placing letters down in a crossword pattern on the board in winning combinations).*

B. Solving a crossword clue

Answer:
— *Initial state: empty squares*
— *Goal state: squares filled with letters making up the word(s) which correctly answer the given clue.*

Problem-solving exercise 1.2 (page 10)

The Chinese tea ceremony

Answer: As stated in the text, this is identical to the Towers of Hanoi in underlying structure, which means that the solution is also the same.

If we arrange it in the same way, the solution becomes easier to work out: use host (H), senior guest (SG) and junior guest (JG) as the three poles (1, 2, and 3 respectively) and the three tasks – stoking, which is the least noble (S), pouring, of medium nobility (P) and reciting, most noble (R) – as the three rings (small, medium and large respectively) (see Fig 1.4).

It is now easy to work out the solution:

— *stoking to senior quest*
— *pouring to junior guest*
— *stoking to junior guest*
— *reciting to senior guest*
— *stoking to host*
— *pouring to senior guest*
— *stoking to senior guest.*

Problem-solving exercise 1.3 (page 13)

See text

REFERENCES

Higgs J 1992 Developing clinical reasoning competencies. Physiotherapy 78(8):575–581
Kahney H 1993 Problem solving: current issues, 2nd edn. Open University Press, Buckingham

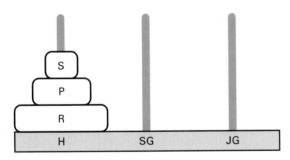

Key: H = Host, SG = Senior guest, JG = Junior guest,
S = Stoking fire, P = Pouring tea,
R = Reciting poetry

Figure 1.4 The underlying structure of the Chinese tea ceremony problem and its similarity to the Towers of Hanoi.

Lindsay P H, Norman D A 1977 Human information processing – an introduction to psychology, 2nd edn. Academic Press, London

May B J, Newman J 1980 Developing competencies in problem solving: a behavioural model. Physical Therapy 57(7):807–813

Morris J 1993 An overview of and comparison among three current approaches to medical and physiotherapy undergraduate education. Physiotherapy 79(2):91–94

2

Changes in the musculoskeletal system

■ Development ■ Ageing ■ Physiological changes ■ Musculoskeletal system

Objectives

By the end of this chapter you should:

1. Have an awareness of the development of the musculoskeletal system and its relationship to the development of the cardiovascular and neural systems.
2. Understand the changes that occur in the mature adult through the ageing process of the musculoskeletal system.
3. Be able to differentiate between the changes due to ageing and those which occur in osteoarthrosis.

Prerequisites

Before reading this chapter you should revise the basic anatomy of muscle, bone, and synovial joints and the pathology of osteoarthrosis. The background knowledge you obtain from this reading will augment the information presented in this section and will help you to answer the questions posed.

INTRODUCTION

The musculoskeletal system provides the gross components of movement and function and is composed of two main sections: the skeletal structure, which provides a scaffolding for muscle attachment, protection to soft sensitive organs and the formation of moveable links (joints), and the muscular system which gives a means of controlling the motion at the joints for function.

The musculoskeletal system cannot work in isolation and is totally dependent on the normal functioning of the other body systems, that is, the central and peripheral nervous systems and the cardiovascular system. These are also influenced by psychological and emotional responses. The initiation and control of movement is governed by the central and peripheral nervous systems and the cardiovascular system provides nutrition and oxygenation to the bones, joints and muscles.

The main emphasis of this chapter will be on the development of the musculoskeletal system, bones, joints and muscle, and, particularly, on the changes associated with ageing. Where appropriate, the related changes in the neural and cardiovascular systems will be considered, as this may clarify the overall picture.

As illustrated in Figure I.1 (p. 3), a knowledge of the progression from the normal state, and its possible ranges, to the abnormal is essential to your understanding of problem solving in orthopaedics. This chapter identifies and defines 'normal' in relation to the changes that naturally occur in the body systems, thus providing you with a grounding from which to explore the 'abnormal'.

DEVELOPMENT

The body develops throughout childhood and adolescence, then reaching a point of maturity after which it slowly declines towards death (Fig. 2.1).

Of course this is a very general overview and the timing of events will vary from person to person. However, there are definite stages in the developmental cycle during which the maturity of each of the body systems is altered (Bell et al 1980):

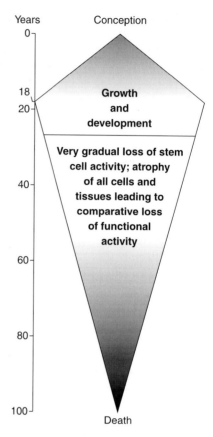

Figure 2.1 Growth, development and atrophy during the ageing process. (Adapted with permission from Govan et al 1991.)

- birth
- puberty (around 10–14 years)
- adolescent growth spurt (around 12–15 years)
- menopause (around 45–55 years).

For example the adolescent growth spurt, which occurs at a slightly later age for boys (around 14–15 years) than girls (around 12–13 years) is responsible for many of the gross changes in body form and structure which in turn are associated with changes in the cardiovascular system, so the latter system does not reach maturity until after this time (Russo 1990). This may also be true for all other systems.

You can see from Figure 2.1 that growth continues until around the age of 18 years and the major development processes continue until the mid-twenties.

This does not mean that a person cannot develop and refine skills and abilities after this time, but generally that the body systems have reached their point of maturation resulting in maximal control of motor performance at that time. The level of this control is individual and the ability to perform maximally is also dependent on other factors, such as lifestyle, exercise and fitness (Govan et al 1991).

More specifically, there are recognisable patterns of change in muscle strength which appear to be predetermined by hereditary factors, but the intervals at which they occur are variable (Hinderer & Hinderer 1993). It is also recognised that the ongoing control of motion is dependent on the parallel development of the musculoskeletal and the neural systems which should evolve in tandem, each acting as a precursor to the development of the other (Hinderer & Hinderer 1993).

In the infant, neuromuscular system development progresses in a predictable sequence, from the control of gross antigravity movements, enabling the growing child to gradually assume and maintain an erect posture, to the fine control of the extremities (Hinderer & Hinderer 1993). It has been shown that age, sex and body proportions have an effect on muscle strength throughout development but particularly after the onset of puberty (Methany 1941, Monotoye & Lamphiear 1977). There are other factors that influence strength, such as motor learning and seasonal and diurnal variation, but these are as relevant to the mature adult as to the developing child.

It is important for therapists to know about the evolution of muscle strength in order to recognise these changes as normal, as opposed to those due to some pathology or abnormality.

Muscle changes during development

Skeletal muscle eventually constitutes 40–45% of total body weight, providing motion, strength and protection to the skeleton by absorbing forces and distributing loads (Nordin & Frankel 1989). Each muscle is composed of a large number of muscle fibres (each containing numerous myofibrils) that form bundles (fascicles) which are in turn surrounded by a sheath of connective tissue (perimysium). A fibrous connective tissue then overlays the whole muscle (epimysium) which, along with the perimysium, forms a continuation of the collagen tissue of tendons, the normal mechanism for attaching muscle to bone.

Each myofibril consists of fibrous filaments of actin and myosin in repeating bands called sarcomeres, throughout the length of the fibril, and it is the delicate strands of the myofibrils which are the functional contractile units of the muscle.

Developmental muscle changes occur at a very early point, with the neuromuscular system developing from the 5th week after conception when pre-muscle masses are formed. The muscles have well established innervation by the 8th week and muscular movements can be detected in utero as early as the 16th week (Espenschade & Eckert 1980). Changes continue throughout the gestation period, and at birth the baby is able to perform reflex movements and some gross activity patterns but is unable to perform controlled voluntary movements. This is due to the immaturity of the nervous system, i.e. the nerves and muscles are connected but much more refinement is needed before smooth controlled movement is possible (Thelen 1985).

After birth there is a large increase in muscle length and diameter, with the number of myofibrils rising markedly. This occurs because the existing myofibrils split longitudinally (Goldspink & Williams 1990). As muscle strength is known to be directly proportional to the cross-sectional muscle area (Rutherford & Jones 1992, Young 1984, Young et al 1984, 1985) and the number of myofibril units (Goldspink & Williams 1990), this would explain the natural increase in strength during development.

The increase in length of the muscle is necessary to allow for the growth of long bones. This is accomplished by the addition of serial sarcomeres enabling a continued overlap between the actin and myosin filaments (in myofibrils), thus retaining the ability to generate force (Goldspink & Williams 1990). These changes in the muscle must be accompanied by adaptations to the neural and vascular supply to permit normal function, that is, control and initiation of muscle contraction and the removal of the resultant waste products.

The development of muscle in the growing child is dependent on the rate of development of the neurological system. During the first year of life, as myelination progresses, the child gains control of its body, first from the neck down and from proximal to distal areas. Thus gross control of the neck, scapular and shoulder movements occurs before that of the hands and all of these are acquired before fine movement and precision is gained. Upper limb control is therefore gained before that of the lower limb, and gross antigravity control develops prior to accuracy (Hinderer & Hinderer 1993).

As neural control increases then muscle strength is gained and refined, but only attains its full magnitude if this control is complemented by the addition of more myofibrils.

One other factor can influence muscle strength: the skill and coordination of a movement. In both developing and mature muscle the learning and repetition of a task can greatly influence the performance of it (Hinderer & Hinderer 1993). Thus muscle strength can be increased due to the learning of the task, with more complicated tasks, such as precision movements, walking and so on, demonstrating an even greater effect.

Self-assessment questions

- **SAQ 2.1.** Which parts of a muscle constitute the contractile units?

- **SAQ 2.2.** Outline which types of movement can be performed at birth.

- **SAQ 2.3.** What does muscle strength directly depend upon?

- **SAQ 2.4.** How does a muscle maintain the generation of force as it lengthens during the developmental sequence?

Bone and joint changes during development

Bone is a specialised connective tissue that provides a solid but flexible structure for support and protection. It has a high content of inorganic material, i.e. mineral salts such as calcium and phosphate, which provides the rigid structure, and of organic material (such as collagen fibres, glycosaminoglycans (GAGs) and water) which gives bone its flexibility (Nordin & Frankel 1989).

As bone stores a significant proportion of the body's mineral salt content, particularly calcium, it therefore plays a major role in mineral homeostasis, but the mechanism involved is not clear (Bland 1993).

In general the length and shape of bones are genetically determined, but it is known that bone mass increases with activity and also that bone structure can alter to accommodate weight-bearing stresses (Nordin & Frankel 1989). This constant response to the demands of weight bearing, by change in the infrastructure of bone and connective tissue to accommodate altered stress, was first recognised by Wolff who stated that: 'bone will alter its size, shape, and trabecular pattern in both the subchondral and cortical bone according to the lines of physical stress' (Wolff's law of bone remodelling; Bland 1993). Therefore bone can constantly change shape to accommodate the structural demands made on it by weight bearing, muscle pull, stress and so on during continuous normal everyday activity.

Biomechanically bone combines strength and stiffness, allowing a certain amount of load to be applied, within the bone's elastic limit, with no permanent deformation taking place. During loading the bone stores the energy transferred and when the load is reduced the bone returns to its normal shape. If the load is taken past the elastic limit of the bone ('yield point') then permanent deformation will take place. If the loading continues then failure (fracture) occurs (Nordin & Frankel 1989).

The growth and development of bone occurs in two ways: the long bones (femur, humerus, tibia, etc.), the vertebrae, the sternum and the ribs, develop from rods of cartilage (endochondral ossification, see below), and the shorter, flatter bones such as the clavicle, skull (parietal, frontal bones), nasal bone, maxilla/mandible, etc. are formed from membranes (intramembranous ossification, see below).

In the fertilised egg, two layers of tissue devel-

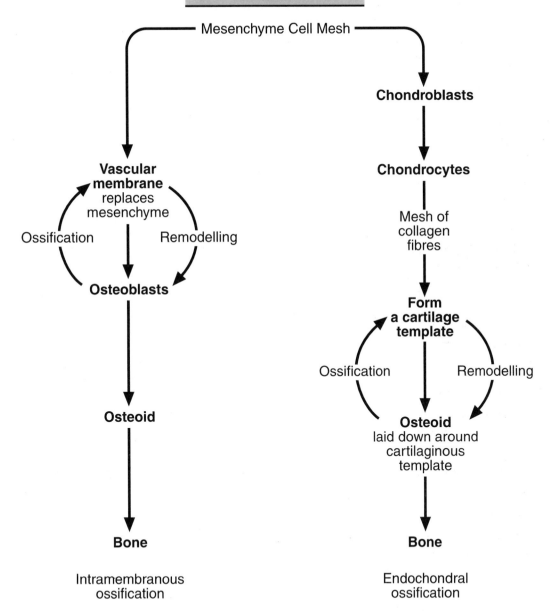

Figure 2.2 From mesenchyme to bone.

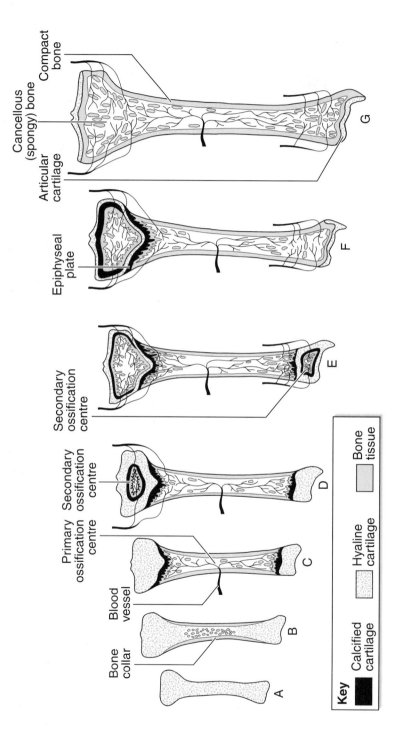

Figure 2.3 Formation and growth of a long bone (tibia) on a cartilage template. A. Hyaline cartilage template surrounded by perichondrium. B. Appearance of bone collar. Hypertrophy of central cells which then die to leave lacunae whose walls calcify. C. Appearance of capillaries. Perichondrium converted to periosteum. Osteoid produced around shaft. The primary ossification centre appears in the middle of the bone (the diaphysis). D. Shaft ossifies and grows by resorption on the inner surface and apposition on outer (see Fig. 2.4 and text for explanation). Osteoclasts break down calcified cartilage centrally. Secondary ossification centres start to appear in epiphyses. E. Development continues and another secondary ossification centre appears in the lower epiphysis when it is invaded by capillaries. Growth is radial here as opposed to the longitudinal growth in the primary centre. F. As the bone approaches adult size, the diaphysis and epiphyses gradually fully ossify, but are still separated by epiphyseal plates (cartilage). When the epiphyseal plates cease to grow there is no further longitudinal bone growth. G. Skeletal maturity is achieved when the epiphyseal plates are replaced by bone. The only cartilage remaining is the layer of hyaline cartilage on the articular surfaces.

op around the 9th day: ectoderm which eventually becomes the superficial layers of skin, hair, nails, some glands and the central nervous system, and the endoderm which develops into the lining of the pulmonary and digestive systems, and so on. Cell proliferation from the ectoderm forms a loose connective tissue which becomes the mesenchyme, a thin layer of tissue between the ectoderm and the endoderm (Shipman et al 1985).

From this mesenchyme, the mesoderm cell layer develops from the 16th day post-fertilisation, and the gradual condensation or proliferation of these cells results in either intramembranous or endochondral ossification (Fig. 2.2).

Intramembranous growth and ossification

The proliferation of the mesenchyme eventually forms a highly vascular membrane. Three months after fertilisation the mesenchyme cells progress to osteoblasts (major bone-forming cells responsible for producing large quantities of osteoid), which ossify and then remodel the already formed membranous tissue. As the condensed mesenchyme is replaced by bone the thick membrane is left surrounding the growing bone tissue, eventually becoming the periosteum, the outer fibrous cover of bone which provides nutrition and the main means of attaching tendon to bone (Shipman et al 1985, Vaughan 1981).

Endochondral growth and ossification

This is the more common type of ossification and starts at the 4th to 5th week of fetal life (Shipman et al 1985).

Once again endochondral development starts from the formation of the mesenchyme cells which proliferate and then turn into chondroblasts (young immature cartilage cells), rather than osteoblasts as in intramembranous ossification (Fig. 2.2). The chondroblasts turn into chondrocytes (mature cartilage cells) which secrete a mesh of collagenous fibres, which in turn surround and separate the cells (Vaughan 1981) forming a matrix. This matrix is basically a cartilage template around which bone is generated. The mesenchyme cells and the collagenous fibres together form the future centres for ossification

and are again enveloped by a layer of tissue, the perichondrium, which is similar to the periosteum in intramembranous ossification (Fig. 2.3A).

Hypertrophy of the chondrocytes occurs and the matrix around the centrally positioned chondrocytes becomes thinner and starts to disappear leaving large empty gaps ('lacunae'). Thus the cells in the centre of the 'cartilage template' enlarge and die, losing their transverse walls whilst the longitudinal walls calcify (Vaughan 1981). The chondrocytes on the periphery do not hypertrophy compared with those in the middle (Shipman et al 1985) (Fig. 2.3B).

As the chondrocytes die in the constant cycle of regrowth, capillaries carrying osteogenic cells, in particular osteoblasts and osteoclasts, overrun the dying cells. From this time the osteoblasts lay down osteoid (uncalcified organic bone matrix) around the cartilaginous cells which slowly become calcified, and turn to true bone (Fig. 2.3C).

The death of the cartilaginous cells allows proliferation of calcification which occurs especially in the long bones at three centres of growth: the middle of the bone (diaphysis) and at either end of the bone (epiphysis), with the diaphysis being the primary centre (Shipman et al 1985) (Fig. 2.4).

Even when the diaphysis and epiphyses are ossified, the cartilaginous epiphyseal plates are still developing and the process of ossification continues, by the constant reabsorption and deposition of bone material, until the growth in bone length is complete.

The width of bone is determined by apposition. In this process, osteoblasts lay down a further matrix of bone minerals on the existing bone surface, and the generation of new bone increases the bone width.

Patterns of ossification

At birth the epiphyseal plates of the long bones are still cartilaginous and some remain like this until bone maturity (Shipman et al 1985) (see Fig. 2.5). The pattern of epiphyseal ossification has been identified as progressing from the elbow (13–15 years), to the hip (13–16 years), to the ankle (13–18 years), to the knee (14–18 years), to the wrist (18–20 years) and eventually the

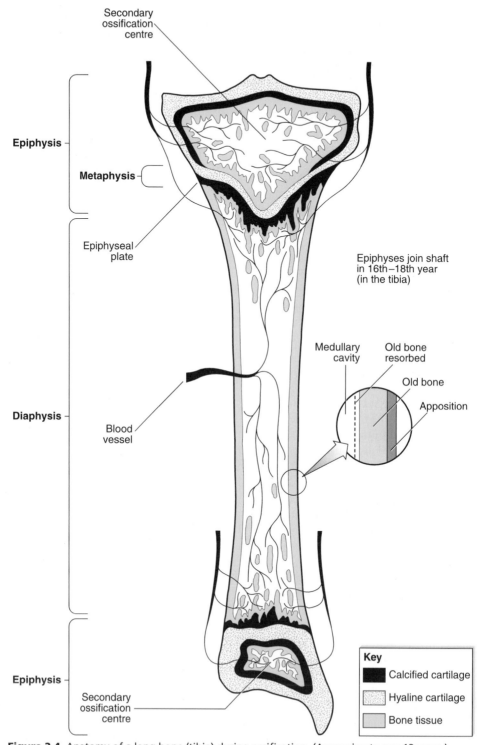

Figure 2.4 Anatomy of a long bone (tibia) during ossification. (Approximate age 12 years.)

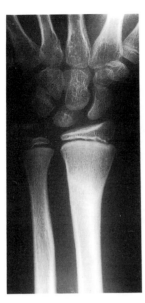

Figure 2.5 X-ray of the non-ossified distal radial epiphyseal plate. (From Dandy 1993 with permission.)

shoulder (15–20 years) with the medial end of the clavicle being reported as incompletely fused as late as 30 years of age (Shipman et al 1985). These timescales encompass both the primary and the secondary ossification timescales.

At birth ossification of the skull is still incomplete, with much of the base remaining cartilaginous. Six large membranes, fontanelles, separate the cranial vaults and these ossify at various times from 2 months to 2 years after birth (Shipman et al 1985) (Fig. 2.6).

Once the fontanelles have ossified there still remain linear sutures between the vault bones. These again ossify at various times, but the process should start at around 17 years of age and be completed by the thirties (Shipman et al 1985).

Often the degree of ossification of the fontanelles, the epiphyses and the sutures is used as an indication of skeletal maturity; the greater the degree of ossification the more advanced is the skeletal maturity.

If either of the epiphyseal plates or fontanelles is damaged or fails to develop, thus not allowing normal growth, then the bone will continue to grow straight (from the diaphysis) but will be shorter than it should be. If only one side of the epiphyseal plate or part of the fontanelle is damaged then the bone will develop an angular deformity (Dandy 1993).

Other features of bone growth and development

Bone length and shape constantly change during the developing years but the bone remains both flexible and elastic throughout its life. This malleability does gradually reduce but is at its greatest in the very early years. In the developing skeletal tissue of the baby, then, only slight stress is needed to deform bone. For example, too small a size of a baby's elasticated cotton suit can deform the feet, and the traditional binding of feet in China made them small. As bone reaches maturity (25 years plus) its flexibility remains high, 'with cortical bone being much stiffer than cancellous, thus withstanding greater stress but less strain before failure' (Nordin & Frankel 1989).

Bone growth and development continue through the first two decades of life, with the length and width still increasing whilst the three-dimensional geometry remains the same (Shipman et al 1985). The timing of the adolescent growth spurt, which starts at 10.3 years in girls and 12 years in boys (Tanner et al 1976), is crucial in determining skeletal height, and the delay of the growth spurt in males gives boys a full 2 years to continue growing before the sudden growth spurt takes place. As a result boys have a mean 28 cm further growth from the start to the end of the spurt, whilst girls have a mean growth of only 25 cm (Vaughan 1981). Bone growth stops some time after the peak velocity of growth, which occurs in girls at around 12 years and in boys at around 14 years. However remodelling by resorption and deposition of bone still continues, ensuring the strength of the overall skeletal structure (Shipman et al 1985).

The main factors that alter the normal skeletal balance, even after bone maturity, are the following:

- *Hormonal level changes* of oestrogen, testosterone, parathormone, growth hormone and thyroxine.

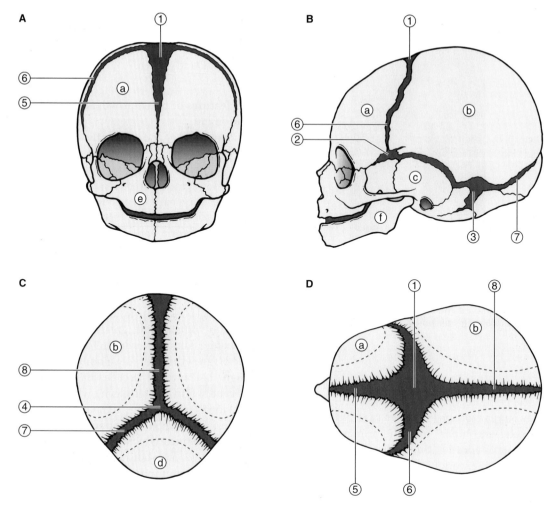

Figure 2.6 Skull of a full-term fetus showing bones, sutures and fontanelles. A From front. B From the left. C From behind. D From above. a, frontal bone; b, parietal bone; .c, temporal bone; d, occipital bone; e, maxilla; f, mandible; 1, anterior (or bregmatic) fontanelle; 2, sphenoidal fontanelle; 3, mastoid fontanelle; 4, posterior (or lambdoid) fontanelle; 5, frontal suture; 6, coronal suture; 7, lambdoid suture; 8, sagittal suture.

- *Mechanical changes*: from altered muscle pull or fracture. Gradually increased muscle pull will stimulate new bone growth and strengthen the bone; loss of muscle strength will reduce the pull on the bone and therefore diminish the local bone strength.
- *Stress and pressure changes*: bone grows in areas of increased weight bearing and reduces in areas where this is decreased.

As the child/adolescent develops, often the soft tissue and the bone growth do not advance at the same rate, resulting in pain or aching due to tissue being pulled at its extreme. Once all tissues catch up with each other the pain/ache will disappear.

Self-assessment questions

- **SAQ 2.5.** Name the main functions of bone.
- **SAQ 2.6.** What does Wolff's law state and what does this imply?
- **SAQ 2.7.** Name the types of ossification of bone.

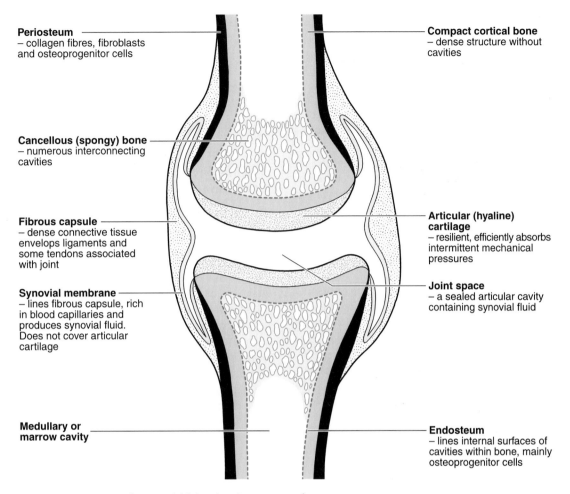

Periosteum
– collagen fibres, fibroblasts
and osteoprogenitor cells

Cancellous (spongy) bone
– numerous interconnecting
cavities

Fibrous capsule
– dense connective tissue
envelops ligaments and
some tendons associated
with joint

Synovial membrane
– lines fibrous capsule, rich
in blood capillaries and
produces synovial fluid.
Does not cover articular
cartilage

**Medullary or
marrow cavity**

Compact cortical bone
– dense structure without
cavities

**Articular (hyaline)
cartilage**
– resilient, efficiently absorbs
intermittent mechanical
pressures

Joint space
– a sealed articular cavity
containing synovial fluid

Endosteum
– lines internal surfaces of
cavities within bone, mainly
osteoprogenitor cells

Figure 2.7 Anatomy of a synovial joint showing common features.

- **SAQ 2.8.** Name the parts of a long bone.

- **SAQ 2.9.** Describe the pattern of timing of epiphyseal ossification.

- **SAQ 2.10.** Name the fontanelles and sutures in the skull and state the ages at which they ossify.

- **SAQ 2.11.** The adolescent growth spurt starts at 10.3 years in girls and 12 years in boys. What factors may influence this growth?

Joints

There are three major types of joint in the human body: fibrous, cartilaginous and synovial. Each type of joint is generated as bone and connective tissue mature, but joint formation is not completed until the normal forces acting across the articulating surfaces provide the stimulus for final development (Shipman et al 1985) (Fig. 2.7).

After the primary centres of ossification (in the shaft) have completed their calcifying process, new bone tissue is stimulated at the interface of the metaphysis and the epiphysis, the epiphyseal plate, until the cartilage tissue is replaced by bone. Each type of joint has developed through the growth and eventual fusion of the secondary centres of ossification in the epiphysis. As the two immature bone ends meet and start to be stressed by forces across the joint, a constant remodelling then occurs and the bone ends generate hyaline cartilage tissue at the force-bearing surfaces.

Tendons and ligaments

Three non-active components of joints are necessary to provide and maintain contact and stability: the fibrous joint capsule (see Fig. 2.7), tendons and ligaments.

The tendons are responsible for the attachment of muscle to bone and as indicated earlier they are often a continuation of the epimysium and perimysium, the fibrous covers of muscle. Ligaments within the joint capsule help to control the degree of motion allowed at a joint, add stability to the joint and prevent excessive motion.

Tendons and ligaments are dense connective tissue, composed of collagen (fibrous protein) and having a meagre blood supply. Collagen gives strength and flexibility and makes up over 75% of the structure of tendons and ligaments. Tendons have more collagen than ligaments particularly in the periphery, where the dry weight of collagen can constitute up to 99% of the total material (Amiel 1984). Collagen contains numerous fibrils and gains its strength from the cross-linking of these fibrils within the structure, giving the ability to withstand high stress levels (Carlstedt & Nordin 1989).

The collagen fibres in tendons lie in parallel so that they can endure the high uniaxial tensile loads which they have to withstand during activity. In contrast, ligaments have to bear stresses in many directions and therefore their collagen fibres are not all parallel but are interfaced with each other in a pattern relating to their functional needs (Amiel 1984).

As the tendons and ligaments mature, the collagen fibrils increase in diameter and the number of cross-links between the fibrils increases, giving the structures greater tensile strength (Carlstedt & Nordin 1989).

Like bone, the tendons, ligaments and capsule remodel to accommodate the stresses put on them. Therefore these tissues all respond to the stimuli of growth, increased weight bearing and increased muscle pull which accompany normal skeletal development.

Self-assessment questions

■ **SAQ 2.12.** Where is the secondary centre of ossification in bone?

■ **SAQ 2.13.** Why are epimysium and perimysium important in muscle attachment?

■ **SAQ 2.14.** What is the difference between the collagen in tendon and ligaments?

Articular (hyaline) cartilage and joint lubrication

Structure of cartilage

Articular cartilage is a highly specialised tissue that is designed to withstand the stresses and strains of weight bearing and constantly altering joint mechanics. It has no vascular supply, lymph channels, or nerves, but has two very important roles: 'distributing joint loads over a wide area thus decreasing the stresses sustained by contacting joint surfaces, and to allow relative movement of the opposing joint surfaces with minimal friction and wear' (Nordin & Frankel 1989).

Cartilage is composed of two layers: the deeper layer, immediately next to the cortical bone is constructed of long columns of chondrocytes arranged perpendicularly to the surface of the bone. These chondrocytes are fat and thickened at the end nearest the bone; at the other end they are thinner, healthier and still produce new cartilage (Shipman et al 1985). The more superficial layer, the 'tangential zone', is a fibrous cover that has fingers of collagen which go vertically down between the chondrocytes to the underlying subchondral bone (Shipman et al 1985).

Cartilage consists of collagen (10–30%), water and inorganic salts, including glycoproteins and lipids (60–87%), and proteoglycans (Pgs) (3–10%) (Nordin & Frankel 1989). The latter are large protein polysaccharide molecules that form a concentrated solution enmeshing the collagen fibrils. Thus the cartilage is often viewed as a 'water-filled sponge' having two distinct parts: the 'fluid' or interstitial part (approximately 75% by wet weight) and the 'solid' part (approximately 25% by wet weight) (Nordin & Frankel 1989).

Synovial fluid

Articular cartilage plays a vital role in the lubri-

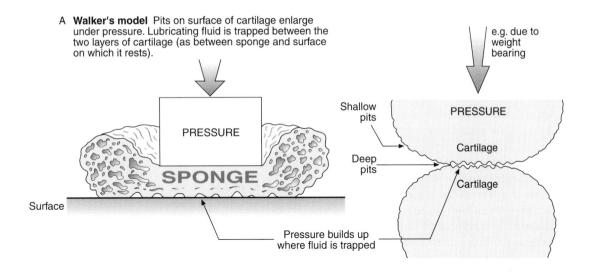

A **Walker's model** Pits on surface of cartilage enlarge under pressure. Lubricating fluid is trapped between the two layers of cartilage (as between sponge and surface on which it rests).

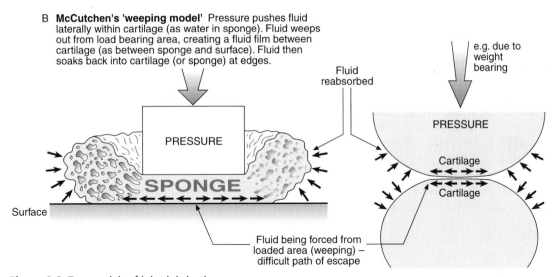

B **McCutchen's 'weeping model'** Pressure pushes fluid laterally within cartilage (as water in sponge). Fluid weeps out from load bearing area, creating a fluid film between cartilage (as between sponge and surface). Fluid then soaks back into cartilage (or sponge) at edges.

Figure 2.8 Two models of joint lubrication.

cation of synovial joints, together with synovial fluid, which in turn is essential for free joint motion, chondrocyte nutrition and reduction of stresses across the joint. Synovial fluid is produced from the synovial membrane of the joint and is composed of a thick serum (clear watery part of blood) and two additional substances: hyaluronic acid, for viscosity and slipperiness, and a double glycoprotein.

Mechanisms of lubrication

Although many mechanisms of lubricating the synovial joints have been suggested (McCutchen 1966, Walker et al 1968, 1970), Nordin & Frankel (1989) state that a combination of mechanisms is probably involved (Fig. 2.8). Thus as there is normally a cyclic function when loading a joint, lubrication will occur in two main ways:

- When a joint is subjected to a low load and is moving, a film of synovial fluid is maintained between the joint surfaces: as some load is applied to the joint an extra supply of fluid lubricant is produced by squeezing out the fluid lying between the chondrocytes of the articular cartilage (see the deep pits in Fig. 2.8A). Thus a fluid film is generated in front of and beneath the articular surface, which is reabsorbed once the load bearing is reduced (Nordin & Frankel 1989).
- If loading is continued, this will cause complete expulsion of the fluid, reducing the quantity of fluid held by the articular cartilage, which will be replaced once the load is removed. A thin film of fluid will always remain but the fluid being squeezed out from the 'boundaries' will be primarily responsible for lubrication. When the load is removed the fluid can then soak back into the articular cartilage as in a sponge (Fig. 2.8B; McCutchen 1966).

Deterioration of cartilage

The mechanical response of cartilage to load is highly complex. It is regarded as a viscoelastic response, i.e. similar to that produced by a combination of a viscous fluid and an elastic solid. The main result of this combination of mechanical properties is that the cartilage can usually withstand the high forces generated by compression, stress, and tension.

Cartilage undergoes continual alteration of load-bearing stress which enhances regeneration of the cartilage. However as this is only a limited capacity, then damage may occur.

It is not until there is substantial damage to the collagen and proteoglycans and removal of the cartilage from the underlying solid bone by constant mechanical stresses (wear) that articular cartilage begins to fail. Once the cartilage starts to decrease in thickness and has small defects then it becomes softer, more permeable, starts to flake and becomes fibrillated (deep vertical clefts appear between the chondrocytes). Therefore the lubricating fluid from between the articular surfaces starts to leak away, allowing direct contact of the surfaces (interfacial wear) and an abrasion process is aggravated.

With alteration in the weight-bearing forces, repeated and added strain on the cartilage surfaces causes fatigue wear. This type of wear is often seen when the ageing joints, with increasing loss of muscle strength, are no longer undergoing the usual biomechanical stresses, and it can take place even if there is good lubrication of the joint (Nordin & Frankel 1989).

Self assessment questions

- **SAQ 2.15.** What are the functions of articular cartilage?

- **SAQ 2.16.** What are proteoglycans and what is their role in cartilage?

- **SAQ 2.17.** Why is cartilage often described as a 'water-filled sponge'?

- **SAQ 2.18.** How does a synovial joint maintain the nutrition of its components?

LIFESTYLE

The normal development of any child and the ageing process in any adult is dependent on a number of external stresses which may impinge at different times, or which may remain constant throughout life. These stresses are essentially due to lifestyle, defined as the particular attitudes, habits or behaviours associated with an individual or group (Collins 1982). But because lifestyles can be so diverse, varying from person to person, or for the same person at different times in life, they will inevitably have differing effects on the changes that occur in the body. Lifestyle, in the very wide-ranging definition given above, will obviously affect the body in a number of ways, but our main concern is how lifestyle variations influence the body's structure, form and function during development and ageing.

Peer and family influences will dictate the environment in which a child is brought up and in which an adult lives. These influences may well involve geographical, cultural and/or religious factors together with social class, and may affect social interactions, family size and occupation (Shephard 1980).

An illustration of this could be the range of

dietary habits seen in our multiclass and multi-cultural society. The particular example of a diet with too much carbohydrate resulting in obesity or an increase in the risk of arteriosclerosis is seen in many cultures or geographical regions. Conversely, there also seems to be an increase in the number of people with vitamin deficiencies due to poor diet. Both these instances would result in characteristic but different morphological changes in the populations involved.

To give another example, the growth and development of a fetus is directly influenced by the amount of nourishment it obtains and if this is diminished at any time then the internal organs undergoing cell division at that period will be prone to damage (Barker 1993). Further to this, if the newborn baby is undersized then it will have an increased risk of coronary heart disease, stroke and diabetes in adult life; therefore the size of the newborn infant can be used as a predictor for adult health (Barker 1993). The strong implication of these points is that external influences on the womb, especially diet, can change the future health and longevity of the unborn (Barker 1993).

A strong influence on the structure and function of the body is the level of activity, which can encompass occupation and hobbies. Both of these may entail varying amounts of physical exercise ranging from that of the sedentary worker to the almost continual activity of the manual labourer, postal delivery worker, professional or amateur sportsperson and so on.

Motivation, either from within the individual or as a result of peer pressure, obviously plays an important part in the level of activity and the quality of physical performance achieved (Smith et al 1989). Verbal encouragement has been shown to enhance performance; Bickers (1993) demonstrated a 33.5% increase in performance of a muscle endurance task with verbal encouragement, when compared with the results attained from same group without encouragement.

AGEING

Stiffness, increased connective tissue, reduced muscle mass, selective atrophy of type II fibres, diminished proprioception, loss of motor neurones, decreased exercise motivation, inactivity and decreased appetite and food intake are age-related changes affecting neuromuscular function and strength (Frontera 1989).

These natural muscular, skeletal, and neural changes occurring with age, are not in themselves detrimental to the capabilities of the systems, but do limit the absolute control of motor performance. This limitation is characterised by a slowing down of movements, a decrease in maximum strength and a loss of fine coordination (Skinner et al 1982). These changes are only gradually noticed by individuals, especially if they have maintained a relatively high standard of health, but will present problems if they reach a degree of severity which causes pain, deformity and/or loss of motor control, or if injury and disease predominate. The natural phenomenon of ageing and, in fact the theoretical concept also, when considered within the real environment, is accelerated and aggravated by extrinsic factors of increased pathophysiological stresses. This is amplified by the intrinsic decrease in the body's ability to respond to these stresses (Govan et al 1991). Malkia (1993) states that it is very difficult to differentiate between the natural effects of ageing on muscle, and the factors causing change which are related to environmental differences and lifestyle. This may equally be true for the other systems in the body.

Although the decline of body systems does not truly present until the fifth decade is reached, the skeletal, muscular and neural systems start to depreciate in the fourth decade (Lexell et al 1988) (Fig. 2.9).

Ageing and the muscular system

The first changes in the muscular system present as a result of alterations in the microscopic muscle structure leading to loss of muscle mass (atrophy) and loss of strength and speed of contraction (Grimby & Saltin 1983, Larsson et al 1979, Vandervoort et al 1986, Young 1984, Young et al 1984, 1985). These changes also appear to arise in conjunction with impaired cardiovascular function and inactivity. Goldspink & Williams (1990) indicate 'that there is a an increase in the

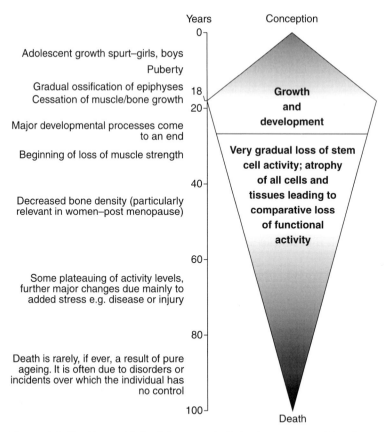

Years   Conception

0

Adolescent growth spurt–girls, boys
Puberty
Gradual ossification of epiphyses   18
Cessation of muscle/bone growth   20

**Growth
and
development**

Major developmental processes come
to an end

Beginning of loss of muscle strength

**Very gradual loss of stem
cell activity; atrophy
of all cells and
tissues leading to
comparative loss
of functional
activity**

40

Decreased bone density (particularly
relevant in women–post menopause)

60

Some plateauing of activity levels,
further major changes due mainly to
added stress e.g. disease or injury

80

Death is rarely, if ever, a result of pure
ageing. It is often due to disorders or
incidents over which the individual has
no control

100

Death

Figure 2.9 The 'rise and fall' of the musculoskeletal system: matching the normal physiological changes in the musculoskeletal system to the ageing process. Adapted with permission from Govan et al (1991).

collagen content of muscle with age with associated thickening of the endomysium and the perimysium'. This is more noticeable in slow muscle (Konanen 1989) and causes an increase in the tensile strength, stiffness and elastic efficiency (Hinderer & Hinderer 1993). Therefore the loss of the full contractile capabilities in conjunction with alterations in neurotransmission (Knortz 1987) in ageing muscle also affect the performance of that muscle.

Atrophy

Prior to discussing the effects of muscle atrophy with age, some knowledge about the different muscle fibre types is needed. A brief overview is given in Table 2.1.

Atrophy has been defined as the loss of muscle mass or a decrease in whole muscle cross-sectional area (St Pierre & Gardiner 1987). Jones &

Round (1992) indicate that there is a loss of up to 30% in muscle mass by 90 years of age. Atrophy of ageing is the result of loss of both muscle fibre types, but with a reduction in the size of mainly type II fibres (Grimby & Saltin 1983, Lexell et al 1988). The selective atrophy of type II fibres is thought to be due to accompanying inactivity and denervation. In the later stages of ageing there tends to be disuse due to a general decrease in activity levels which constitutes a reduced demand for muscle contraction. Extended reduction in activity will mainly affect the antigravity muscles such as soleus muscle because they require stimulation by repeated normal functional patterns (Goldspink & Williams 1990).

Thus changes occur within the tissue, which include diminished capillary density, and a fall in the amount of muscle proteins and of substances involved in energy release. Consequently there is

Table 2.1 Characteristics of skeletal muscle fibre types (adapted from Harris & Watkins 1993)

	Type I (red)	Type II (white)
Diameter	27 micrometres	44 micrometres
Myoglobin content	High	Low
Mitochondria	High	Low
Blood supply	Extensive	Less extensive
Motor end plate	Smaller	Larger
Nerve fibre diameter	Smaller	Larger
Motor unit size	Small	Large
Nerve conduction velocity	Low	High
Contraction time	85 milliseconds	25 milliseconds
Tension	Low	High
Endurance	Long sustained contraction	Fatigues easily
Function	Walking, long-distance running, most functional activities of daily living	Rapid, high power, sudden contractions, such as heavy lifting activities

decreased endurance, force and aerobic/anaerobic capacity, as well as a loss of elasticity due to thinning of connective tissue (St Pierre & Gardiner 1987). Electromyographical studies have demonstrated that, as well as the reduction in muscle fibres in the motor units, there is also a reduction in the number of motor units (Campbell et al 1973). This is substantiated by Tomlinson et al (1969), Aniansson et al (1981) and Tomlinson & Irving (1997) who suggest that the changes in muscle are of neurological origin, rather than simply arising from within the muscle tissue itself.

Strength

Specific decline of muscle strength occurs after the age of 50 years (Lexell et al 1988), although some decline does present after 30 years of age. Rutherford & Jones (1992) demonstrated that there is a 40% loss of strength in the quadriceps muscle alone between the third and the fourth decade, with the cross-sectional area being reduced by 23% and therefore the force-generating capacity of the muscle being diminished by 20%.

This has also been shown by Young et al (1984, 1985), who found that the loss of muscle strength was proportional to the reduction in the cross-sectional area of the muscle. One explanation for

this could be the reduction in levels of hormones such as oestrogen and growth hormone, which does lead to general musculoskeletal atrophy which may be modified at particular sites by superimposed patterns of muscular activity (Rutherford & Jones 1992).

Ageing muscle strength is very often tested by using isometric contraction only, but Malkia (1993) questions this and indicates that muscle performance in ageing should only be tested in 'certain controlled movement conditions of speed, duration and load via energy pathways in movement'. The advance of isokinetic measurement systems has assisted in this.

Fatigability

With ageing there is greater atrophy of type II muscle fibres compared with type I. This leaves the non-fatigable type I muscle fibres predominating, and therefore there is a greater loss of muscle strength than endurance (Stokes & Cooper 1993). O'Connor et al (1993) have shown, with a small sample of active elderly (63–80 years) and young (21–33 years) people, that although the younger age group could generate higher torques (mean of 175.21 newton-metres (Nm) compared with 102.21 Nm), the elderly group could sustain their contraction for a longer period of time, thus demonstrating that elderly muscle does not fatigue as quickly as younger muscle.

This can be explained by looking at the pattern of recruitment of muscle fibres in the normal subject during maximal voluntary contraction (MVC). Initially all muscle fibre types are recruited at a high firing rate, the fast type II fibres being initiated first then the slower type I fibres coming in. The firing rate reduces as the type II fibres fatigue. The type I fibres maintain their input but as they cannot produce the same force as the type II fibres this will be at a reduced magnitude. Therefore in elderly people the average magnitude of the MVC is reduced but the average length of time for which it can be sustained is greater than in younger people (O'Connor et al 1993). It has also been noted that muscle endurance declines with age more in males than in females (Lennmarken et al 1985).

Functional performance and training

Malkia (1993) demonstrated in a cross-sectional survey on physical performance that muscle strength is related to subjective perception of physical ability and hypothesises that the perceived decline in physical ability in the elderly may have an effect on overall muscle strength and vice versa.

In animal and human studies (Konanen 1989) has shown that muscle fibre types can be changed and that with endurance training there is a change from fast to slow muscle fibres.

Elderly muscle can demonstrate a similar trend in gaining strength as younger muscle (Vandervoort et al 1986) but trained athletes between the ages of 30 and 70 years can maintain greater strength than untrained people of similar ages (Sipila & Suominen 1991).

Thus, lifestyle does have an effect on the ability of muscle to perform, but appropriate exercise is essential (Astrand 1986) in maintaining and retraining elderly muscle.

Ageing and non-contractile tissue

The maturation of collagen in the non-contractile tissues occurs around the age of 20 years and after that the magnitude of the tensile properties seem to plateau. Then, after a variable period of time, the cross-links between and within the collagen decrease in number and quality. The tensile strength and stiffness of collagen then decreases and the tissues cannot withstand deformation (Carlstedt & Nordin 1989).

Self-assessment questions

- **SAQ 2.19.** Outline the first changes in ageing muscle.

- **SAQ 2.20.** Define atrophy.

- **SAQ 2.21.** During ageing the type II muscle fibres are lost to a greater extent; what does this imply for muscle performance?

The cardiovascular system and total body fitness

The capacity for whole body exercise, particularly aerobic capability, declines first, despite relatively normal muscle metabolism and this decline occurs before any morphological changes in muscle are evident (Grimby & Saltin 1983).

This loss of aerobic power is thought to be due to cardiopulmonary changes, in particular to reduced maximal cardiac output and maximal heart rate (Mahler et al 1986). It should be noted that the reduced cardiovascular fitness is not completely irreversible, and useful changes through fitness training can be attained (Smith 1989) regardless of age.

It must be stressed that improvement in performance is just as feasible in the elderly as in the young, for both specific muscle function (Frontera et al 1988, Moritani & De Vries 1980) and whole body endurance exercise, which leads to an increase in maximum oxygen uptake (Makrides 1986). However the changes associated with ageing cannot be stopped, only postponed.

Ageing of bone and joints

After bone has matured the amount of stress which it can endure slowly reduces, for a number of reasons. During the normal ageing process, bone becomes progressively less dense with the longitudinal trabeculae becoming thinner and the transverse trabeculae being reabsorbed (Nordin & Frankel 1989). This reduction in bone density (osteoporosis) is greater in women than in men and is accelerated 5–10 years after the menopause (Rutherford & Jones 1992). Rutherford & Jones (1992) also note that bone mass reductions with age vary at different sites, with the mass of the distal femur decreasing after the third decade and the decrease in mass of the spinal vertebrae and the middle of the femur being delayed until the fifth or sixth decade. Therefore bones are prone to fracture or alteration from added stress, at different ages.

Thus the bone is reduced in size, strength and stiffness, as the total amount of bone tissue diminishes, particularly cancellous bone. Burstein et al (1976) demonstrated that the amount of strain older bone can withstand is only half that of younger bone, signifying increased brittleness and a possible loss of energy storage capacity.

The loss of bone in the elderly is dependent on the amount of bone that was present at the point of bone maturity. Therefore as the amount of bone is extremely variable between different individuals, and in the various parts of the skeletal system, the total amount of bone lost in old age is very hard to predict (Shipman et al 1985).

Bone loss after maturity is also dependent on dietary factors and is enhanced by the normal reduction in the amount of calcium that can be absorbed, particularly after the age of 70 years (Vaughan 1981). The reduction of mineral content in bone means that the normal homeostatic balance has to be reestablished; therefore if there is an added loss of calcium due to reduced uptake of minerals this balance will be more difficult to maintain.

As we get older, generally, lesser demands are made on bone, with muscle strength and weight bearing being reduced (from a reduction or loss of weight-bearing activity), thus periosteal and subperiosteal bone is reabsorbed resulting in the loss of strength and stiffness, as mentioned earlier (Nordin & Frankel 1989). However locally, as muscle strength decreases with age, the resulting altered biomechanical alignment and stresses across bone and joints cause changes (usually an increase) to the size and shape of the joint surfaces. Thus the cartilaginous tissue at the joint surface and the underlying bone proliferates, as described by Wolff's law. So, the joint dimensions may increase in size with the subchondral bone appearing thicker on X-ray.

The loss of muscle strength and therefore altered muscle/tendon pull, along with hormonal changes to the bone of ageing females, induces a loss of bone density (osteoporosis). Hence the bone is much more prone to fracture and/or collapse (Bland 1993). The altered pull of the muscle/tendon may also cause initial trauma to its bony attachment resulting in a proliferation of new bone, forming a cartilaginous or bony spur. This usually occurs at the bony attachment of the tendons. With a reduction in muscle strength in ageing, there may be an inability to control the normal joint stresses, leading to a change in the weight-bearing forces across the joint. The weight-bearing surfaces of the joints start to fail due to 'either repeated application of high loads over a relatively short period or with the repetition of low loads over an extended period, even though the magnitude of those loads may be much lower than the material's ultimate strength' (Nordin & Frankel 1989).

These changes are not necessarily noticed until further external stresses such as injury, infection or inflammation occur. Often, in fact, it is not until the additional stresses on the hyaline cartilage at the bone ends and the underlying subchondral bone progress to eburnation (polished state) and excessive signs of 'wear and tear' are shown, with the subsequent diagnosis of osteoarthrosis, that it becomes obvious that these mechanical changes have been occurring for some time.

Self-assessment questions

- **SAQ 2.22.** What is osteoporosis and why does it occur to a greater extent after the menopause?

- **SAQ 2.23.** Which type of bone is reduced most during the ageing process?

- **SAQ 2.24.** How does the operation of Wolff's law affect ageing bone?

COMPARISON OF THE MUSCULOSKELETAL CHANGES DUE TO AGEING AND THOSE DUE TO OSTEOARTHROSIS

Problem-solving exercise 2.1

The results of the ageing process have been outlined in this chapter and there has been no attempt to compare them with the effects of osteoarthrosis. Meachim (1969) outlined the comparison between the two processes for bone, joint and articular cartilage. The changes in the ageing process are given in the table below. In the prerequisites for this chapter you were asked to revise the pathology of osteoarthrosis. Therefore you should be able to answer the following question.

■ **A.** From your reading can you fill in the comparable changes that occur in articular cartilage, bone, joint and muscle in the pathology of osteoarthrosis?

Osteoarthrosis	Ageing
	Normal metabolism
	Normal enzymatic modelling
	Cartilage changes only
	No chondrocyte mitosis
	Normal rates of synthesis of collagen and proteoglycans
	No change or a reduction in the water content of cartilage
	Fibrillation, non-progressive, non-weight-bearing sites of cartilage
	No eburnation of cartilage
	Osteophytes at joint edges only, with excessive use
	Increased collagen cross-links
	No inflammation
	No joint effusion
	Normal pigment in cartilage
	Reduction in type II muscle fibres
	No sclerosis of subchondral bone
	Minimal loss of joint space, may occur at the periphery. There should be no loss of joint congruity
	No ongoing joint/muscle pain

(List modified and adapted from Bland 1993.)

Summary

Development and ageing involve all the components of the musculoskeletal system: muscle, bone, joint capsule, tendons, ligaments and articular cartilage. The musculoskeletal system cannot survive in isolation and is dependent on the development, maturation and ageing effects of the neural and cardiovascular systems.

All the changes that occur throughout the 25–30 years of development of muscle, bone, tendon, articular cartilage and ligaments are slowly reversed at the start of the ageing process, but the timescale for ageing is much longer (from around 30 years of age until death). But the effects of ageing are most significant after 55 years of age, especially around the time of the menopause in women.

The effects of ageing will be influenced by the lifestyle and fitness of the person throughout their active years, with the onset of the effects of ageing being less evident in the fitter and healthier individual.

The normal effects of ageing do not necessarily cause problems to the individual but may reduce their functional level, speed and performance. It is not until the effects of the stresses on the musculoskeletal structures cause failure that the changes of ageing develop into pathological signs and symptoms.

ANSWERS TO THE QUESTIONS AND EXERCISE

Self-assessment questions (page 22)

■ **SAQ 2.1.** Which parts of a muscle constitute the contractile units?

Answer: Myofibrils, consisting of sarcomeres with filaments of actin and myosin, are the main contractile units.

■ **SAQ 2.2.** Outline which types of movement can be performed at birth.

Answer: Reflex movements and some gross activity patterns.

■ **SAQ 2.3.** What does muscle strength directly depend upon?

Answer: Muscle cross-sectional area and the number of myofibrils.

■ **SAQ 2.4.** How does a muscle maintain the generation of force as it lengthens during the developmental sequence?

Answer: By the addition of serial sarcomeres, so that there is a continued overlap of actin and myosin filaments.

Self-assessment questions (pages 28–29)

■ **SAQ 2.5.** Name the main functions of bone.

Answer: Support, protection and mineral homeostasis.

■ **SAQ 2.6.** What does Wolff's law state and what does this imply?

Answer: Bone will alter its size, shape, and trabecular pattern, in both the subchondral and cortical bone, according to the line of physical stress. This implies that bone is constantly remodelling to accommodate the natural stresses on body tissue.

■ **SAQ 2.7.** Name the types of ossification of bone.

Answer: Endochondral (cartilage) ossification and intramembranous ossification.

■ **SAQ 2.8.** Name the parts of a long bone.

Answer:
— *Epiphysis: distal part*
— *Metaphysis: start of the secondary centre of ossification; the site of the epiphyseal plate*
— *Epiphyseal plate: junction of the epiphysis and the diaphysis; the growth plate*
— *Diaphysis: shaft of the bone*
— *Medullary cavity: cavity in the centre of the shaft of the bone*
— *Cancellous bone: open weave, lighter and spongier bone*
— *Cortical bone: hard crust of bone tissue forming the exterior layers.*

■ **SAQ 2.9.** Describe the pattern of timing of epiphyseal ossification.

Answer: Elbow (13–15 years); hip (13–16 years); ankle (13–18 years); knee (14–18 years); wrist (18–20 years); shoulder (15–20 years), and the medial end of the clavicle up to 30 years of age.

■ **SAQ 2.10.** Name the fontanelles and sutures in the skull and state the ages at which they ossify.

Answer: Fontanelles: anterior (bregmatic), sphenoidal, mastoid, posterior (lambdoid). Sutures: frontal, coronal, lambdoid, sagittal. Fontanelles ossify from 2 months to 2 years. Sutures ossify between 17 years and 30 years

■ **SAQ 2.11.** The adolescent growth spurt starts at 10.3 years in girls and 12 years in boys. What factors may influence this growth?

Answer: Alterations to the hormone level, mechanics and stress and pressure.

Self-assessment questions (page 30)

■ **SAQ 2.12.** Where is the secondary centre of ossification in bone?

Answer: The epiphysis.

■ **SAQ 2.13.** Why are epimysium and perimysium important in muscle attachment?

Answer: They combine with the collagen of the tendon to join the muscle to the bone.

■ **SAQ 2.14.** What is the difference between the collagen in tendon and ligaments?

Answer: The collagen fibres in tendons lie parallel; however, in ligaments some of the fibres are parallel but they also lie in a functional pattern which can give multidirectional strength.

Self-assessment questions (page 32)

■ **SAQ 2.15.** What are the functions of articular cartilage?

Answer: To distribute joint loads over a wide area, reduce friction between opposing joint surfaces and help in the lubrication of the joint.

■ **SAQ 2.16.** What are proteoglycans and what is their role in cartilage?

Answer: They are large protein polysaccharide molecules, which form a concentrated solution enmeshing the collagen fibres.

■ **SAQ 2.17.** Why is cartilage often described as a 'water-filled sponge'?

Answer: It is constructed of a solid part (collagen) and a fluid part (water and inorganic salts), and acts in a similar way to a sponge in performing its functions.

■ **SAQ 2.18.** How does a synovial joint maintain the nutrition of its components?

Answer: Synovial fluid is generated by the synovial membrane and it is distributed with the aid of the articular cartilage; either the fluid is pushed ahead of the motion and reabsorbed when the pressure is reduced, or the direct pressure squeezes out the fluid from the articular cartilage.

Self-assessment questions (page 36)

■ **SAQ 2.19.** Outline the first changes in ageing muscle.

Answer: Microscopic changes with resulting loss of muscle mass, strength and speed of contraction.

■ **SAQ 2.20.** Define atrophy.

Answer: Loss of muscle mass; therefore a reduction in the cross-sectional area of the muscle.

■ **SAQ 2.21.** During ageing the type II muscle fibres are lost to a greater extent; what does this imply for muscle performance?

Answer: A relatively greater reduction in the strength which can be generated and slighter loss of endurance.

Self-assessment questions (page 37)

■ **SAQ 2.22.** What is osteoporosis and why does it occur to a greater extent after the menopause?

Answer: Reduction in bone density. It is worse after the menopause because of the changes in hormone levels.

■ **SAQ 2.23.** Which type of bone is reduced most during the ageing process?

Answer: Cancellous bone.

■ **SAQ 2.24.** How does the operation of Wolff's law affect ageing bone?

Answer: The weight-bearing stresses across the joint change with age. Therefore where there is added pressure, the underlying cartilage and bone first proliferate to accommodate for the increase, but where the pressure is reduced the cartilage and bone are not stimulated to remodel and there may be a loss of tissue.

Problem-solving exercise 2.1 (page 38)

■ **A.** From your reading, can you fill in the comparable changes that occur in articular cartilage, bone, joint and muscle in the pathology of osteoarthrosis?

Answer:

Osteoarthrosis

Highly anabolic and synthetic process

Enzymatic destruction of hard tissue

Remodelling of all tissues about joint (articular and periarticular)

Chondrocyte mitosis

Intense increased synthesis of collagen and proteoglycan

Increased water content of cartilage

Fibrillation, focal and progressive at weight-bearing sites

Eburnation, ivory-like

Osteophytes occur with other joint changes

No increased collagen cross-links

Inflammation

Joint effusion present on occasions

No pigment-cartilage

Reduction in type II and type I muscle fibres

Sclerosis of subchondral bone

Narrowing of the joint space and loss of joint congruity, particularly at the surfaces bearing the greatest weights

Joint and/or muscle pain

REFERENCES

Amiel A 1984 Tendons and ligaments: a morphological and biochemical comparison. Journal of Orthopaedic Research 1:257

Aniansson A, Grimby G, Hedberg G et al 1981 Muscle morphology, enzyme activity and muscle strength in elderly men and women. Clinical Physiology 1:73

Astrand P-O 1986 Exercise physiology of the mature athlete. In: Sutton J R, Brock R M (eds) Sports medicine for the mature athlete. Benchmark Press, Indianapolis, ch 3, p 3–15

Barker D 1993 What makes them grow into healthy adults? Medical Research Council News 60:8

Bell G, Emslie-Smith D, Paterson C 1980 Textbook of physiology. Churchill Livingstone, Edinburgh

Bickers M 1993 Does verbal encouragement work? The effect of verbal encouragement on a muscular endurance task. Clinical Rehabilitation 7:196

Bland J H 1993 Mechanisms of adaptation in the joint. In: Crosbie J, McConnell J (eds) Key issues in musculoskeletal physiotherapy. Butterworth Heinemann, Oxford, p 88–113

Burstein A, Reilly D, Martens M 1976 Aging of bone tissue; mechanical properties. Journal of Bone and Joint Surgery 58A:82

Campbell M J, McComas A J, Petito F 1973 Physiological changes in ageing muscle. Journal of Neurology, Neurosurgery and Psychiatry 36:174

Carlstedt C, Nordin M 1989 Biomechanics of tendons and ligaments. In: Nordin M, Frankel V (eds) Basic biomechanics of the musculoskeletal system, 2nd edn. Lea & Febiger, Philadelphia, ch 3, p 59–74

Collins 1982 The New Collins Concise English Dictionary. Collins, London

Dandy D 1993 Essential orthopaedics and trauma. Churchill Livingstone, Edinburgh

Espenschade A, Eckert H 1980 Motor development, 2nd edn. Charles E Merrill, Columbus, Ohio

Frontera W R 1989 Strength training in the elderly. In: Harris R, Harris S (eds) Physical activity, aging and sports. CSA, Albany, p 319

Frontera W R, Meredith C N, O'Reilly K P et al 1988 Strength conditioning in older men: skeletal muscle hypertrophy and improved function. Journal of Applied Physiology 64:1038

Goldspink G, Williams P 1990 Muscle fibre and connective tissue changes associated with use and disuse. In: Ada L, Canning C (eds) Key issues in neurological physiotherapy. Butterworth Heinemann, Oxford, ch 8, p 197–218

Govan A, McFarlane P, Callender R 1991 Pathology illustrated, 3rd edn. Churchill Livingstone, Edinburgh

Grimby G, Saltin B 1983 The ageing muscle. Clinical Physiology 3:209

Harris B A, Watkins M P 1993 Muscle performance: principles and general theory. In: Harms-Ringdahl K (ed) IPPT8 Muscle strength. Churchill Livingstone, Edinburgh

Hinderer K A, Hinderer S R 1993 Development and assessment in children and adolescents. In: Harms-Ringdahl K (ed) IPPT 8 Muscle strength. Churchill Livingstone, Edinburgh

Jones D, Round J 1992 Skeletal muscle in health and disease. Manchester University Press, Manchester

Knortz K A 1987 Muscle physiology applied to geriatric rehabilitation. Topics in Geriatric Rehabilitation 2(4):1

Konanen V 1989 Effects of ageing and physical training on rat skeletal muscle. Acta Physiologica Scandinavica 135 (suppl 577)

Larsson L, Grimby G, Karlsson J 1979 Muscle strength and speed of movement in relationship to age and muscle morphology. Journal of Applied Physiology 46:451

Lennmarken C, Bergman T, Larsson J et al 1985 Skeletal muscle function in man: force relaxation rate, endurance, and contraction time – dependence on sex and age. Clinical Physiology 5:243

Lexell J, Taylor C C, Sjostrom M 1988 What is the cause of the ageing atrophy? Journal of the Neurological Sciences 84:275

McCutchen C W 1966 Boundary lubrication by synovial fluid: demonstration and possible osmotic explanation. Federation Proceedings 25:1061

Mahler D A, Cunningham L N, Curfman L D 1986 Ageing and exercise performance. Clinical Geriatric Medicine 2:433

Makrides L 1986 Physical training in young and older healthy subjects. In: Sutton J R, Brock R M (eds) Sports medicine for the mature athlete. Benchmark Press, Indianapolis, p 363

Malkia E 1993 Strength and aging: patterns of change and implications for training. In: Harms-Ringdahl K (ed) IPPT 8 Muscle strength. Churchill Livingstone, Edinburgh

Meachim G 1969 Age changes in articular cartilage. Clinical Orthopaedics 64:33

Methany E 1941 Breathing capacity and grip strength of preschool children. Child Welfare 18(2):1

Monotoye H J, Lamphiear D E 1977 Grip and arm strength in males and females, aged 10–69 years. Research Quarterly 48:109

Moritani T, De Vries H W 1980 Potential for gross muscle hypertrophy in older men. Journal of Gerontology 35:672

Nordin M, Frankel V 1989 Basic biomechanics of the musculoskeletal system, 2nd edn. Lea & Febiger, Philadelphia

O'Connor M, Carnell P, Manuel J, Scott O M 1993 Contractile characteristics of human quadriceps femoris muscle in active elderly and young adults. Proceedings of the Physiological Society, London

Russo P 1990 Cardiovascular responses associated with activity and inactivity. In: Canning C, Ada L (eds) Key issues in neurological physiotherapy. Butterworth Heinemann, London, ch 6, p 127–154

Rutherford O, Jones D 1992 Relationship of muscle and bone loss and activity levels with age in women. Age and Ageing 21:286

Shephard R J 1980 Population aspects of human working capacity. Annals of Human Biology 7(1):1

Shipman P, Walker A, Bichell D 1985 The human skeleton. Harvard University Press, Cambridge, Massachusetts

Sipila S, Suominen H 1991 Ultrasound imaging of the quadriceps muscle in elderly athletes and untrained men. Muscle and Nerve 14: 527

Skinner J, Tipton C, Vailas A 1982 Exercise, physical training and the aging process. In: Viidik A (ed) Lectures in gerontology. Vol I: On biology of aging. Part B. Academic Press, London, p 407

Smith G A, Nelson R G, Sadoff S J, Sadoff A M 1989 Assessing sincerity of effort in maximal grip strength tests. American Journal of Physical Medicine and Rehabilitation 2:73

Smith W D F 1989 Fitness training in the elderly: Canadian experience. Geriatric Medicine 19:55

Stokes M, Cooper R 1993 Physiological factors influencing performance of skeletal muscle. In: Crosbie J, McConnell J (eds) Key issues in musculoskeletal physiotherapy. Butterworth Heinemann, Oxford, ch 2

St Pierre D, Gardiner P 1987 The effect of immobilisation and exercise on muscle function: a review. Physiotherapy Canada 39:24

Tanner J M, Whitehouse R H, Marubini E, Resele L F 1976 The adolescent growth spurt of boys and girls of the Harpenden growth study. Annals of Human Biology 3:109

Thelen E 1985 The developmental origins of motor coordination; leg movements in human infants. Developmental Psychobiology 18(1):1

Tomlinson B E, Walton J N, Rebeiz J J 1969 The effects on ageing in and cachexia upon skeletal muscle. A histopathological study. Journal of Neural Science 9:321

Tomlinson B E, Irving D 1977 The numbers of limb motor neurones in the human lumbosacral cors throughout life. Journal of Neural Science 34:213

Vandervoort A A, Hayes K C, Belanger A Y 1986 Strength and endurance of skeletal muscle in the elderly. Physiotherapy Canada 38:167

Vaughan J 1981 The physiology of bone. Clarendon Press, Oxford.

Walker P, Dowson D, Longfield M, Wright V 1968 'Boosted lubrication' in synovial joints by fluid entrapment and enrichment. Annals of the Rheumatic Diseases 27:512

Walker P, Dowson D, Longfield M, Wright V 1970 Mode of aggregation of hyaluronic acid protein complex on the surface of articular cartilage. Annals of the Rheumatic Diseases 29:591

Young A 1984 The relative isometric strength of type I and type II muscle fibres in the human quadriceps. Clinical Physiology 4:23

Young A, Stokes M, Crowe M 1984 Size and strength of quadriceps muscle of old and young women. European Journal of Clinical Investigation 14:282

Young A, Stokes M, Crowe M 1985 Size and strength of quadriceps muscle of old and young men. Clinical Physiology 5:145

3

Recognition of change in the musculoskeletal system: assessment

■ Assessment ■ Change and its measurement ■ Physiotherapy management
■ Health models

CONTENTS

Objectives

By the end of this chapter you will:

1. Have an awareness of the different philosophies underlying assessment.
2. Have an understanding of the different changes measured by different assessments and be aware of the suitability of different types of assessments for differing situations.

Prerequisites

Before reading this chapter you should revise the different assessment techniques and schedules you have used up to now for assessing musculoskeletal changes.

INTRODUCTION

The Code of Conduct of the Chartered Society of Physiotherapy (1990) charges its members with the absolute need to assess each patient before treating him or her.

The assessment acts as the baseline for the decisions we subsequently take. It is therefore of ultimate importance for our patient as his or her future management will depend on it. By looking in detail at different facets of assessment and developing a good rationale based on a sound theory base, the physiotherapist will become flexible in using only those aspects of the very detailed assessment apparatus that are relevant for the particular patient about to be assessed. This is true for the subjective as well as the objective assessment. Time spent on acquiring good and flexible assessment skills always pays off in terms of treatment outcome: a poor assessment cannot be compensated for by a technically excellent treatment as one would not be able to ascertain the extent of the possible change.

The first question we need to ask is 'assessment of what'? Do we assess change or do we assess needs? Is the assessment aimed at for instance, a change in range of movement, or is it geared towards establishing what would be necessary to enable the patient to be as independent as possible?

Physiotherapists are experts in recognising when change has taken place. We realise the wide variety of what is normal but also have an understanding of what changes are beyond the realm of normal. This specialised discernment is something our particular training/education can bring to the assessment procedure.

Demonstrating and measuring this change is the underlying core of assessment. The recognition and validation of change has been central to physiotherapists becoming recognised as independent and autonomous practitioners. This identification and measurement of change is being authenticated by slowly expanding research efforts (Parry 1985).

HEALTH MODELS

Before this discussion goes any further we need to consider different models of health and the resulting roles of physiotherapist and patient within these. As will be seen, the model in which the practitioner works has a considerable defining influence on the role of the patient. The different paradigms feed the assessment philosophy and hence are directly related to outcome.

The biomedical model

In a strict biomedical model the patient's referring problem is defined in terms of a system breakdown. His or her body is seen as a biological entity which has developed a fault. The role of the practitioner is therefore to identify the area of breakdown while the role of the patient is to cooperate with the treatment and to get better. Years of 'the fracture in bed 5' or 'the total hip replacement in the side ward' give evidence of the ultimate starkness of this approach. It is believed that the body is governed by certain natural laws which can be predicted and which assume a vaguely linear pattern.

Within this model, the purpose of assessment clearly is to identify the pathological or mechanical change rather than to try to understand the impact of the current happening on the patient's life. Questions about the patient's personal life, hobbies, profession and general perceptions about his or her problem and so on, seem to be less important if not irrelevant within this model as they will not influence the treatment avenue. As long as physiotherapists saw themselves more as doctors' assistants than as autonomous practitioners, working within this model was appropriate and congruent with our treatment approaches.

In strict terms, however, this model suggested that, as we all shared bodies that reacted along similar physiological lines, we would react similarly to therapeutic advances. This is clearly not so: all of us will be able to recall situations that demonstrated how differently we all respond to the same stimulus. Even though the noxious insult may be the same, the level of pain it causes is likely to be quite different in different people. On the other hand, two patients with the same orthopaedic diagnosis might recover at completely different rates. Using the biomedical model, it is hard to generate acceptable explanations for these happenings and it has been felt not to be altogether congruent with the different therapies.

However, it is difficult to fully explore other models as long as we work within a referral system that is still steeped in the biomedical approach. I do not want to be too critical about this model though, as there are clear situations within which this is the most appropriate structure to assess and work. Remind yourself of your experiences in ITU settings.

The biopsychosocial model

Over the past years, therefore, health professionals in general and physiotherapists in particular have moved away from the very powerful biomedical mind set and have shifted more towards a model that incorporates the patient as a partner and does not just look at him or her as a biological system which has broken down. This biopsychosocial model views the patient as presenting with a problem which could lie in the spheres of his body, psyche or social environment. Here the role of the health professional is to empower the patient to deal with the existing problem in an individual way. This automatically assumes that the patient and the therapist have to negotiate goals in a collaborative effort (rather than the therapist informing the patient of his/her objectives).

The treatment outcome as well as the assessment does not merely deal with the identification of a biological breakdown but also with the meaning this has for the patient and the influence this has on the patient's lifestyle.

This model takes into account the fact that all of us are different and that we are affected quite differently by events, hence allowing for our vulnerability factors. Remember how some patients do not want to know anything about their clinical diagnosis and just want to leave it up to the professional to get on with it and 'cure' them, while others ask a lot of very detailed questions and wish to be in a situation where they can make an informed choice about their future. This might include the decision not to avail themselves of our treatment.

You can see how different the assessments would need to be for these two types of patient in order to get the best result for them. It is therefore vital that you search your physiotherapist's

soul and become aware of how you tick within certain physiotherapy situations. Do you lean more towards a biomedical or biopsychosocial approach in your patient assessments? Are your assessments geared to elicit 'hard' measures only (measurable signs) or do you include 'soft' measures which are more focused on the individual? This will clearly be different according to the setting you usually work in. It is essential that we consider these points before the assessment is planned and executed.

ASSESSMENT IN GENERAL

The physiotherapy assessment usually falls into two or even three components (Parry 1985).

- a subjective examination, that is an interview, listening to the patient's story;
- an objective examination, the measuring of hard findings, and
- interpretations.

Physiotherapists spend much time becoming accomplished in these three elements of assessment and have developed a certain thoroughness in this. One thought which comes to mind is that although the patient shares a disorder with others (i.e. his biological system has failed in a predictable way), his or her needs are individual and therefore the priorities that are set must be individual priorities, incorporating an individual potential for response (Watts 1985).

The assessment is carried out with scientific rigour and follows predictable and strictly ordered thought processes. As mentioned earlier we set much store by this approach and base the right to be autonomous practitioners on this element of our practice and education.

Watts (1985) links the decision-making process, which is really the consequence of assessment, to having a vision which is clearly related to the physiotherapist's understanding of her role and responsibility in this interaction. Is she meant to be the powerful healer or does she see herself more as the patient's partner who is able to empower him?

Watts refers further to the possible danger of a narrowness of vision if the choices in assessment and decision making are made in an unconscious way. How can we make these choices explicit and hence conscious? Self-awareness, as previously mentioned, can be a considerable step in this direction. The implementation of regular peer supervision amongst physiotherapists as a routine means of ensuring good practice is an excellent avenue to achieve this. Are there some assessment, and hence management options we never consider and why is that? The disadvantage of having a predictable and well structured route through the information-gathering process is the possible lack of safeguards concerning the recognition of something different as relevant. The rapidly expanding study of the processes of clinical reasoning might help us to make our thought processes explicit, and hence might allow us to develop in breadth rather than just in depth.

Do we use all the information gained in an assessment? Is our assessment aimed only at picking out the useful information for this patient? Watts (1985) stresses the importance of exploring what our assessments are based on. Are they based on theory or really on professional anecdotes? Are we aware of where this theory comes from? Is it borrowed from the fields of medicine or sociology or is it based on physiotherapy observations? What markers do we use in our assessments? Do we use the concepts of normal/abnormal or stability/mobility or disorder pathways (for instance, osteoarthritis versus rheumatoid arthritis, and so on)? How do we report change? Do we report it in terms of judgemental statements or descriptions of state or in any other way? How do we ensure the relevance of this information that we collect? Hislop (1985) states that evaluation/assessment by the physiotherapist must display a recognition of the uniqueness of the relationship of the patient as a person on the one hand and a disorder of the social context of society or community in which the person or the patient lives on the other. This is a very taxing standard. This, Hislop says, cannot be taught but can only be achieved through continuous practice and of course reflection on these decision-making processes. Every individual clinician seems to attain this by recognised routes but it seems clear that a critical stance and self-awareness, rather than conformity, are vital ingredients.

Four ingredients for the achievement of clinical excellence have been stated to be memory, knowledge, competence and performance (Hislop 1985). As previously mentioned, change can only be evaluated if one has an accurate knowledge of the normal variations in people which then allows the clinician to decide when something is beyond the normal range. The same is true, of course, concerning the predictability of treatment effects. Once again, therefore, a sound knowledge base is demanded.

Two approaches to assessment

Ramsden's model of assessment

Elsa Ramsden (1985) looked at the different stages influencing the decision-making process in an assessment. She subdivided these into seven subcategories which she feels identify individuals' differing roles and responsibilities in the assessment process.

1. receiving
2. inferring
3. feeling
4. feeling about feeling
5. determining
6. deciding
7. acting.

Self-assessment question

- **SAQ 3.1.** Which of the above categories are you aware of as a physiotherapist? Do you put these into the same order?

This model takes it for granted that people process data, decode the information which comes via the senses and encode the messages they send.

Ramsden (1985) again proposes the following four strategies for change resulting from this assessment.

1. Identify the need for change.
2. Establish goals for change.
3. Select means for the attainment of change (equals a goal).
4. Evaluate the results of change.

These four stages are at the heart of each and

every assessment but they do not automatically occur. For this to happen, she says, three things have to happen in the change process. First, there has to be a need for change; secondly the necessary relationship between patient and therapist needs to be established; lastly, an appropriate course of action working towards the desired change or goal needs to be established. These things sound clear and straightforward but the level of skills involved in this is obviously considerable.

Self-assessment question

■ **SAQ 3.2.** Does this sound familiar to you? Can you try to verbalise and identify your own implicit structure of assessments?

Work on the relationship of patient and therapist must be the focus for assessment or treatment if progress or cooperation is to be achieved. The quality of this relationship is of paramount importance if we want to achieve the very best results in our assessment and hence it must be included in our scrutiny of our own practice.

Ramsden (1985) argues that a model for change must be placed within the context of a problem-solving analysis. Again, she identifies several stages: first recognising the problem, then identifying and locating resources, and finally by proposing alternative courses. Only then does she embark on selecting the course of action, initiating it and starting to collect data. These are followed by the evaluation process.

Paris' approach to assessment

Stanley Paris (1985) approaches assessment from a different angle. Rather than being immersed in the process of assessment as Ramsden is, his concerns are more focused on outcome and hence on our understanding of the underlying causes for the patient's distress and the course our assessments will take.

He challenges our understanding of pathology leading to pain which in turn leads to spasm. This cycle would keep our assessments firmly within the realms of the biomedical model, leaving us with the problem of how we would identify the needs for change in terms of disease process. Paris' own thinking had led him to iden-

tify a triad consisting of dysfunction, which in turn creates or contributes to a noxious stimulus which will then lead to an involuntary muscle holding. Should the involuntary muscle holding not resolve, it will automatically cause a circulatory problem (stasis) which leads to the retention of metabolites and hence, once again, to pain. Paris' point (1985) is that an assessment therefore should not try to identify a syndrome but rather symptoms which when treated will relieve the syndrome and hence the pain.

In this concept the need for change is couched in terms of function and this, by definition, must result in an individually differing goal.

Paris (1985) reminds us that while most physicians will wait or need to wait for laboratory results to confirm the suspected diagnosis, physiotherapists tend to feel that they need to be able to come to an instant opinion on which to base judgements about treatment and further management. This often leads to premature decisions and to incorrect information being given to the patient. It is necessary to postpone the first treatment of the patient until after the assessment has been evaluated properly.

Should you use examination sheets or not?

There are obviously clear advantages in using examination sheets, such as neatness, speed, consistency and easy transferability. However, the disadvantages should not be minimised. Are all patients going to need the same kind of questioning or approach; with some might it be possible to branch off much earlier into a particular area of the interview and assessment? This will depend largely on the experience, or lack of it, of the examiner.

It seems important that their usefulness should be gauged for each assessment setting (see also Ch. 7). They should be used in a flexible way and the reasons for using them must be clear to the user. In team settings examination sheets can surely be regarded as a standard way of documenting a baseline and subsequent change, and therefore might be regarded by the team members as a useful and necessary tool.

On the other hand examination sheets are

surely less helpful if they act purely as a prompt for the assessor. In that case a standardised method might automatically mean a non-individualised approach to the patient's problem. Clearly then, a patient-centred problem-solving approach would be impossible and therefore this could be regarded as poor practice.

How should you go about assessing a patient?

Paris (1985), who is committed to considering symptoms rather than syndromes, divides his evaluation into the following 15 points:

1. interview with receptionist
2. pain assessment
3. initial observation
4. history and interview with physiotherapist
5. structural observation
6. active movements
7. upper and lower extremity evaluation
8. neuro assessment
9. palpation for condition
10. palpation for position
11. palpation for mobility
12. X-rays and other medical findings
13. summary of objective findings
14. plan of treatment for objective findings, and
15. prognosis.

Self-assessment question

■ **SAQ 3.3.** Reflecting on the Ramsden and the Paris approaches to assessment, where does your own thinking fit in? In order to be a good assessor it is important that you become aware of your own thinking patterns.

Assessment and problem solving

The physiotherapy assessment has so far been firmly linked to problem solving.

Is it possible to predict who is going to be a good problem solver and who is not? Newble et al (1995) suggest that problem solving is not a separate skill and therefore it is impossible to predict individuals' problem-solving abilities in one area by having observed them solve prob-lems in another. It appears therefore that this skill is very context-specific. A marvellous illustration of this was provided by De Groot (1965) who observed the problem solving of chess grand-masters. These subjects were unable to transfer their exceptionally highly developed skills from chess to another area. Problem solving in assess-ments, therefore, needs to be linked to very spe-cific knowledge of the theories underpinning the area of muscular skeletal problems and recogni-tion of the specificity of that particular context.

What is needed for a good assessment?

The function of the assessment is to make sense of the examination findings. Grieve (1981) defines the role of the examination as being: 'to understand fully how the patient is troubled and then to seek a physical basis for these symptoms in terms of objective signs'. He continues: 'Assessment is the judgement that is necessary to make sense of these findings; hence to identify a relationship between the symptoms reported and the signs of disturbed function'.

This makes it very clear that the assessor needs highly specific knowledge and also speci-fic skills. But it seems that the interdependence of these two ingredients, knowledge and skills, is the vital ingredient. This interdependence, though, is not an abstract thing but a continually changing entity fed by our attitudes (Newble et al 1995). Self-awareness, which has already been mentioned several times, is an essential part of being a physiotherapist and this needs as much training and continual development as the more technical side of our profession. Partici-pation in experiential learning (that is, in or through clinical practice) is essential. More about this can be found in the literature on clinical rea-soning in physiotherapy (Carr et al 1995).

Remember the patient with whom you were unable to forge any relationship? Who seemed to bring out your most impatient side? Have you any idea why that was? Do the patients whom you cannot help have anything in common? Are you aware of what or of whom they remind you? Or are you aware that the very angry patient who seems unable to cooperate with you has project-ed his feelings onto you, though they really belong to a totally different setting, and retaliation on your part is therefore going to be the most damaging reaction? This is clearly not only true for negative happenings but also for really successful encounters. What was it in your patient that made it so easy for you to get onto the same wavelength as him? Unless these factors are clearly understood, their impact on the assessment might be harmful and unhelpful.

Skills and knowledge are enhanced by experience. The less experience the assessor has with patients, the more the therapist will have to stick to very clear-cut signposts. Feltovich & Barrows (1984) refer to that as following 'illness scripts'. At the other end of the continuum, the experienced clinician has in his or her mind a vast bank of previous experiences or memories on which he or she can draw quickly and efficiently. It is therefore much easier for the experienced clinician to recognise patterns and to extrapolate information from them (Brooks et al 1991). They are able to perceive relations between different bits of information. The expert therefore seems to do less problem solving than the novice as the former has already stored solutions to many everyday problems he or she may be confronted with in clinical practice (Kahney 1993). The student, on the other hand, may be quite daunted by the sheer number of demands of this process.

ASSESSMENT OF ORTHOPAEDIC PATIENTS

Having reviewed the background to assessment per se, it is now time to look at how assessment may be addressed for an orthopaedic patient.

What is the role of the physiotherapist in an assessment?
Hertling & Kessler (1990) believe this to be to 'clarify the nature and extent of the lesion, to assess the extent of resulting disability and to recover significant data in order to establish a basis against which to judge progress'.

Self-assessment question

■ **SAQ 3.4.** Do you agree with the above statement or would you add to it or qualify it?

As mentioned earlier physiotherapists have to come to their opinion by evaluating first the purely subjective data offered by the patient, and secondly the objective data as elicited by a clinical examination. In this they are quite different from, for example, doctors, who on the whole have the benefit of laboratory results.

The setting of the assessment
Many well-known orthopaedic surgeons (e.g. Dandy 1993) and physicians (e.g. Cyriax 1982) as well as physiotherapists (e.g. Grieve 1981) have suggested their own assessment schedules.

However the actual sequence of your assessment plan will depend a lot on the setting you work in. Do you work in an outpatient department with independent patients coming with a well defined problem or do you work on a ward with bedbound patients who have undergone surgery or experienced the diagnosis of a progressive disease? Or perhaps you work in the community with patients in their own home, coping with a chronic and perhaps disabling disease.

Self-assessment question

■ **SAQ 3.5.** How do you think the assessment might change with the setting you work in and why?

The aim of the assessment
The aim of the assessment – whichever way you elicit the information – is to establish what the patient's problem is, what it means to the patient (i.e. which aspect of it is the most disturbing to the patient) and what clinical objective findings can be found to narrow down the possible clinical diagnosis.

The subjective examination

How should we and can we elicit the information needed for the professional judgement (assessment) that we discussed earlier?

Jones et al (1994) remind us of the need to use open-ended questions rather than just yes/no questions, to use the patient's words as much as possible when investigating the problem and to repeat part of the patient's story for clarification. How many times, though, do we put words into the patient's mouth in order to clarify a point our way or hurry him or her towards a solution that we anticipate?

What is your favourite way of structuring the initial interview? Do you allow the patient to tell his or her own story in a semi-structured way or do you lead him or her along a very strictly controlled path? Are you aware of your reasons for that?

For a more detailed discussion of the skills needed for the subjective assessment refer to Thomson (1992, 1998).

Certain information has to be elicited, and the sort of things that you would need to find out are:

1. Why is the patient here?
2. What is the problem?
3. Where is the problem?
4. How does it behave?
5. Are there any contraindications to treatment by a physiotherapist?

Why is the patient here?

Was she referred by her general practitioner, consultant, another health professional or did she refer herself to you? This might give you an insight into how the patient thinks about her health. Does she feel responsible for her health, and able to influence it; does she indicate that she would be quite prepared and happy to work towards the solution of her problem? Or does she give the impression that she expects you to solve all her problems?

Perhaps she already hints to you that she has no faith in medicine in general and physiotherapy in particular. As you know past experiences will influence the cognition of the present. If the patient therefore has had a good or an unsatisfactory experience with physiotherapists in the past this will influence her present expectations of you as well as of herself.

Why now?

What else is going on in the patient's life?

What is the problem?

Self-assessment question

■ **SAQ 3.6.** What sort of physiotherapy problems do you know or have you dealt with?

On the whole patients get referred to physiotherapists for pain, loss of function and associated signs such as swelling. If the patient is able to describe a very clear incident (for example, trauma, disease onset) it is important to discover as much as possible about this incident and to get a feel for the patient's own assessment of the situation. What is the meaning for him of all that has happened? Make sure to be open to all the subtle intimations and not only to listen to the obvious. Listen to the patient's metaphors. A lot of very pertinent but hidden meaning is conveyed in this part of the patient interview.

How does the patient's lifestyle contribute to or detract from his problem? Are you dealing with a very fit and independent person who has a good understanding of how his body works or are you treating a person whose lifestyle is such that he is under continual mental stress without the necessary time to relax or even to feel what his body is telling him.

What else would you want to know about the problem?

You have established how it happened and the meaning of it for the patient, and you now need to find out if this was the first occurrence of this particular trouble or not. This is important when you are trying to make sense of the patient's words and non-verbal cues, as it will again link in with his and your expectations.

Where is the problem?

It is important to ascertain whether the patient can be precise about the site of the pain. The physiotherapist tries to understand the location of the pain; for example, does it cover a large area or a very specific narrow area? Can the area of the pain be identified as a recognisable anatomical or neurological segment? If not does it remind you of a description of disease (for instance, diabetes can mirror musculoskeletal problems) and if so which one?

Self-assessment questions

■ **SAQ 3.7.** You will remember from your previous reading and experience that some anatomical entities have a very precise pain distribution. Where do muscles, ligaments, bones, nerves, blood vessels and capsules refer pain to?

- **SAQ 3.8.** Can you remember the mechanism they use for referral?

- **SAQ 3.9.** Are you clear why some of them refer pain locally and others are able to refer pain away from their anatomical position?

Kellgren (1938, 1939) did some of the pioneering work in this field. He managed to map pain referrals by irritating pain-sensitive structures, such as ligaments, and recorded the subjects' pain distribution once he had manipulated these structures.

Once you have established whether the pain is limited to a specific area or not, you then must want to find out if it ever changes its position or extent when it is relieved or exacerbated.

How does it behave?

In many ways this question could be the linchpin of this part of your examination. As physiotherapists we deal mainly with problems that incorporate a mechanical element rather than purely disease. This means that we are looking for a behaviour pattern indicative of this mechanical aspect.

Self-assessment questions

- **SAQ 3.10.** How would you expect the behaviour of symptoms to differ between someone who had a mechanical problem and someone who was suffering from a disease process?

- **SAQ 3.11.** What cues would you be looking for from the patient?

The first thing to establish therefore is if this problem changes with movement or rest. Most pain problems that we can treat will have an element of 'being helped by rest'. It is less likely that someone with unremitting pain will be helped by physiotherapeutic, hence mechanical or electrical techniques. Persistent night pain is much more suggestive of a malignant, inflammatory or metabolic cause than a mechanical one.

Once you have established that there is a movement element to the problem you need to find out as much as possible about this relationship. The first question is: precisely what movement increases or decreases the pain?

You then need to know how quickly the pain comes on once the exacerbating movement has occurred, how severe it is in comparison with the 'normal' level and for how long it persists once the aggravating movement has been stopped. These three points will help you to evaluate the irritability of the problem, and this information will then guide you when you are thinking about the objective examination which is to follow. How aggressive will you be able to be in this part of the examination? This helpful concept of irritability has been around for a long time and has been explored in physiotherapy by Maitland (1964).

Contraindications to physiotherapy treatment

Clearly, as in all aspects of physiotherapy there are contraindications to this type of treatment which should be looked or listened for when examining a patient with an orthopaedic or musculoskeletal problem. As at the beginning of this chapter you will have scanned your memory, often not in a conscious way, for possible theories underpinning the patient's story while you were listening to him or her. By now, therefore, you might already have some ideas as to the nature of the problem (i.e. which structure could be responsible).

What alternatives to your vague and not yet fully developed hypothesis do you need to exclude or include?

We said earlier that a hallmark of a musculoskeletal problem is its reaction to movement and rest. Thus, in someone complaining of unremitting pain that is unchanged by either rest or movement one would suspect serious disease processes which would need to be explored.

The following questions could be asked:

- Have you had any significant weight loss? Remember, that patients with malignant disease often exhibit marked weight loss.
- What sort of tablets are you on? While it is important to chart the rhythm of painkillers

and anti-inflammatory drugs when assessing the patient's pain levels, it is essential that you investigate the long-term use of systemic steroids or anticoagulants. These medications can be associated with osteoporosis.

- Has any member in your family suffered from rheumatoid arthritis? Remember the possible hereditary nature of this disease.
- Have you noticed any change in your bladder or bowels? Naturally, the lack of exercise resulting from pain or injury or the use of painkillers interferes with these functions, but you need to explore whether either retention or incontinence have been present as this could be a sign of cord or cauda equina involvement. This would clearly not be a problem primarily for a physiotherapist but require investigation by an orthopaedic or neurosurgeon.

Results of the subjective examination

At the end of this first part of the assessment you should now have gained a thorough insight into:

- the patient's problem and how he or she views it
- the patient's expectations of you and himself
- the history, nature and behaviour of the problem
- irritability.

You should be aware of:

- possible contraindications to physiotherapy treatment
- other possible contributing factors

and you should have:

- a working hypothesis about which structures might be involved
- a sound theoretical reason for planning particular investigations.

The objective examination

You are now ready to start the second and equally important aspect of the assessment process: you need to identify the extent of the disturbed function. Objective findings will help you to establish a firmer relationship between the patient's symptoms and your own hypothesis. While we mostly do not diagnose a condition in the medical sense, we continually check our memory bank for recognition of previous groupings of symptoms that might help us in the planning of the tests to be done on and with the patient's problem. An assessment has to be carefully prepared and will depend totally on the findings of the subjective assessment.

Part of the preparation might include the revision of basic facts from the fields of anatomy, physiology, kinesiology and pathology and the way in which these are influenced by psychosocial considerations. For example, in the case of a young woman with an ankle injury you might ask yourself: what is the anatomy of the ankle joint? What are the biomechanical features of the ankle joint? Does her lifestyle contribute to the problem experienced at the moment?

It becomes clear that without a good knowledge base it would be difficult to make sense of the clinical presentation, a management plan would be extremely shaky and it would be virtually impossible to make a good prediction about the outcome.

The questions to ask yourself now are the following:

- What are the essential findings of the assessment so far?
- What tests or investigations are needed to 'firm them up' and harden your hypothesis?
- What findings are red herrings, or 'tombstones' of previous incidents as Grieve (1981) called them; i.e. which findings do not directly or immediately contribute to this current problem.
- What do you know about the problem so far and what do you need to look up?

An extensive objective examination will include aspects of:

1. observation
2. active movements
3. passive movements
4. resisted or repeated movements

5. palpation of the area
6. neural tension testing
7. neurological testing (if indicated).

Clearly only the most potent tests are going to be employed and only those that are going to shed most light onto the problem. For a more detailed discussion on the various tests to be considered refer to other orthopaedic texts (e.g. Hertling & Kessler 1990).

The novice examiner will often tend to employ an 'overkill' strategy. He or she will do every test in the book in order to find objective data to confirm the very vague hypothesis. This is because he or she is new to the game and therefore has not yet collected the multitude of information and knowledge that allows for speedy pattern recognition. With growing experience the examiner will be able to tailor investigations more specifically to his or her needs.

Problem-solving exercise 3.1

A 25-year-old woman has been referred with a 2-week history of intense left-sided low back pain radiating into her left calf after gardening.
A 56-year-old man has been referred with a history of several years of repeated bouts of general backache and stiffness without a specific onset.

■ Would you employ the same objective examination on these two patients, both complaining of low back pain? What is different in the two scenarios?

If you need to, refer back to the chapter on problem solving.

Differences between the two scenarios
Some differences are:

1. age of patient
2. time since onset of problem
3. description of onset
4. location / specificity of pain
5. intensity of pain.

Age of patient. What is the diagnostic relevance of the age of the patient? Degenerative processes (hence a more generalised problem) are less likely in a 25-year-old in contrast to a 56-year-old. That might lead you to a very localised testing procedure for the woman while you might want to test the male patient's movements more generally. What do you know about the mechanisms of degeneration of joints?

Time since onset of problem. On the one hand there is a very short time span with a 'fresh' injury and on the other there is a long-standing problem appearing in repeated bouts of pain. You would expect to find the previously mentioned 'tombstones' of old pain events in the older patient but would not anticipate this in the younger one. Therefore your investigations need to be much more far-reaching in the man than in the woman when it comes to movement tests. Are you happy with your knowledge of the differences between acute and chronic pain and the associated effects on mood and motivation?

Description of onset. The big difference here is the exact mechanical nature of one (lifting) in contrast to the unknown onset of the other. The anatomical and neurological entities that are stressed by hyperflexion and perhaps twisting need to be fully concentrated on with respect to the young woman, while others might be excluded. Clearly the man, with his more generalised and vague history, needs a more general movement examination in order to narrow down the multitude of possibilities.

Location of pain. What anatomical entity do you know of that refers pain to the calf? You need to remind yourself of the different patterns of referral and their relevance. For example, a specific pattern below the knee often hints towards nerve root involvement, while more general referred pain can be a symptom of muscle or ligament involvement though these rarely refer pain below the knee. This differentiation clearly narrows down the examination options in our two patients: the woman patient's must have a focus on possible nerve root involvement while the man's needs to include examinations of joints, muscles and ligaments because of the unspecific nature of his problem. General aching rarely is a symptom of nerve root involvement and hence this does not have to be given a priority in the initial assessment of the man.

Intensity of pain. Again, authors such as Grieve (1981) will be able to help you with the differentiation of certain pain descriptors which hint at the anatomical source. We mentioned earlier the importance of the concept of irritability and the role intensity of pain plays in its definition. Clearly the more irritable a patient's problem seems, the less aggressive the objective examination has to be.

So, at the end of your preparation for the objective examination what are you left with in terms of necessary tests and investigations? Which procedures do you need to employ to clarify the nature of these patients' back pain?

Objective examination of the 25-year-old woman

1. *Observation*
   Is there evidence of her avoiding flexion?
2. *Active movements*
   Gentle testing of extension (is this pain-free?) and then flexion (is this painful?).
   Testing of side flexion and rotation most probably have little extra to offer, and therefore can be left out, initially.
3. *Passive movements*
   Muscles and ligaments are not suspected as a cause for her pain, hence this will not add anything to test the provisional hypothesis (nerve root involvement); put onto a 'reserve list' to come back to later.
4. *Resisted movements*
   Again these would not add anything to our provisional knowledge about this lady's problem. Also far too painful.
5. *Repeated movements*
   These could clearly be indicative of a joint or ligamentous problem, which is not our hypothesis for this patient, but they can also have decisive information to offer if one remembers McKenzie's (1981) ideas about nerve root involvement in derangements. Hence there might be an increase of pain when repeating flexion (her hypothesised mode of injury) and a possible decrease when repeating extension (the opposite of her hypothesised mode of injury).

6. *Palpation*
   It will be useful to get an insight into the degree of soft tissue agitation but any passive intervertebral joint movement will have nothing to offer; this is not part of our hypothesis so far. Again, far too painful.
7. *Neural tension*
   Clearly in someone with a suspected nerve root involvement the neural tension needs to be tested, as a positive test would really help to firm up the hypothesis. A reduced straight-leg raise test between 30° and 70° would indicate reduced movement of the nerve root and hence possible compression.
8. *Neurological testing*
   In anyone with pain radiating away from the midline, muscle strength, sensation and reflexes need to be checked as they are directly related to nerve root involvement. Look for areas of classic wasting (e.g. wasted extensor digitorum brevis is a good indication for a L5 lesion).

Objective examination of the 56-year-old man

What would this examination look like for the 56-year-old man with generalised back pain?

As this is a general and repetitive problem it is more difficult to come up with a working hypothesis for him. This means that the examination needs to include more tests rather than focusing on a particular anatomical apparatus. Revision of pain referral patterns (Grieve 1981) and bearing his age in mind will indicate however that he is less likely to be suffering from a nerve root problem caused by an intervertebral disc. Therefore, investigations that are particularly aimed at that diagnosis can be left out (at first) of the battery of intended tests as they will not be able to help the investigator with his or her struggle to confirm the working hypothesis.

At the moment one would have to say that the cause of his problem might be a degenerative process. This will lead to tests that stress spinal joints, the intervertebral discs, the surrounding muscles and ligaments.

1. *Observation*
   Is there any movement, position, etc. that he seems to dislike? This will help you to

narrow down the vast possibilities for his back pain. Are you able to discern that perhaps a particular movement direction seems to be worse than others?

2. *Active movements*
Unless a clearer picture has emerged by observing him undress or get on/off a chair or plinth, you need to test all movements in the hope that you will be able to discern a particular movement pattern that is more troublesome than the others (e.g. are you able to identify a compression, hence joint, or stretch, hence soft tissue, pattern?). This is still in line with the hypothesis of joints, muscles or ligaments being involved in the cause of his problem as active movements test all of these.

3. *Passive movements*
These might add a little insight with regard to joint involvement (he will not be able to protect a possibly painful range muscularly), but can add a lot of knowledge concerning his muscle and ligament length or tightness.

4. *Resisted movements*
These will have little information to offer unless a suspicion has arisen that his muscles are the prime reason for the problem; the other anatomical entities do not really respond to this kind of testing in a clear way.

5. *Palpation*
This is necessary to localise the problem as much as possible; the soft tissue condition (swelling, fibrosis, spasm, etc.) must be identified, but the palpation findings from the individual spinal joints provide the most potent objective data as they help to narrow down the anatomical possibilities as well as the actual location.
The biggest danger here is the identification of 'tombstones' (remnants of previous episodes which have burnt themselves out but resulted in stiff or painful joints). It is important therefore to link the findings to the patient's present problem rather than just identifying a painful spot unrelated to the patient's current pain. (One could identify such areas in most of the asymptomatic population.)

6. *Neural tension*
Nerve root involvement has been previously excluded, and although we do not need more

information along that line, we are dealing with a repetitive problem which quite reasonably might have affected nervous structures (by inflammatory processes?) as they travelled, for instance, through the layers of affected soft tissues or passed joints that might have been inflamed and swollen. Steadily increasing evidence (Butler 1991) makes it imperative to test the length of the neural tissues.

7. *Neurological testing*
We have decided that this problem is unlikely to be caused by nerve root involvement; thus data collected under this heading would be unhelpful and confusing.

Recognition of patterns

Now you have finished the initial data collection and you need to come up with a reasoned hypothesis which can result in a management plan. It is here that a lot of problems occur. You have ended up with an enormous amount of information, not all of it meaningful, and you are left needing to identify certain patterns which you have got to recognise as belonging together in a relevant way. It is obvious that you will not be able to recognise these patterns unless you have actually experienced them at some point. This has been discussed in more detail and depth by Cox (1988). If you are a beginner you may have jumped to the wrong conclusion (i.e. decided on the wrong hypothesis). It is therefore important that you keep an eye on your 'reserve list' of tests and results to help you to change your mind if necessary.

Finally, you might want to test yourself on how far you have travelled on the road to pattern recognition. The test given below has been researched by Case et al (1988).

Self-assessment

What are the various options you might want to consider as the cause of back pain? Remember to include referred visceral pain which could mimic back pain. Some possible causes are listed below:

A Intervertebral disc prolapse
B Muscular sprain

C Ligamentous sprain
D Postural strain
E Spondylosis
F Arthrosis of spinal joints
G Fracture of a vertebra
H Kidney problem
I Spondylolisthesis
J Hypermobility syndrome
K Spinal tumour
L Scheuermann's disease
M Dysfunction
N Osteoporosis.

For each of the following patients with back pain, select the most likely diagnosis and make sure that you have a rationale for it (otherwise testing for the diagnosis can be difficult).

■ **SAQ 3.12.** A 35-year-old computer analyst has back pain after a some heavy gardening work; he developed leg pain after about 2 days; flexion is most painful.

■ **SAQ 3.13.** A 18-year-old student developed back pain after falling 10 metres through a snow bridge; all movements are equally painful; rest relieves pain somewhat.

■ **SAQ 3.14.** A 25-year-old ballet dancer complains of severe back pain; it is aggravated by end-range positions; more than seven joints (!) seem to have excess movement.

■ **SAQ 3.15.** A 15-year-old boy noticed a dull central back ache which is aggravated by loading his spine and mostly relieved by rest.

■ **SAQ 3.16.** A 48-year-old mother of five has had a long history of episodic back pain, which for the first time has travelled down her leg and into her foot; she presents with a hyperlordosis in her spine.

■ **SAQ 3.17.** A 39-year-old man complained of a dull central backache on prolonged sitting which is on the whole relieved by walking around and getting up from a chair; flexion is limited and painful, but repeated flexion eases his pain and range increases.

■ **SAQ 3.18.** A 58-year-old bus driver complained of central sharp back pain which is worse at the end of the day and is helped by rest; no particular movement makes his pain worse.

■ **SAQ 3.19.** A 30-year-old woman felt a sharp twinge on the left side of her back while playing tennis; she was able to continue to play but felt totally 'seized up' after she had stopped playing.

■ **SAQ 3.20.** A 40-year-old machine operator after years of repetitive bending to the left noticed a sharp and very localised pain on the left side of her back; extension and left-side bending increased her pain.

■ **SAQ 3.21.** A 70-year-old woman started to notice a generalised and sharp pain around the centre of her back; extension seemed to make it worse.

■ **SAQ 3.22.** A 28-year-old accountant experienced sharp general pain in his back after pulling a surprisingly heavy weight; passive movements are pain-free but active extension is very painful.

■ **SAQ 3.23.** A 20-year-old student complained of general back pain after sitting in front of a computer for more than 1 hour; pain is relieved once he gets up; all movements are pain-free.

■ **SAQ 3.24.** A 25-year-old man complained of severe central back pain which is unrelieved or aggravated by any movement or position; night pain is persistent; general malaise was noticed.

■ **SAQ 3.25.** A 57-year-old woman started to complain of severe colic-like pain in her central back which was unrelieved or aggravated by any movement; certain unpredictable positions seemed to affect it, as well as going to the toilet.

Summary

This chapter has introduced you to various ideas concerning assessment, the skills needed for it and how to acquire them, and finally has offered you the opportunity to work through an example of testing hypotheses.

The examples have focused very much on pathology. Fleming (1991) in her 'three-track mind model' focuses on the three different strands of reasoning going on in the therapist's mind:

- Procedural reasoning: this focuses on the disease or pathology (e.g. the examples above).
- Interactive reasoning: the face-to-face encounters and the ensuing relationship are at the centre here; the experience the particular problem has engendered is looked at.
- Conditional reasoning: this takes into consideration both the patient as a social being as well as the condition he or she complains of and hence is a much more involved multidimensional thinking process.

(For a fuller discussion of the 'three-track' model see Chapter 4, p. 69.)

Clinical reasoning is obviously one of the hallmarks of an autonomous health worker and the assessment is an early opportunity to put this into practice.

ANSWERS TO QUESTIONS

Self-assessment questions 3.7–3.9 (pages 50–51)

See information in text.

Self-assessment questions 3.10, 3.11 (page 51)

See information in text.

Problem-solving exercise 3.1

See information in text.

Problem-solving exercise 3.2

See information in text, and section following the exercise.

Self-assessment questions (page 56)

- ■ **SAQ 3.12.** *A, intervertebral disc prolapse.*
- ■ **SAQ 3.13.** *G, fracture of a vertebra.*
- ■ **SAQ 3.14.** *J, hypermobility syndrome.*
- ■ **SAQ 3.15.** *L, Scheuermann's disease.*
- ■ **SAQ 3.16.** *I, spondylolisthesis.*
- ■ **SAQ 3.17.** *M, dysfunction.*
- ■ **SAQ 3.18.** *E, spondylosis.*
- ■ **SAQ 3.19.** *C, ligamentous sprain.*
- ■ **SAQ 3.20.** *F, arthrosis of spinal joints.*
- ■ **SAQ 3.21.** *N, osteoporosis.*
- ■ **SAQ 3.22.** *B, muscular sprain.*
- ■ **SAQ 3.23.** *D, postural strain.*
- ■ **SAQ 3.24.** *K, spinal tumour.*
- ■ **SAQ 3.25.** *H, kidney problem.*

REFERENCES

Brooks L R, Norman G R, Allen S W 1991 The role of specific similarity in a medical diagnostic task. Journal of Experimental Psychology: General 120: 278–287

Butler D S 1991 Mobilisation of the nervous system. Churchill Livingstone, Edinburgh

Carr J, Jones M, Higgs H J 1995 Teaching towards clinical reasoning expertise in physiotherapy practice. In: Higgs H J, Jones M (eds) Clinical reasoning in the health professions. Butterworth Heinemann, Oxford, ch 19, p 235

Case S M, Swanson D B, Stillman P S 1988 Evaluating diagnostic pattern recognition: the psychometric characteristics of a new item format. Proceedings of the 27th Conference on Research in Medical Education. Association of American Medical Colleges, Washington

Chartered Society of Physiotherapy 1990 Code of

professional conduct. Chartered Society of Physiotherapy, London

Cox K 1988 How to teach clinical reasoning. In: Cox K, Ewan C E (eds) The medical teacher, 2nd edn. Churchill Livingstone, Edinburgh, ch 14, p 102

Cyriax J 1982 Textbook of orthopaedic medicine. The diagnosis of soft tissue lesions, 8th edn. Baillière Tindall, London, vol 1

Dandy D 1993 Essential orthopaedics and trauma, 2nd edn. Churchill Livingstone, Edinburgh

De Groot A 1965 Thought and choice in chess. Monton, The Hague

Feltovich P J, Barrows H S 1984 Issues in generality in medical problem solving. In: Schmidt H G, De Volder M L (eds) Tutorials in problem-based teaching. Van Gorcum, Assen, Maastricht, p 128

Fleming M 1991 The therapist with the three-track mind. American Journal of Occupational Therapy 45(11): 1007–1014

Grieve G 1981 Common vertebral joint problems. Churchill Livingstone, Edinburgh

Hassenkamp A 1998 Clinical reasoning: a student's nightmare. British Journal of Therapy and Rehabilitation 5:75–78

Hertling D, Kessler R 1990 Management of common musculoskeletal disorders. Physical therapy principles and methods, 2nd edn. J B Lippincott, Philadelphia

Hislop H J 1985 Clinical decision making: educational, data and risk factors. In: Wolf S L (ed) Clinical decision making in physical therapy. F A Davis, Philadelphia, ch 2, p 25

Jones M, Christensen N, Carr J 1994 Clinical reasoning in orthopaedic manual therapy. In: Grant R (ed) Clinics in physical therapy. Physical therapy of the cervical and thoracic spine, 2nd edn. Churchill Livingstone, New York, ch 6, p 89

Kahney H 1993 Problem solving: current issues, 2nd edn. Open University Press, Buckingham

Kellgren J H 1938 Observations on referred pain arising from muscle. Clinical Science 3: 175

Kellgren J H 1939 On the distribution of pain from deep somatic structures with charts of segmental areas. Clinical Science 4:303

Maitland G 1964 Vertebral manipulations. Butterworths, London

McKenzie R 1981 The lumbar spine. Mechanical diagnosis and therapy. Spinal therapy. Waikanae, New Zealand

Newble D, van der Vlenten C, Norman G 1995 Assessing clinical reasoning. In: Higgs H J, Jones M (eds) Clinical reasoning in the health professions. Butterworth Heinemann, Oxford, ch 13, p 168

Paris S V 1985 Clinical decision making: orthopaedic physical therapy. In: Wolf S L (ed) Clinical decision making in physical therapy. F A Davis, Philadelphia, ch 10, p 215

Parry A 1985 Physiotherapy assessment, 2nd edn. Croom Helm, London

Ramsden E L 1985 Bases for clinical decision making: perception of the patient, the clinician's role and responsibility. In: Wolf S L (ed) Clinical decision making in physical therapy. F A Davis, Philadelphia ch 5, p 91

Thomson D J 1992 Counselling. In: French S (ed) Physiotherapy – a psychosocial approach. Butterworth Heinemann, Oxford, ch 26, p 364

Thomson D J 1998 Counselling and clinical reasoning: the meaning of practice. British Journal of Therapy and Rehabilitation 5:88–106

Watts N T 1985 Decision analysis: a tool for improving physical therapy practice and education. In: Wolf S L (ed) Clinical decision making in physical therapy. F A Davis, Philadelphia, ch 1, p 7

4

Decision making and clinical reasoning in orthopaedics

■ Orthopaedics ■ Decision making ■ Clinical reasoning
■ Hypothetico-deductive model ■ Pattern recognition
■ Knowledge–reasoning integration

CONTENTS

Objectives

By the end of this chapter you should:

1. Have an overview of the areas covered in orthopaedics.
2. Have a basic understanding of problem solving within the clinical situation.
3. Be able to relate this to the process of decision making and clinical reasoning in the orthopaedic setting.
4. Start to appreciate how you can use problem solving and clinical reasoning in your decision making in orthopaedic practice.

Prerequisites

In order to obtain most benefit from this chapter, you should have read Chapters 1 to 3.

INTRODUCTION

The chapters up to and including this one are introductory. Later you will be looking at the more specific areas of orthopaedics and will develop your skills in problem solving – at least in the theoretical sense.

By now you should have a general idea of the changes that occur naturally in the body during ageing, and how in some cases they can become severe enough to cause problems for the individual, usually manifesting as pain and loss of function. There are also situations where the body is affected by diseases or injuries which can cause problems in themselves and/or aggravate the changes due to ageing. It may be at this point, where 'changes' turn into 'problems', that people seek some form of help from health professionals, and thus physiotherapists may have contact with them. However, physiotherapists may be involved before this stage if part of their role is in the education of individuals or groups regarding the avoidance and prevention of injury. Of course it is not possible to stop the normal changes of ageing or prevent disease. But it is possible to reduce the risk of accident or exacerbation by attempting to influence everyday activities, such as lifting techniques or habitual postures adopted for work situations, and in some cases, certain elements of lifestyle such as levels of exercise.

In both educational and treatment situations, the knowledge of normal and pathological change is needed. In education, it is important to explain the reasons behind advice regarding any exercises or changes of activity that are recommended. More importantly, in the treatment setting, the physiotherapist must be aware of the underlying changes and how they may affect the patient physically, psychologically and socially, as discussed in Chapters 2 and 3. This will facilitate the making of informed decisions when problem lists, goals and treatment plans are formulated. These processes are closely related to the issues discussed in Chapter 3 where the recognition of change in the musculoskeletal system was considered and how that knowledge could be used during subjective and objective assessment.

If you are able to remember these important points in your dealings with patients, you will already be going through the problem-solving process. As you will recall from Chapter 1, the best way to become skilled in problem solving is to actually do it, and the case studies in this book have been designed to start you off. Then by practising and reflecting on your performance, both with the case studies and when you deal with real patients, you will gradually enhance your ability to make clinical decisions.

THE RANGE OF ORTHOPAEDICS

Physiotherapists come into contact in virtually all areas of health care with patients who have orthopaedic problems. Usually these problems are of primary importance on orthopaedic wards or in the outpatient setting. But the incidence of patients with orthopaedic problems is much more common than this, and physiotherapists could be called upon to deal with them even if they are specialists in other areas such as intensive care, neurology or care of the elderly. In fact orthopaedic problems span the whole spectrum, cutting across all ages and specialities. In some cases they may be secondary issues, but they can have an impact upon overall outcome for the patient if they are not addressed. This is why it is important to have a good grounding in the subject.

It is perhaps also true to say that although orthopaedics is very wide ranging, it is one of the fundamental fields for the physiotherapist. It is often seen as being rather more straightforward and easier to understand than other areas, and so is covered early on in the syllabi of most courses. This unfortunately can cause an underestimation of its importance.

Fractures

This is probably the area that most people would think of if they were asked to explain the term 'orthopaedics', i.e. the loss in continuity of a bone. It can be due to many different causes such as trauma, repeated small stresses or pathological change such as neoplasia.

In this area, the physiotherapist is usually

involved at a slightly later stage once the fracture has been reduced and fixed.

Soft tissue injury

This is the area of orthopaedics that covers damage to tissues such as ligament, tendon or muscle. Again there can be various causes of this damage: for example, a single traumatic event such as a fall or sports injury, or a longer-term stress on a structure such as inflammation of the synovial lining of a tendon sheath after many repetitions of the same movement.

Here the physiotherapist may be the first-line contact for the treatment of the patient.

Rheumatology

This area of medicine deals with patients with rheumatic diseases, also known as connective tissue diseases. These conditions are often thought of as affecting only the joints, but in fact they can affect connective tissues throughout the body and so can also influence systemic function. On the whole these are incurable, chronic diseases of unknown causation. But they are subsumed with orthopaedics as patients in both areas present with many similar problems, for instance pain, swelling and loss of function. However, the approach of the physiotherapist may vary because of the long-term nature of rheumatic diseases and the reliance on pharmacological management.

Usually, the physiotherapist is part of a team of health care workers who are involved with the management of each patient.

Bone disease

This area of orthopaedics returns to skeletal problems. The diseases are many and varied, such as those acquired due to previous trauma like osteomyelitis (infection of bone post-fracture), those of unknown causation such as neoplasm (e.g. osteosarcoma), or those possibly having some connection with the changes of ageing, like osteoporosis.

Here again, the physiotherapist will be part of the team involved in the management of these patients. The overall approach to each patient may differ depending on the disease, but the skills and techniques used by the physiotherapist will be similar to those in the previously mentioned areas of orthopaedics.

Congenital and paediatric deformities

This is the area of orthopaedics dealing with particular deformities in children, which could be due to trauma, for instance a fracture through the epiphyseal growth plate which affects the development of the bone, or congenital conditions such as congenital dislocation of the hips.

Once more, the approach of the physiotherapist will be similar to that in the previously mentioned areas, working with other members of the health care team and with special consideration for the age of the patients. However, it is extremely important to address these problems as early as possible in order to avoid further complications later in life.

Joint replacement

A number of the above-mentioned injuries and diseases can lead to a patient's needing a joint replacement. For example, many patients with rheumatic disorders which can seriously damage the joints will eventually require a replacement in order to be able to function effectively. This may also be necessary after certain fractures, such as those that divide the neck of the femur. In this injury the blood supply to the head of the femur can be compromised and it may subsequently die, so it is often decided to replace it with a metal implant. Some centres specialise in replacements of large areas of bone that have been affected by neoplasia. These areas are usually carefully measured and replacements are custom made for each patient.

Joint replacement can therefore span a wide variety of patients with problems due to injury or disease. Here again the physiotherapist will be part of a team dealing with the patient. Quite often orthopaedic surgeons prescribe very specific regimes that patients must follow postoperatively. In the ideal situation the physiotherapist will have been involved in the design of these regimes, but this is not always the case.

Orthopaedic problems: general points

All of the areas of orthopaedics discussed above are covered in the following chapters. It is useful to remember that any of the conditions mentioned may be complicated by damage to other structures such as blood vessels or nerves. Also, as the physiotherapist involved, you must be prepared to take all necessary points into consideration during your assessment and subsequent clinical decision making, and this will involve physical, psychological and social factors. You also need to remember that the patient and any carers involved are part of the team, and their opinions and needs should give direction to the rehabilitation process.

Now you have a clear picture of the content of the following chapters, it is hoped that it will be a little easier for you to transfer the earlier information on problem solving into that setting. The remainder of this chapter will now focus on the issues of decision making and reasoning in the clinical and, particularly, the orthopaedic situation.

DECISION MAKING AND CLINICAL REASONING IN ORTHOPAEDICS

In Chapter 1 you thought about problem solving in very general terms, as it begins in childhood and continues throughout life on a daily basis. This must now put into the context of physiotherapy and related to the decisions you make and the clinical reasoning that occurs in order to reach those decisions.

Clinical reasoning can be defined as: 'A process attempting to structure meaning from a mass of confusing data and experiences occurring within a specific clinical context and then making decisions based on this understanding' (Higgs 1996).

This is not a purely logical process as it is dealing with 'messy' human data – so it is not possible to use an algorithm (see Ch. 1) to reach a conclusion. It is not like attempting a maths prob-

lem but more like arranging a wedding (Higgs 1996). Here, some logistics are involved (e.g. 'Look at the size of the church: how many guests can be fitted in?' or 'What menu shall we choose for 82 guests and how much will it cost?') but there are also the messier issues, such as who will be offended if they are not invited — and does it matter? The seating plan might also cause some headaches! So a mixture of problem-solving and reasoning methods must be applied to deal with both the logic and the 'mess'.

To be an effective practitioner you must develop your problem-solving skills. It is essential that you are able to look at the large amount of information you obtain from an assessment and then organise it and identify specific patient problems. From this point it is then possible to formulate goals and treatment plans. If the goals and treatments are appropriate, then in order to get to this stage you must have used clinical reasoning to come to these decisions.

Clinical reasoning involves thinking about what you do, talking to others about the way you work and essentially giving reasons for your thoughts and actions. It forms the basis of your physiotherapy practice and underpins problem solving (Alsop & Ryan 1996). So, it is very important that you grasp the basic concept. Obviously those processes that lead to problem solving will go on at a certain level almost without you noticing, as discussed in Chapter 1, because everyone starts to use them very early in life. But it is not until you consciously acknowledge these processes that you can start to think about them and work to improve your skills. This is especially true in the clinical setting. 'Once you have mastered clinical reasoning ideas you can start to develop the processes that will help you to become proficient at reasoning, and this will improve your practice' (Alsop & Ryan 1996).

But it is important to remember that what you already know influences the decisions you make. So a well organised knowledge base, gleaned from background theoretical work as well as from your experiences, will help you to make decisions more efficiently. 'Reasoning is only as good as the information on which it occurs ...' (Jones 1992).

Self-assessment question

■ **SAQ 4.1.** Why is it not possible to use algorithms to solve problems in the clinical setting?

It seems fairly widely accepted in the available literature that knowledge is essential if decisions are to be made on solid reasoning. This applies to both the expert and the novice. In the clinical situation this knowledge will be gained from a myriad of sources. A good starting place is reading relevant books and papers. But when a patient is attending for assessment, then other sources of information include:

- patient notes and X-rays (if available)
- reports from other members of the health care team
- talking to the patient and/or carer (in both an informal and a formal way)
- observation from the moment the patient appears
- palpation of affected parts
- examination/specific tests and measurement, if appropriate
- observation of specific functional activities
- patient responses to health and well-being indices (which can be well recognised, published questionnaires if appropriate, or simple ones designed specifically by the physiotherapist for patients in that area).

These ways of obtaining information involve the senses, mainly vision, hearing and touch. It is essential that the physiotherapist keeps an open mind, looking carefully at the patient, listening to what is being said, as well as noting non-verbal messages and using the hands to feel for physical problems. As part of the ongoing process, this information has to be analysed to ascertain which parts are relevant. The physiotherapist must also consider both the reliability and the validity of these data (Higgs & Jones 1995). This information can then be used to 'solve' practical clinical problems through a reasoning process. This information-gathering process has already been discussed in Chapter 3, dealing with assessment.

In order to improve in these skills the physiotherapist should reassess the whole procedure and reflect on which parts worked successfully and which did not, and why this happened. This is summed up by Higgs & Jones (1995) as the use of knowledge, the act of thinking and the process of metacognition which is the awareness and monitoring of the thinking process.

Self-assessment question

■ **SAQ 4.2.** When you know you are about to see a new patient, you will need information about that person. List as many sources of this information as you can.

Models of clinical reasoning

A large amount of work has been carried out on clinical reasoning in a number of the health professions, particularly that of medical practitioners and occupational therapists, and more recently on clinical reasoning by physiotherapists. This work ranges from studies of different methods of reasoning to theoretical discussions. A number of models have emerged from this, some of which will be briefly summarised here. The general process of clinical reasoning and the steps involved are shown in Figure 4.1. Look back at this from time to time as you read the next section.

The hypothetico-deductive model

This model of clinical reasoning originated from research in the medical field. It is a method often used in scientific work, where hypotheses are generated from observations, the hypotheses are tested through the collection of more data and then they are modified accordingly (Jones 1992). This translates to the clinical field when a physiotherapist generates an hypothesis about a particular patient from initial observation, tests this hypothesis by collecting more data (in the ways mentioned above) and modifies the hypothesis as necessary. This model has been commonly used for a number of years either alone or as one of a number of strategies in medicine, physiotherapy,

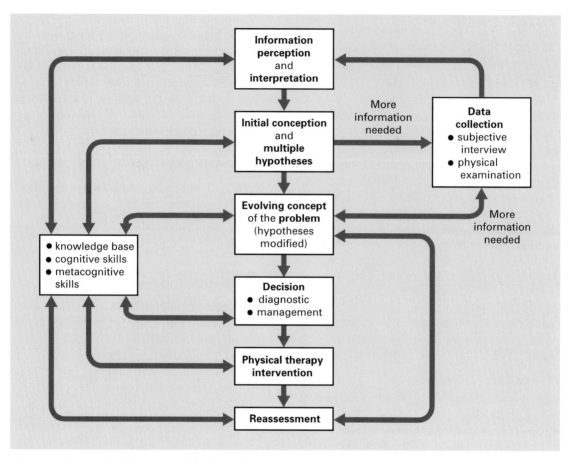

Figure 4.1 Factors involved in the clinical reasoning process.

occupational therapy and nursing (Higgs & Jones 1995).

Jones (1992) describes an 'initial concept' which the physiotherapist develops on first coming into contact with the patient; for instance in the outpatient setting this would occur on greeting the patient, listening to any comments made and observing general points such as posture, build, movement, facial expression, age, and so on. As part of this process the physiotherapist is also devising a 'preliminary working hypothesis' (or more than one) which will be considered and modified as the assessment takes place.

For example, consider a patient with rheumatoid arthritis. The physiotherapist watches her as she gets up from the chair, walks to the cubicle, gets undressed ready for examination and sits on the plinth. During this time there should already

be a formulation of the initial concept and working hypotheses regarding the source of any problems with these activities, i.e. which joints are affected and their degree of involvement. These hypotheses will then be tested as the assessment goes on and additional data are collected.

This idea can be focused further by considering the example of a patient who is referred for physiotherapy because of a shoulder problem. After formulation of the initial concept and working hypotheses by the aforementioned method, the physiotherapist goes on to ask specific questions and examine the patient physically. However, the data gathered here do not support the hypothesis of a damaged shoulder; in fact the evidence points to the symptoms coming from an injury to the neck. So the hypothesis would need to be modified and the line of enquiry changed to collect data referring to the newly identified problem area, and so on. Jones (1992) refers to this process as an 'evolving concept' which will lead eventually to diagnostic and management decisions.

The speed and efficiency with which this process occurs with any patient will depend on a number of factors which have already been mentioned. These include the knowledge base of the physiotherapist, the ability to analyse and synthesise data (i.e. cognitive skills) and the physiotherapist's level of awareness and monitoring of these thinking processes (i.e. metacognitive skills). If he or she has a lot of experience with a particular type of patient then the hypothesis modification should occur more quickly than with someone who is a novice in the field.

Figure 4.2 shows the process of hypothetico-deductive reasoning as explained by Higgs & Jones (1995).

Examples of possible errors in reasoning that could occur during a hypothetico-deductive process are mentioned below.

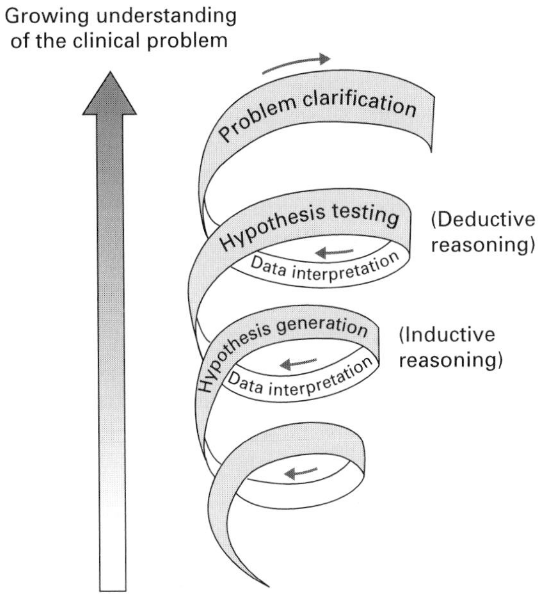

- Making assumptions.
- Prematurely limiting the number of hypotheses; for example, not looking at the joints adjacent to a problem area which could be the cause of referred pain.
- Making a decision based on limited or biased data.
- The physiotherapist only attends to data that support his or her hypothesis while ignoring (probably unconsciously) negating factors. This is another area of bias.
- Failure to understand how factors covary with one another. For example, two symptoms may seem to be related but a full investigation is necessary to see whether or not this interpretation is correct.
- Confusion of covariance and causality, i.e. the two symptoms may indeed covary when investigated, but this does not prove that they are both caused by the same source.

(Adapted from Jones 1992.)

There are many other possible reasoning errors and, generally, less experienced clinicians tend to make more of them. But 'experts' have also been shown to be biased in their use of information obtained from assessment of patients.

Figure 4.2 The hypothetico-deductive model of reasoning; a fairly slow, detailed process. This is illustrated by the loops showing the extra work that needs to be done by the practitioner in order to understand the case fully enough to decide on appropriate action.

> **Self-assessment question**
>
> ■ **SAQ 4.3.** What are the factors involved in the process of improving the skills of problem solving and reasoning (after Higgs & Jones 1995)?

Generally the hypothetico-deductive approach is a reliable method, being both safe and solid. But it is rather slow and related very much to physical disorders. Novices tend to use this method, but experts have usually moved on from this stage. However, if an expert is dealing with an unfamiliar scenario he/she will tend to fall back on this model of reasoning.

Pattern recognition

As already pointed out, the 'expert' physiotherapist has a better organised and greater store of knowledge in memory than the novice. This allows the use of different types of clinical reasoning although there may still be some use of the hypothetico-deductive model in conjunction with these.

Pattern recognition can be defined as 'Direct, automatic retrieval from a well structured network of stored knowledge' (Higgs 1996) and it is, as the term suggests, the physiotherapist's recognition of a particular pattern when observing or examining a patient.

It can also be described in terms of inductive reasoning – 'a method of reasoning by which a general law or principle is inferred from observed particular instances' (Flew 1984). So in very basic terms this means that if on observation A1 has a particular quality, A2 has that quality, and A3 also has that quality and so on, then all As (probably) possess that quality. In clinical parlance, if a physiotherapist observes that patient A1's type of gait is due to OA hip, patient A2's similar type of gait is due to OA hip, patient A3's type of gait, also similar, is due to OA hip and so on, he or she may induce that all patients with that type of gait (probably) move that way because of OA of the hip joint. Hopefully, however, you can see that there are weaknesses to this argument which appears rather simplistic, especially taking into account the 'messy' nature of human data. There is also a danger here that the clinician could make assumptions about the patient when certain signs/symptoms are discovered, and a misdiagnosis could be made if all the evidence is not considered. So it is important to consider the same sorts of possible errors in reasoning here as with the previous model.

Self-assessment question

■ **SAQ 4.4.** Try to remember as many possible errors in the reasoning process as you can. Think back to your clinical experience – have you ever made any of these errors?

There is no doubt that an expert in a particular area does recognise patterns in patient presentation, especially if the type of patient has been seen many times before, so the automatic retrieval of knowledge mentioned above appears to occur. This recognition of a pattern of signs

and symptoms stored in 'clinical memory' happens so quickly as to sometimes be called intuitive (Higgs & Jones 1995).

The information gained from assessment tends to be grouped and categorised and then compared for similarities and differences with previously encountered patients and/or situations. This process is used in a diagnostic sense and is sometimes called 'forward reasoning'; but again in order for the process to take place, a large and well organised knowledge base is necessary (Jones 1992). This type of pattern recognition has been shown in many contexts other than physiotherapy: think back to our example mentioned in Chapters 1 and 3, of expert chess players.

As the expert physiotherapist gains more data during the examination of a patient there are probably repeated instances of pattern recognition going on throughout, not just for initial diagnosis of the condition. Decisions are then made based on the perceived connections between the current case and those previous experiences stored in memory (Higgs & Jones 1995). It has been found that therapists who are more experienced automatically consider a range of options before making their decisions, whereas novices on the whole are not able to do this. Students and newly qualified physiotherapists tend to have a narrower approach, being less able to think more widely due to their rather limited knowledge and experience base. Alsop & Ryan (1996) stress the importance of developing the skill of thinking widely and inductively as this leads on to the ability to generate and actively seek new ideas, and so find possible solutions to problems (Fig. 4.3).

Whereas the hypothetico-deductive approach depends on both inductive and deductive reasoning, the pattern recognition model relies on inductive reasoning as the new information is compared with existing patterns of knowledge (see Fig. 4.4).

This method is not generally used by novices as they do not have such a well organised knowledge base or the automatic ability to categorise data. They also lack the variety of patterns stored in memory that the experts have (Jones 1992). Some of these skills can be developed to a certain extent if the novices consider case studies of typi-

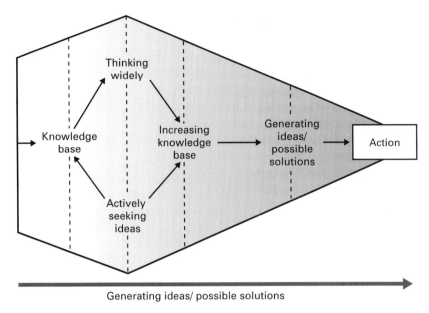

Generating ideas/ possible solutions

Figure 4.3 Inductive reasoning.

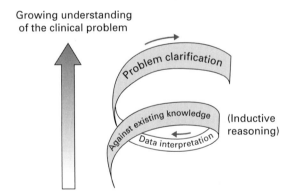

Growing understanding of the clinical problem

Problem clarification

Against existing knowledge

Data interpretation

(Inductive reasoning)

Figure 4.4 The pattern recognition model; a faster and more efficient process than the hypothetico-deductive approach. Here fewer loops are necessary and the physiotherapist can decide on appropriate action more quickly because of the information and experience already 'in storage'.

cal patients in a particular area. Prion & Graby (1995) describe the use of case studies as an instructional method when teaching clinical reasoning. In their situation, with student nurses, it was shown to be a positive step. The students reported that the case studies made the information more 'real' and the tutors found that the students had learned and remembered more than ever before. One of the comments that came up

quite often was that it was very useful to talk ideas through and to see how the instructors were thinking about the particular cases.

When you are using this book to consider case studies, perhaps you might have the opportunity to discuss your ideas with another reader or a colleague. If this is not possible, at least you can compare your thinking with that offered by the authors. When you are working in the clinical situation, try to take every opportunity to discuss cases both with physiotherapists who are at the same level as you, and with those you consider to be 'experts'. This will help you to develop your knowledge base and clinical reasoning skills.

But it would seem that there is no real substitute for experience. Without experience it is possible to get side-tracked during assessment or to attend too much to irrelevant data. Dealing with patients is never straightforward because of the plethora of individual differences that occur.

It is important to note however that the pattern recognition type of clinical reasoning is not particularly useful, even to experts, in unfamiliar situations. If a senior physiotherapist who has specialised in treating patients with sports injuries is suddenly placed in the intensive care situation then he or she will probably fall back on the hypothetico-deductive model.

Knowledge–reasoning integration

This model appears to be an evolution from the previous two models where the knowledge base and clinical skills were looked at almost as separate entities. Higgs & Jones (1995) proposed the knowledge–reasoning integration model, where the two aspects are regarded as being much more interactive and it is thought that they develop in parallel. Knowledge is restructured as it is used in clinical reasoning and it ultimately becomes a store of specific detailed case studies with all the associated information and biomedical knowledge that has been used in past instances. But, as well as this, it also allows for intuitive and interpretative approaches to knowledge and clinical reasoning.

The work of Schell & Cervero

Some researchers in the occupational therapy field have looked at these more integrated ways of clinical reasoning. Schell & Cervero (1993) reviewed the available literature and discuss three different methods of reasoning: scientific, narrative and pragmatic.

1. *Scientific reasoning*

In this type of reasoning effective use is made of research-based theory and technique. This is felt to have helped with the 'professionalisation' of the field.

This 'professionalisation' is still an ongoing process in physiotherapy. The emphasis is on evidence-based practice, setting of guidelines and standards of practice, looking at outcome measures and audit of these outcomes. It is intended that these activities will help to establish physiotherapy more firmly as based on available research. Much of this work is occurring in response to changes in the health care system in the UK, where purchasers and users of the system are asking for evidence that physiotherapy is effective.

However on its own, this scientific reasoning approach is not felt to be a complete description of the complexity of clinical practice.

2. *Narrative reasoning* (Mattingly 1991)

Here clinical reasoning is considered to be 'an imagistic and phenomenological mode of think-ing'. The 'messiness' of human data is again considered in this model, and most clinical reasoning is thought to occur during treatment rather than during assessment.

There are two main ways in which narrative reasoning occurs whilst considering the whole patient: 'through the therapists sharing stories and through therapists creating therapeutic stories with current patients'. These stories can help the physiotherapist to reason through and understand a little of the patients' experience of the biomedical conditions affecting them. It is possible to examine issues around the meaning the disability has for the patient and the motivation that will affect patient performance. This model takes contextual issues into account.

One way to think of this is that the physiotherapist considers the patient as the main character in a book which then allows him/her to form a story or narrative about that person's life. This includes looking at what has gone on in the past, where that person is now and what might occur in the future. This will tend to personalise the approach to practice, with the physiotherapy input at least attempting to mirror aspects of the person's lifestyle. This can in turn increase levels of participation as the treatment seems more meaningful to the patient. But in order for this to happen, it is essential that the narratives of the patient and the therapist are the same (Alsop & Ryan 1996).

This is an area where good communication and interpersonal skills on the part of the physiotherapist are essential. The patient and/or carers must be consulted and considered to be an integral part of the health care team. If this does not occur then the patient's progress could be hindered as he or she may not see the relevance of the treatment. The physiotherapist must consider what the patient perceives to be the main problems or issues. If Mrs White is most worried about whether she will be able to return to her own house or not after her hip replacement, it is essential that the physiotherapist addresses this and not skirt round or avoid the subject altogether.

3. *Pragmatic reasoning*

This takes wider issues into account such as

organisational, political and economic realities. These may well have an effect on practice. This is another example of contextual issues being taken into account, but this time it is not the patient's context but rather institutional issues which could either inhibit or facilitate therapy.

Such questions are definitely becoming more prominent again because of the changes in the health service in the UK. Physiotherapists, although they are autonomous practitioners, may find they have less control over who they treat and when and how they treat them due to financial or policy constraints. This could have a major influence on clinical reasoning processes, whatever the beliefs or attitudes of the individual therapist.

This work by Schell & Cervero (1993) emphasises once again the multifaceted nature of clinical reasoning. Inevitably it is not only about physiotherapist–patient interaction but also involves other issues.

Fleming and the 'three-track mind'

Fleming (1991), who is also from an occupational therapy background, uses this this multifaceted approach to clinical reasoning in her theory regarding the therapist with the 'three-track mind'. Again three types of reasoning are postulated.

1. *Procedural reasoning* guides the therapist when thinking about the physical performance of the patient. This involves knowledge about the condition, pathophysiology, course, prognosis, how long the patient has had the condition, its effects, possible interventions, possible problems, assessment techniques, possible findings and so on. In the physiotherapy setting much of this occurs before the patient is even seen, with an image being formed of what might be expected in each particular case.
2. *Interactive reasoning* is used to help with understanding the patient as a person, and how he or she is managing within the environment. This will tend to occur more as the physiotherapist interacts with the patient during assessment and treatment.

3. *Conditional reasoning* integrates the previous two but also helps the physiotherapist to 'project an imagined future condition or situation for the patient'. It is therefore the imaginative and integrative part of the reasoning. How might that patient progress in the next few weeks/months, depending on all of the factors in the previous categories? This is a very dynamic process.

Problem-solving exercise 4.1

Imagine you are about to see a new patient with rheumatoid arthritis. Try to work through the three tracks of reasoning described by Fleming in considering how you might use your clinical reasoning skills in your contact with her.

■ Procedural reasoning: consider your knowledge of the condition and possible consequences, i.e. signs and symptoms/disability. What problems might you expect? How could you identify them? What might you find out?

■ Interactive reasoning: form an image of the person in your mind. How is she performing within her particular setting?

■ Conditional reasoning: synthesise from the previous two: What should you do? This is how she is now; how might she progress in the next few weeks?

Experienced clinicians are apparently able to shift rapidly from one of the three tracks of reasoning to another, as well as analyse different aspects of the patient problem simultaneously. It is important to point out that not all of these processes are easy even for a very experienced physiotherapist, particularly that of seeing some picture of the patient in the future. But it is a good approach to aim for as it is much more complete than others, putting the patient in context and not focusing on the medical model which tends to miss so much.

Many of these issues are begun to be addressed in the following chapters, during consideration of the case studies. However, it is only when in contact with real patients that the physiotherapist can develop these skills.

CONCLUSIONS

As mentioned earlier in this chapter, a great deal of work is being carried out with regard to clinical reasoning and the steps that occur during the process. It is the foundation of successful problem identification and so in turn, of treatment decisions. It is not simple; it could not be, given the complexity and 'messiness' of humans in general, and more specifically for physiotherapists and others in the health care team, their health problems. This accepted, the solution is to do as much as possible to acquire the knowledge base and the skills for collecting the data, and along with this to develop the ability to think widely and actively seek out new ideas.

It would seem that there is no substitute for experience, but this experience can be guided rather than its being a matter of trial and error. Without a helping hand a student or newly qualified clinician could be making mistakes in reasoning without being aware of it. This is where reflection and critical appraisal of performance become essential, that is, the metacognitive process mentioned earlier, where the physiotherapist actively thinks about his or her thinking and reasoning methods.

The models of clinical reasoning presented here are only examples of the many different approaches identified in the literature; however, they seem to encompass the essential factors involved. Novices are said to utilise the hypothetico-deductive model as it is the one based on the actual condition of the patient and seems most grounded in the medical model of health care. It is perhaps the easiest one to grasp. However, development of reasoning methods is not a stepwise process with the physiotherapist being 'promoted' through the ranks of clinical reasoning levels. Rather, it is more of a flexible scenario where new skills and knowledge are added as experience increases. The novice practitioner may indeed use some elements of the other reasoning methods mentioned at an early stage – but perhaps not as intuitively as an experienced physiotherapist.

The learning process continues throughout life and this is no less true of clinical reasoning. Practice and experience are needed to achieve and maintain competence in this area. Clinical reasoning is a complex and multifaceted process which does take a long time to master. But it is essential to develop a self-aware and self-monitoring approach to attaining knowledge and to the thinking processes that are necessary for sound, clinical problem-solving skills (knowledge, cognition and metacognition).

Summary

This chapter has outlined the areas of orthopaedics dealt with in the later chapters of the book to facilitate the reader in thinking about clinical decision making and problem solving within the specific clinical settings.

A brief outline of clinical reasoning has been given, along with examples of current models: the hypothetico-deductive model; the pattern recognition model, and the knowledge–reasoning integration model. These have been described in outline and related where possible to the orthopaedic situation.

If you are particularly interested in the subject of clinical reasoning, please refer to the texts in the reference list.

REFERENCES

Alsop A, Ryan S 1996 Making the most of fieldwork education – a practical approach. Chapman & Hall, London, ch 14

Fleming M H 1991 The therapist with the three track mind. American Journal of Occupational Therapy 45(11):1007–1014

Flew A 1984 A dictionary of philosophy. Pan, London

Higgs J 1996 Clinical reasoning. Personal communication

Higgs J, Jones M 1995 Clinical reasoning. In: Higgs J, Jones M (eds) Clinical reasoning in the health professions. Butterworth Heinemann, Oxford, ch 1

Jones M 1992 Clinical reasoning in manual therapy. Physical Therapy 72(12):875–884

Mattingly C 1991 What is clinical reasoning? American Journal of Occupational Therapy 45:979–986

Prion S, Graby R P 1995 The case study as an instructional method to teach clinical reasoning. In: Higgs J, Jones M (eds) Clinical reasoning in the health professions. Butterworth Heinemann, Oxford, ch 15

Schell B A, Cervero R M 1993 Clinical reasoning in occupational therapy: an integrative review. American Journal of Occupational Therapy 47(7):605–610

5

Fractures

■ Fractures ■ Classification ■ Management ■ Complications
■ Physiotherapy management ■ Stability

CONTENTS

Objectives

By end of this chapter you should:

1. Have an overview of the classification, management, normal healing times and complications of fractures.
2. Understand the assessment of a patient post fracture, in both the inpatient and outpatient setting.
3. Recognise how to problem solve for patient treatment and assessment, whatever the fracture site, extent or medical management.

Prerequisites

Read Chapter 2 on bone and joint changes during development. Familiarise yourself with fracture healing and medical management, recommended reading: Dandy 1993, McRae 1994, Crawford Adams & Hamblen 1992 (see References).

INTRODUCTION

Fractures or loss of continuity in the substance of a bone (McRae 1994) are a common occurrence and demand considerable treatment time and financial resources, in the accident and emergency (A&E) department through physiotherapy outpatient departments to community care.

Although the human skeletal system demonstrates both strength and a degree of flexibility, unfortunately we subject it to some very difficult trials and mishaps, testing its strength and endurance. When the forces become too great, exceeding the normal stress or strain load of bone, a fracture will occur.

The skeletal system forms a frame to which muscles, tendons, ligaments and connective tissue are affixed, allowing a firm attachment so that they can perform their movement functions. Without this 'solid' frame the soft tissue could not exert the forces needed to perform the functions of motion – a fundamental requirement of human life. Further to this, the skeletal system offers protection to the more vulnerable viscera: lungs, heart, digestive system, bladder and so on, which would otherwise be extremely prone to injury.

In Chapter 2 we have already addressed the role and function of bone as we develop and age. If you have not already reread Chapter 2 go back to it now and refresh your memory.

This chapter does not cover all aspects and types of fractures but will outline their general management and then, through case studies, explore physiotherapy rehabilitation of specific fractures with an approach that may be extrapolated to other skeletal areas.

(Note: '#', which is the sign for fractures, is sometimes used in this chapter.)

CLASSIFICATION OF FRACTURES

Fractures are classified according to several factors:

1. Skin damage
   - Open (compound): the skin is broken either from an external source or as a result of the bone fracturing then piercing the skin (compound from within).
   - Closed (simple): skin remains intact.

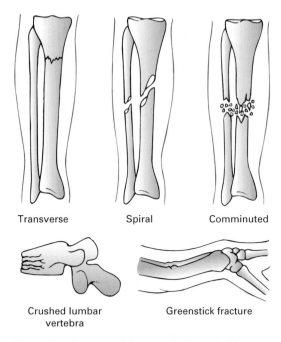

Transverse   Spiral   Comminuted

Crushed lumbar   Greenstick fracture
vertebra

Figure 5.1 Patterns of fracture. (Adapted with permission from Dandy 1993.)

2. Shape or line of fracture (Fig. 5.1).
   - Transverse/horizontal
   - Oblique/spiral
   - Comminuted: many small parts
   - Crush
   - Greenstick: bend in an immature bone, with a break in one of the bone cortices.
3. Displacement
   - Undisplaced: bone ends are still in apposition; although there is a clear break, there is usually no need for reduction.
   - Displaced: bone ends do not meet and reduction is necessary to achieve anatomical position prior to stabilisation, which is always needed. Soft tissue between the bone ends, or muscle spasm, may be causing the displacement and this has to be corrected prior to reduction.
   - Impacted: bone ends have been firmly shunted together so forming a stable but shortened bone. Often minimal external support is needed except for reduced weight bearing in lower limb fractures.

- Stable: fracture where the bone ends are held firmly, either by position or by the surrounding tissues. Thus reduction is often unnecessary and minimal support is needed; for example, an impacted fracture or a fracture of the metacarpals where the surrounding muscle tissue is holding the bone ends in place.

Therefore a fracture can be described, for example, as:

a. an open spiral fracture of the tibia;
b. a closed impacted fracture of the neck of femur.

Self-assessment question

■ **SAQ 5.1.** Outline and/or draw what you understand by the two above descriptions.

Answer:

a. *Open spiral fracture of the tibia: the tibia has a fracture in the shape of a spiral which has broken the skin at the fracture site. This needs manipulation back to the anatomical position prior to stabilisation.*

b. *Closed impacted fracture of the neck of femur: the neck of the femur has been pushed into the head of the femur resulting in a stable fracture which does not need reduction by manipulation but will need some protection from weight bearing. No skin damage.*

See also Figure 5.2.

A fracture can also be classified by its position,

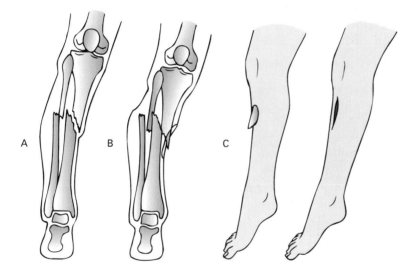

(a)

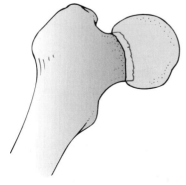

(b)

Figure 5.2 (a) A, spiral fracture of the tibia and fibula with no skin damage; B, open (compound) fracture of the tibia; C, external view of open fracture of the tibia. (b) Closed impacted fracture of the femur. (Adapted with permission from McRae 1994.)

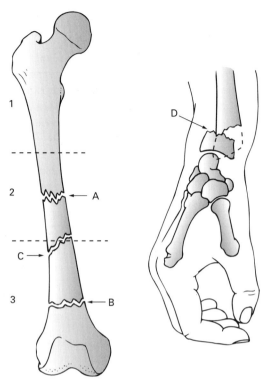

Figure 5.3 Arbeitsgemeinschaft für osteosynthesefragen (AO) classification of fracture position. A, transverse fracture of the middle third of the femur; B, transverse fracture of the distal third of the femur; C, spiral fracture of the distal third of the femur; D, epiphyseal fracture of the distal third of the radius. (Adapted with permission from McRae 1994.)

using the *Arbeitsgemeinschaft für osteosynthesefragen* (AO) classification of proximal (1), central diaphyseal (2) and distal (3) segments (Fig. 5.3) (McRae 1994). Both segments 1 and 3 can include either epiphyseal or intra-articular fractures where the break transverses either the epiphyseal (bone growth) plate of a child or the joint surface. Epiphyseal fractures may be categorised according to the Harris & Salter classification (Fig. 5.4).

Further details of AO classification and the Harris & Salter epiphyseal fracture classification can be found in McRae (1994).

Both epiphyseal and intra-articular (see below) fractures can cause major secondary problems and are regarded as more complex fractures. Epiphyseal fractures may cause a total lack of growth stimulation at the plate, if it has been crushed, thus the bone will be shorter than that on the contralateral side. If the fracture involves only one side of the plate the bone will grow with an anteroposterior or valgus/varus deformity if not corrected.

The term intra-articular describes any fracture that involves the articular surface of a joint (Fig. 5.5). When this occurs it is very important that joint congruity is restored so that no roughened or malaligned surfaces remain, predisposing the joint to excessive secondary wear and tear.

CAUSES OF FRACTURES

Whatever the classification of fractures, there

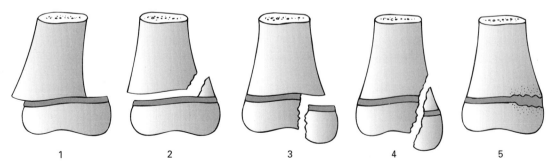

Figure 5.4 Harris & Salter classification of epiphyseal injuries: (1) epiphyseal slip only; (2) fracture through the epiphyseal plate with a triangular fragment of shaft attached to the epiphysis; (3) fracture through the epiphysis extending to the epiphyseal plate; (4) fracture through the epiphysis and shaft crossing the epiphyseal plate; (5) obliteration of the epiphyseal plate. (Adapted with permission from Dandy 1993.)

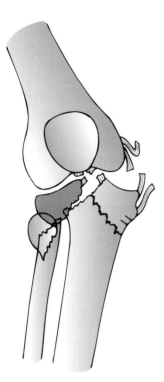

Figure 5.5 Intra-articular fracture. (Adapted with permission from McRae 1994.)

will also be some soft tissue, nerve or vascular involvement, although not necessarily all at the same time except in severe injuries.

Direct trauma

Here fractures are caused by a direct blow, such as:

- a kick on the shin in football
- a car hitting a pedestrian
- a person falling and landing on both calcanei.

In these situations the force of the blow is more likely to cause a transverse or crush fracture, and the layers of tissue from superficial to deep may be affected, that is skin, fascia/connective tissue, muscle, nerves and blood vessels.

Indirect trauma

Examples of indirect trauma include:

- a fall onto the outstretched hand resulting in a rotatory force with a spiral/oblique fracture of the humerus

- football boot studs placed firmly on the ground with the body weight of the person still moving over the foot, leading to a spiral/oblique fracture of the tibia.

These events therefore result in less soft tissue damage but often more displacement of the bone ends. The greater the indirect force, the more extreme the break which can lead to greater soft tissue damage.

Pathological causes

Pathological fractures occur where there is already a weakened area or diseased portion present, for instance with osteoporosis, tumours, cysts or metabolic disorders. The bone fractures from within because its internal structure is weakened or engorged with tissue other than bone. Damage can occur to the soft tissue and muscle attachments surrounding the fracture, either through pressure from the growing tumour/cyst or from the collapse of the bone.

Stress/fatigue fractures

These are caused by repeated excessive loading onto a bone. This results in mechanical bendings of the bone, of small magnitude, which eventually summate to cause a fracture. Therefore, anyone who repeatedly places high forces across a bone is prone to this injury, for example:

- fracture of the second metatarsal in someone repeatedly walking for excessive distances
- fracture of the upper third of the tibia in long-distance runners
- pars interarticularis fractures in fast bowlers.

Avulsion

These fractures arise when either a sudden muscular action of high force 'pulls off' a segment of bone to which the muscle is attached, or when a high traction force occurs across a joint and the ligament or joint capsule remains intact but a small piece of bone attachment is 'pulled off', for example when the medial collateral ligament of the knee pulls off the medial epicondyle of the femur.

Common sites for avulsion fractures through muscle pulls are:

- base of the fifth metatarsal (peroneus brevis)
- tibial tuberosity (quadriceps)
- upper pole of patella (quadriceps)
- lesser trochanter (iliopsoas)
- anterior superior iliac crest (iliopsoas).

Severe avulsion fractures are one cause of joint instability resulting in a fracture dislocation, where the joint surfaces become displaced but there is no ligamentous damage. The fracture usually occurs near to or into the joint surface, thus allowing excessive joint movement to take place with only a slight additional force. Intra-articular fractures may also cause a fracture dis-location where a larger piece of bone, with ligamentous or joint capsule attachment, becomes detached from the main part of the bone.

Fracture dislocations are usually managed as a fracture might be, and with good bone healing, normal joint laxity is restored.

Subluxation and dislocation

Joint surface displacement without a fracture is always accompanied by severe stretching of liga-mentous and capsular tissue resulting in a partial malalignment (subluxation) or, if the soft tissue becomes torn, then a total malalignment or dislo-cation takes place.

Both subluxation and dislocation will be dis-cussed in Chapter 6 on soft tissue injuries, as no fracture is involved.

MANAGEMENT OF FRACTURES

There are three stages in the management of frac-tures:

- Reduction: manipulation of the bone to its correct anatomical position.
- Immobilisation: to hold the bone in the correct reduced position.
- Rehabilitation: returning the person to as full function as possible after the trauma or disease.

Reduction

It could be argued that bone can heal whatever position it is left in so there is no need to reduce the fracture. Unfortunately poor position of bone ends can lead to malunion (union in a poor posi-tion) and thus severe deformity or loss of bone length can occur. With either of these primary problems, secondary changes may ensue:

- shortening of muscle length with resultant loss of force
- altered biomechanics and weight bearing across joints both ipsi- and contralaterally
- alteration in range of motion at all joints in the limb (Dandy 1993, McRae 1994).

Both the primary and secondary factors will predispose the joints above and below the frac-ture site, and possibly all the joints in that limb, to osteoarthrosis (Tetsworth & Paley 1994).

Thus a manipulation of the bone ends is undertaken to reduce them into a position where a minimum of 50% of the bone ends are overlap-ping and in contact with each other. During manipulation a traction (longitudinal) force is exerted distal to the fracture site to pull the short-ened bone ends back to their required length and then an anteroposterior, lateral or rotatory force may be added to gain good correction. This will usually be done either under local or general anaesthetic, but some fractures may need to be surgically reduced.

Too much distraction may cause a disturbance to bone healing, as ideally there needs to be con-tact between the bone ends to stimulate bone growth.

Self-assessment question

- **SAQ 5.2.** Which fractures, by classification, do not need reducing and why not?

    Answer:
    Those that are:
    - *Impacted: the bone ends are held together and usually motionless. These fractures may become loose prior to union, especially if weight bearing begins too soon; therefore they may need to be reduced if the bone end position changes.*
    - *Stable: the bone ends have to be in good apposition for a fracture to be stable, with at least 50% overlap, and they are*

> *held in place by the surrounding soft tissues.*
> - *Undisplaced: there is already a good anatomical position with a minimum of 50% overlap of bone ends, so that the fracture is termed undisplaced.*

Healing times

Before going on to discuss immobilisation and rehabilitation we should consider how long it takes for fractures to heal. In general the healing time of a fracture depends on its position in the body. For full details of fracture healing times please consult any of the books mentioned in the Prerequisites section.

There are two stages to consider.

1. *Union:* the partial repair of the bone, when the initial callus forms around the bone ends so that there is minimal movement. The bone under pressure will still give a little and will be painful. On X-ray the fracture line will still be visible. Full bone maturity has not been reached therefore full weight bearing cannot be undertaken and some external support is usually still needed. This can be moderated as the healing moves from union to consolidation.
2. *Consolidation:* full repair of the bone, where no movement takes place at the fracture site. On X-ray no fracture lines are seen and the bone trabeculae now cross where the fracture used to be. Full function can now commence without damaging the fracture.

Although most references to fracture healing will, rightly, not give exact timescales for fracture healing, there are some basic guidelines (Crawford Adams & Hamblen 1992, Dandy 1993,

McRae 1994). Table 5.1 lists the approximate times for union and consolidation in normal bone.

Union will usually take place anytime between 3 and 10 weeks. Consolidation will take approximately double the union times and full remodelling takes about double the consolidation times. At the consolidation stage the excess bone stabilising the fracture site is fully mature but it is not until the final stage of remodelling that the bone returns to its pre-fracture shape.

In children all the stages are reached more quickly and callus can occur in the first 2 weeks post-fracture; thus all these times must be adjusted accordingly.

Immobilisation

Once reduction has been achieved the bone segments must be held in place by immobilisation. This is achieved by one of three means:

1. conservative: external fixation (plaster of Paris (POP), splints, and so on)
2. external fixators
3. internal fixation.

It is quite common for more than one form of immobilisation to be used in the management of the patient before the fracture has united. The type of immobilisation used depends on a number of factors, such as the type and extent of fracture, and the health or age of the patient. These will not be discussed here as, on the whole, the medical staff make this decision.

The type of immobilisation is important to the therapist as it dictates when therapy commences and the extent of that therapy allowed. All forms of immobilisation, to a greater or lesser degree, will inevitably predispose the affected part to post-immobilisation joint stiffness, muscle weak-

Table 5.1 Approximate union and consolidation times in normal bone

Fracture position	Union time, weeks	Consolidation time, weeks
Proximal third of humerus	3	6
Distal third of radius/ulna	6	12
Proximal third of femur	4–6	8–12
Distal third of femur	6	12
Proximal third of tibia	6–8	12–16
Distal third of tibia	8–10	16–20

ness, alteration in proprioception, slowing down of the circulation and altered sensation through disuse. Thus these become the main issues for the rehabilitation phase.

Conservative: external fixation

Immobilisation in slings, collar and cuff, tubigrip, splinting materials (Plastazote, Orthoplast, etc.), plaster of paris (POP), polymer resin casts and other such methods all fall into this category. Skin or skeletal traction is also included, but this obviously requires hospitalisation and is therefore dealt with at the end of this section. All other forms of conservative immobilisation either need only 1–2 days of hospitalisation or, as in most cases, none at all.

In this category non-surgical means are used to support the fracture and a sling/collar and cuff or POP are the commonest methods used. These are cheap and easy to apply but the choice of appliance within this category is dictated mainly by the anatomical area of the fracture.

Slings and collar and cuff

Obviously slings and collar and cuff are used only in upper limb fractures, and there are four types of immobilisation (Dandy 1993; Fig. 5.6).

1. *A simple triangular bandage* or *broad arm sling* is used to support the weight of the forearm and hand thus relieving the weight on the upper arm. It can therefore be used for fractures or injuries around the shoulder, humerus or elbow.

2. *A collar and cuff* (c&c). Although this can be used to support the whole forearm/arm as with the triangular bandage, above, the main advantage offered by using a collar and cuff is support from the wrist only. Thus the collar and cuff takes the weight of the forearm, but the humerus is left unsupported so that a gravitational traction force is exerted on it allowing longitudinal correction of shaft fractures.

3. *A high sling* supports the whole arm keeping the hand/wrist in elevation so reducing the risk of swelling in the hand. Thus it does not act directly to support the fracture but to eliminate one complication. Therefore this type of sling is used after hand, wrist and forearm fractures when treated either with or without POP, or external splint. It should be remembered that the

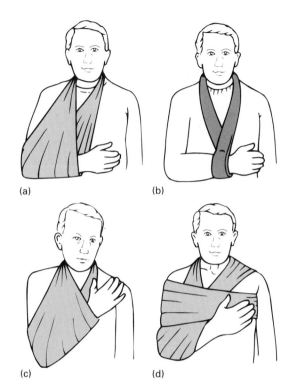

(a)   (b)

(c)   (d)

Figure 5.6 Support for upper limb fractures. (a) A simple triangular bandage; (b) collar and cuff; (c) high sling; (d) swathe and body bandage. (Adapted with permission from Dandy 1993.)

patient should be encouraged to remove the sling to exercise the limb through as full a range as possible, and then return the limb to the elevated support on completion.

4. *A body bandage* is a sling which supports the arm as with the triangular bandage but the arm is then bandaged to the side; thus it can only be worn under the clothes. This is used predominantly to prevent movement of the upper arm especially in the very early stages (1–10 days) after fracture of the neck/head of humerus or after shoulder surgery. The body bandage offers extreme support but does loosen in time and the bandage needs to be reapplied regularly.

With any form of sling or collar and cuff, the patient must keep the non-painful joints moving and, when possible, contract all muscles isometrically to maintain minimal tone. It is also very important that the patient notes any changes in sensation (numbness or paraesthesia), colour (bluish), severe increase in swelling or loss of motor function in the hand / wrist. All of these are signs of complications and will be discussed in the section on POP.

Self-assessment question

■ **SAQ 5.3.** A patient has been issued with a collar and cuff immediately after a fracture of the upper third of the humeral shaft. Which joints would you advise him/her to move?

Plaster of paris (POP) casts

POP is the term used to describe gypsona-impregnated bandages which have been used for many years to maintain bone / joint position. The bandages, after being soaked in cold water, produce a semi-liquid POP and are then moulded to the part, encompassing the joints above and below the fracture. After 20–30 minutes the POP starts to dry and hold its shape, but full drying takes up to 24 hours, thus weight bearing must be delayed until after this time.

The advantages of POP are that it is cheap, easy to apply, useful in immobilising most fracture sites, can be easily reinforced / replaced and can be placed over small wounds or scars after they have been dressed. The disadvantages include potential vascular occlusion, pressure sores, undiagnosed infection and joint stiffness after POP use. The main disadvantages to the patient are: the weight of the cast, especially in the lower limb; that it can be quite warm and itchy; if wet it will disintegrate; and children especially can get items caught between the skin and the cast, which could cause undetected pressure sores and / or infections.

When they dry POP bandages become rigid and brittle and are therefore prone to cracking particularly with overuse, thus skin irritation or rubbing can ensue.

The advantages far outweigh the disadvantages and this would be the first choice of immobilisation for most simple fractures.

If the patient is elderly and would benefit from a lighter support; if the fracture is in a young patient who continues to lead an active life, or if a patient has more than one fracture, polymer resin casts may be applied, such as Hexolite or Baycast. To make the cast lighter, polymer resin-impregnated bandages are used instead of POP. To increase the durability of the cast or to stop it disintegrating when wet, then a normal POP is applied but with a polymer resin overcoat. The main disadvantage of using polymer resin is that it is twice as expensive as POP bandages. Polymer resin is also much more brittle than POP when dry and can cause skin rubbing or cuts.

POP- or polymer resin-impregnated bandages must be applied carefully and instructions on how to do this can be found in McRae (1994).

Both of these types of bandage will shrink as they set, and given also the natural tendency for the soft tissue around the fracture site to swell 24–48 hours after the fracture, this means that the bandage should not be applied too tightly and that a cotton sleeve and then wool covering must be placed over the limb prior to application of the POP. The cast may also be split after setting to ensure adequate room for swelling to occur without causing additional pressure to the vascular tissues. A crepe bandage is then applied over the cast to hold it in place.

A dynamic brace can also be applied using POP or polymer resin or plastics such as Orthoplast (Pesco & Altner 1993) or Plastazote. etc. The dynamic (cast) brace has the benefit of allowing controlled movement at a joint, whilst maintaining the position and stability of the fracture (Fig. 5.7). Fractures of the shaft of femur are very often treated with POP or polymer resin braces, either after traction or internal fixation when extra fracture support is needed. Thus patient hospitalisation time is reduced and function and joint mobility can start earlier. Dynamic braces can also be used for fractures of the tibia, radius and ulna and lower humerus. Plastic materials can be used to brace these fractures, but as they are very expensive they should be used sparingly.

Self-assessment question

■ **SAQ 5.4.** How would the patient know if the POP was causing too much pressure, and what advice would be given to them? (See end of chapter.)

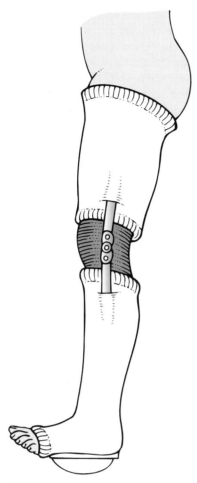

Figure 5.7 A cast brace.

Case study 5.1

Mrs Andrews, immediately post-injury (1)
Mrs Andrews, a 67-year-old lady arrives at the A&E department at her local hospital following a fall onto her outstretched (R) hand. After X-ray and orthopaedic assessment she has been diagnosed as having a (R) Colles' fracture. Following reduction under local anaesthesia, a dorsal POP back slab has been applied and she is to return in 5 days' time to attend the fracture clinic.

Self-assessment questions

■ **SAQ 5.5.** What is a Colles' fracture?

Answer: Colles fractures occur predominantly in older people, following a fall onto the outstretched hand. Similar mechanics in a younger person would be more likely to cause fractures of the forearm or humerus. There is a common belief that there is an association between this fracture and osteoporosis, as it is much more common in postmenopausal women. It is a fracture of the distal radius within 2.5 cm of the wrist; the classic 'dinner fork' deformity which results is due to the dorsal and radial displacement of the distal fragment of bone.

■ **SAQ 5.6.** How long will this fracture take to reach union and consolidation? What do these terms mean?

Problem-solving exercise 5.1

■ What type of support will the patient be given for the arm, and what instructions should she carry out prior to review in 5 days' time?

(See end of chapter to check your answer or if you have problems.)

Skin and skeletal traction
The changing management of patients with fractures means that long-term traction is not often used as an individual treatment. It is more routinely used as a temporary holding immobilisation until: skin wounds are healed; muscle spasm has reduced so that correct limb length can be achieved; other injuries are treated; the patient is fit enough for surgery or operation time becomes available, and in young children (who heal more quickly anyway).

There are two basic types of traction: skin and skeletal.

Skin traction (Fig. 5.8). Tape or elastic adhesive bandages are placed around the limb distal to the fracture and weight is suspended from the end to apply traction. The commonest form of

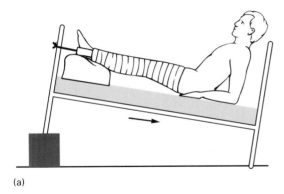

(a)

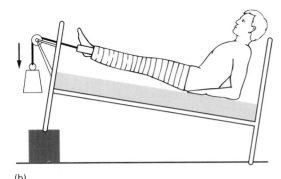

(b)

Figure 5.8 Skin traction. (a) Fixed traction: the weight of the patient provides traction. (b) Sliding traction: the weight of the patient still applies traction but his own weight is counterbalanced by a weight attached to a cord running over a pulley. (Adapted with permission from Dandy 1993.)

this is sliding skin traction before internal fixation of a fractured neck of femur in an elderly patient. The tape is wrapped around the leg and weights are suspended from a D sling at the end, the bed is raised and the patient's weight yields a counterbalance traction at the fracture.

This type of traction can also be used in patients with back pain who are being kept on bed rest.

For fractures of the shaft of femur in children under 3 years of age, gallows traction can be used. Here both legs are suspended vertically by strong tapes, thereby lifting the buttocks off the bed; thus traction is applied to the femur (Dandy 1993).

The only time traction is used in the upper

limb is for a displaced supracondylar fracture, which is more common in children. Dunlop traction is then used, where the forearm is held in the vertical position with the humerus in 90° of abduction and clear of the bed.

Skeletal traction. The commonest form of skeletal traction is that used to manage fractures of the femoral or tibial shaft, but it can also be used to provide stabilisation to unstable cervical spine fractures.

In fractures of the cervical spine, two screws are inserted into the skull and weights (1–5 kg, depending on the location of the fracture) are attached to callipers to distract and realign the cervical segments, reducing pressure on the spinal cord (Grundy et al 1993).

(This chapter will not explore spinal fractures and their consequences in detail. If you want to find out more about this, try reading Bromley 1991, Grundy et al 1993, and McRae 1994.)

In femoral shaft fractures the leg is placed in a Thomas splint for support and then either a Steinmann or Denham pin is surgically inserted behind the tibial tubercle, so that an appropriate weight can be attached to it. A longitudinal force is exerted through the tibia onto the quadriceps, hamstrings and the knee joint. Thus the lower end of the femur is pulled into correct alignment. If too much weight is applied the femoral length will be overcorrected and a gap will occur between the bone ends. Canvas straps and pads are placed around the leg and attached to the Thomas splint to ensure correction of the fracture in the anteroposterior and lateral planes. X-rays of the femur in traction will ensure correct alignment. Finally the Thomas splint is then suspended from an overhead 'Balkan' beam, with counterbalance weights, to allow free movement of the leg (Fig. 5.9).

A similar set-up can be used to supply traction to the calcaneus when severe tibial fractures are present.

General points concerning traction. Traction allows the free joints to be mobilised and the free muscles to be contracted much earlier than either POP or other external splints. The main disadvantage is that the patient is kept on bed rest, although only for a few days in most cases using skin traction. Thus, as with anyone on bed rest,

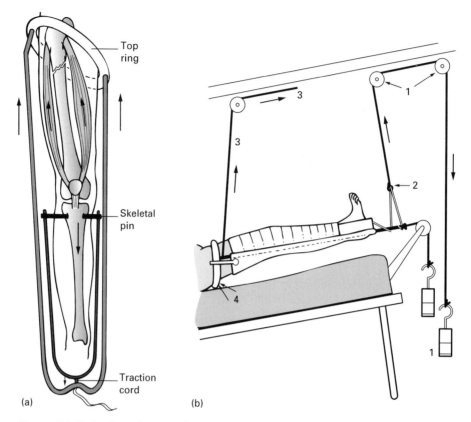

Figure 5.9 Skeletal traction provided by a Thomas splint. (a) The top ring provides one point of traction. The traction cord is attached to the skeletal pin and to the end of the Thomas splint. (b) A 'lively' system may be preferred, which may be achieved in various ways, for instance by weights and a system of pulleys (1). The suspension cord may be arranged in Y-fashion to straddle both irons of the Thomas splint (2). Although it is often attempted, support for the proximal end of the splint (3) is less clearly of benefit as it may cause extra pressure beneath the ring (4). (Adapted with permission from McRae 1994.)

care must be taken to ensure good bed mobility, skin care and respiratory function.

With either skin or skeletal traction, during exercise or general body movements rubbing can occur under the tapes or canvas supports, particularly during muscle contraction as this causes localised movement. Therefore the underlying skin must be inspected with great care if the patient complains of either soreness or rubbing. Pressure areas should be checked by all staff especially the area of the Achilles tendon at the end of the tape or the canvas of the Thomas splint, the patella and the ring top of the Thomas splint.

Self-assessment question

■ **SAQ 5.7.** What are the specific disadvantages of bed rest and which groups are most at risk?

Answer: Loss of motion either of the affected limb or generally which can give rise to a number of other problems:

— Slowing down of circulation which may predispose to vascular problems (deep vein thrombosis, pulmonary embolism).

— Loss of ability to maintain full respiratory function due to lack of mobility and compression of the bases and posterior

lobes of the lungs; therefore more risk of chest infections.
— Increased risk of pressure sores through extra pressure being exerted over greater trochanters, ischial tuberosities, sacrum, calcanei, Achilles tendons, elbows, scapulae and the back of the head.
— Loss of generalised muscle tone.
— Loss of independence.
— Poor posture, as patient tends to be in a half-lying or slumped lying position; therefore, over time, back pain or stiffness can ensue.

The groups most at risk: the elderly; those with a previous medical history which would make them more prone to the complications above, and those with multiple injuries.

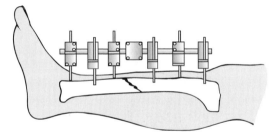

Figure 5.10 External fixator. (Adapted with permission from Dandy 1993.)

All of the above complications can occur even if patients are not in traction, but because traction grossly limits movement and patients are already in shock from the trauma, then they are even more at risk of these occuring. A report on the incidence of pressure sores in a single NHS trust hospital, showed that 10.3 patients per 100 admissions to orthopaedic wards developed pressure sores; this was 6% higher than on other wards (Clark & Watts 1994). Although this rate was for all patients and not just those on traction, it is still important to note that there is a very high incidence of patients with pressure sores on orthopaedic wards, and many of these will be elderly patients who will inevitably spend some time in skin traction following a fracture of the neck of femur.

External fixators

With this type of immobilisation, the bone fragments are held by an external scaffolding attached to up to six pins (Fig. 5.10) which are inserted percutaneously, either to one side of the bone (monofixator using cantilever construction, e.g. Orthofix Dynamic Axial fixator®) with a strong external rigid support, or completely through the bone and skin at both sides with a ring scaffolding at the top and bottom of the frame (ring fixator, e.g. Ilisarow®).

The monofixator is more commonly used; Hessman et al (1994) report that tibial fractures are the fractures most commonly fixed this way. Pelvic, femoral, humeral, ankle, foot (Hessman et al 1994) and Colles' (Pesco & Altner 1993) fractures are also reported to have been treated using external fixators (monofixator).

Halopelvic traction (Fig. 5.11) was one of the first forms of external ring fixator to be used in the management of spinal correction or after operation (Calliet 1975). Here a ring is placed around the skull and two or four screws are inserted, rods are surgically implanted through the pelvis and two or four strong external uprights support the upper and lower fixation points. A modification of this device is still used in the stabilisation of cervical fractures after skeletal traction, that is the halopelvic jacket, where a POP or polymer resin jacket replaces the pelvic rods.

The advantage of using external fixation in the management of long bone fractures is that it can be used in patients with severe skin loss or infection (Dandy 1993) or soft tissue or vascular injury (Hessman et al 1994). It also allows easy alteration, under X-ray control, to the alignment of the bone fragments and, particularly, either compression or traction can be added as necessary (Dandy 1993). The greatest disadvantages are that the pin tracks can become infected and therefore there is a risk of osteomyelitis or osteitis, and that refracture may occur if the fixation is removed too quickly.

These devices are quite unsightly to look at and many patients and relatives or friends may find it difficult to come to terms with the sight of the fracture scaffolding.

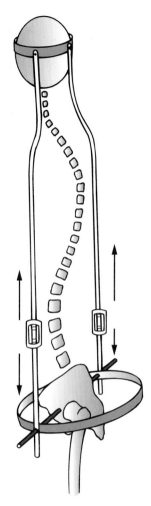

Figure 5.11 A halopelvic device. (Adapted with permission from Calliet 1975.)

General points

The bone pins of the external fixator are inserted through the soft tissue and muscle making the latter painful to contract, and thus the soft tissue around the joints distal to the fracture may contract causing loss of motion, often reducing function severely. This is particularly so in tibial fractures where the ankle is held in plantarflexion because it is very difficult to dorsiflex. Some surgeons will attach a footplate to the external fixator to try to stop plantarflexion taking place. Even if this is present then dorsiflexion exercise (active and passive) must take place to restore strength.

Thus the role of the physiotherapist must be to:

- Maintain the soft tissue length of the plantar flexors by passive or active assisted movement, i.e. place a sling around the distal part of the foot and gently pull the sling towards the body. This will stretch the posterior calf muscles: the gastrocnemius with the knee straight and the soleus with the knee bent; the spring ligament and the plantar aspect of the foot will also be stretched.
- Mobilise the subtalar joint (inversion and eversion), the distal joints (pronation and supination) and long and transverse arches of the foot.
- Maintain full knee extension as the tight plantar flexors will tend to pull the knee into flexion.
- Maintain isometric contraction of the dorsiflexors as much as the patient is able.
- Keep the skin from sticking to the pin sites by encouraging gentle oscillatory joint movements.
- Maintain venous return to prevent swelling and vascular problems, by gentle ankle movements with good strong contraction of the long toe flexors/extensors whilst in elevation.
- Encourage the patient to check the skin distal to the fracture daily to keep it hydrated with moisturiser.

External fixation which does not pierce large muscle groups, such as halopelvic traction, the halobody jacket or pelvic fracture fixation is much easier to maintain and produces far fewer muscle problems. Pelvic external fixation does however bring problems of its own, as the pins can damage the internal organs within the pelvis such as the urethra or bladder. All other types of external fixation, for instance of the humerus and radius and so on, will incur similar muscle or joint problems.

Operative internal fixation

In the patient's operation notes you will often see the abbreviation 'ORIF'; this stands for 'Open

Reduction Internal Fixation' and therefore describes the act of reducing the fracture prior to fixing it internally. Thus you know that the patient has had some form of internal fixation but not the specific details.

The type of internal fixation will again depend on the position and extent of the fracture, and the size, texture and strength of the bone (McRae 1994). Therefore there is a huge variety of internal fixation devices which the surgeon can insert to stabilise the reduced fracture. These include screws, plates, intramedullary nails, locking nails, wires or nailplates (sliding or compression) (Figs 5.12–5.16). They can be used in combination in severe fractures (Fig. 5.17).

Further information about the various kinds of internal fixation can be obtained from Dandy 1993, ch. 6, and McRae 1994, ch. 4.

Internal fixation is indicated when:

- Fractures cannot be controlled in any other way, i.e. other methods of immobilisation have failed.
- Patients have fractures of more than one bone.
- The blood supply to the limb is jeopardised by the fracture and the vessels must be protected (Dandy 1993).
- Bone ends cannot be reduced without opening the fracture site to remove muscle and soft tissue debris.

Internal fixation is very often used with multiple fractures, providing the patient is suitable for a general anaesthetic. Internal fixation provides the quickest form of stability to the fracture stop-

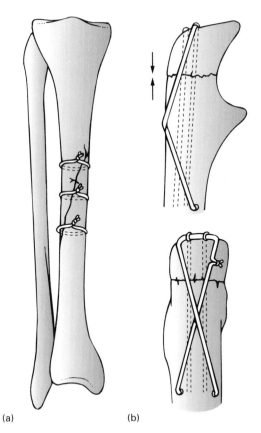

(a)   (b)

Figure 5.12 Internal fixation: wire. (a) Cerclage wiring of the tibia; (b) and (c) tension band wiring of the olecranon. (Adapted with permission from Dandy 1993.)

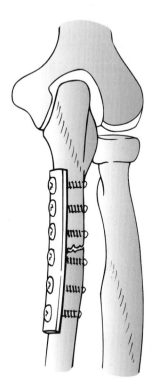

Figure 5.13 Internal fixation: plate. (Adapted with permission from McRae 1994.)

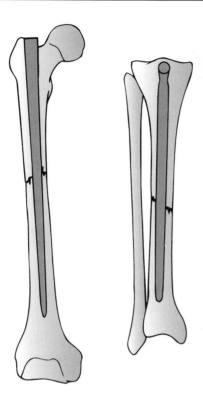

Figure 5.14 Internal fixation: intramedullary nails. (Adapted with permission from Dandy 1993.)

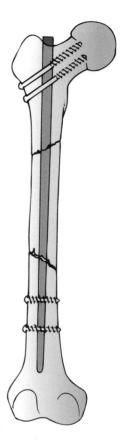

Figure 5.15 Internal fixation: locking intramedullary nail. Screws are passed into the fragments above and below the fracture to hold the bone out to length. (Adapted with permission from Dandy 1993.)

ping the blood loss which automatically occurs when a bone is broken. Severe loss of blood can increase the shock experienced by the patient and, left uncontrolled, can be fatal. Internal fixation will also provide early stability to multiple fractures thus reducing pain and increasing function to the patient.

The advantages include:

- Better chances of obtaining good reduction and union (McRae 1994).
- Early mobilisation both generally and specifically.

The disadvantages are:

- Risk of infection.
- Additional trauma of surgery to bone and surrounding tissue.

Internal fixation, like splints/casts and exter-

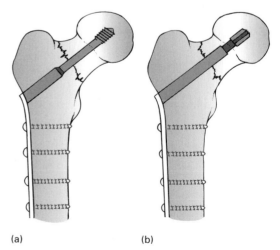

(a)   (b)

Figure 5.16 Internal fixation with nail-plates: (a) compression; (b) sliding. (Adapted with permission from Dandy 1993.)

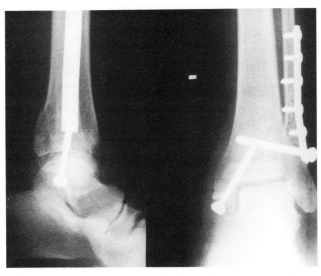

Figure 5.17 Internal fixation: combination of screws and plate. (Adapted with permission from Dandy 1993.)

nal fixators, acts as an immobilisation device until fracture healing takes place, but unlike the other devices internal fixation is not visible. Thus there is often a misunderstanding with patients and junior staff alike, that the internal fixation device will be strong enough to support the normal stress or strain loads of bone. This is not the case and extra support with reduced loading must be given to the internal scaffolding until initial callus formation occurs. Thus a patient with an internally fixed fracture of the humerus should have a broad sling or collar and cuff in the early stages, to help support the weight of the arm and reduce function. Or the patient with an internally fixed femur or tibia must remain non-weight-bearing until initial callus forms, to ensure no excess loading occurs across the fracture site.

Normally after internal fixation, only limited joint movement will take place in the initial stages because of pain, swelling, bruising and apprehension. But when these reduce after 10–14 days the patient may be tempted to use the limb normally. It is important that at this time the patient is seen again by either medical or therapy staff to remind them of the basic 'do's and 'don't's.

Postoperative care

As the patient has had a general anaesthetic then alongside the physiotherapy aims of treatment for the fracture site, are those for postoperative care. The physiotherapist must assess the respiratory and vascular performance and general mobility. These will be discussed in the rehabilitation section.

Rehabilitation

Initial rehabilitation instructions after the injury

Rehabilitation starts as soon as the fracture has been reduced. From the first contact with the patient, the physiotherapist must ensure that the patient fully understands the rehabilitation process to aid full recovery.

It has been well documented that complications can commence immediately after the fracture if the patient or care staff are not aware of potential problems. Thus suitable instruction to all concerned is absolutely necessary. All members of staff are still involved at this stage and any of the medical, nursing or therapy staff may contribute this information depending on the policy at specific hospitals.

Basic instructions

The instructions to Mrs Andrews described earlier (Problem-solving exercise 5.1, Answer) should be given to all patients, with upper limb fractures. Therefore to refresh your memory revise Problem-solving exercise 5.1.

Self-assessment question

■ **SAQ 5.8.** What instructions should be given to a patient with a fracture of the lower third of tibia and fibula, who is being sent home, non-weight-bearing, in a long leg POP cast from thigh to toes?

These basic instructions underpin the process of rehabilitation. The overall objective of post-fracture rehabilitation is to aid fracture healing in the appropriate timescale, returning the patients to their functional norm, with as few complications as possible.

Complications of fractures

Some of the complications of fractures have been mentioned before, but need to be highlighted again before addressing rehabilitation.

Long-term complications

Alteration to the healing rate

Delayed union. The fracture takes a longer time to heal than usual, accompanied by abnormal bone changes. This is usually managed by having a longer immobilisation time.

Non-union. The fracture does not unite in the recognised time frame. Bone infection or excessive movement at the bone ends are examples of causes of non-union. Non-union is usually managed initially by a longer time of immobilisation, then if it persists surgical management by internal fixation with excision of bone ends and bone grafting is used. In very severe cases of non-union, with long-standing pain and/or infection, amputation of the limb may be necessary.

Mal-union. The fracture unites but with an unacceptable degree of angulation or rotation. If severe, the bone can be re-aligned by manipulation if un-united, or if union or consolidation has occurred then an osteotomy may be performed to correct the malalignment.

Shortening

As a result of mal-union the bone ends may heal in an overlapped position thus shortening the bone length. This is particularly important in the lower limb where a resultant leg length imbalance of greater than 1.25 cm may cause secondary low back pain and greater loading across the hip joint, possibly leading to secondary osteoarthrosis.

Joint stiffness

There may be loss of full joint range of motion from either periarticular or intra-articular causes.

Periarticular causes. These may be pain, swelling, haemorrhage, reduced muscle function or muscle tethering, capsular or ligamentous damage.

Intra-articular causes. These include joint adhesions, malalignment of joint surfaces, excessive callus formation with intra-articular fractures, or loose bodies.

Avascular necrosis

The blood supply to the bone has been interrupted and therefore the bone dies and crumbles, and the joint involving that bone become painful and stiff. This commonly occurs with fractures of the neck of femur, scaphoid, talus, lunate or in segments of a comminuted fracture where the blood supply has been totally severed.

Autonomic problems: Sudeck's atrophy or reflex sympathetic dystrophy

'Sudeck's atrophy' refers to hand symptoms which may occur after a Colles' or wrist fracture and 'reflex sympathetic dystrophy' is a term used when symptoms occur in the foot after ankle fractures.

In Sudeck's atrophy the Colles' fracture is fully united but on X-ray there is patchy osteoporosis. There is severe post-traumatic pain with autonomic changes including swelling of the hand and fingers. The skin is warm, pink and has a polished shiny appearance. Excessive pain along with the swelling increases, preventing movement of the fingers and wrist.

Myositis ossificans

This is usually seen at the elbow, after a supracondylar fracture but can occur at any joint especially the hip, shoulder or knee. It is especially seen in paraplegic or head injury patients where passive movements or stretching is carried out regularly, often against increased muscle tone. A calcified mass develops in the soft tissues of a joint after severe trauma and may be associated with intense haematoma. As there is a strong belief that passive movement or stretching predisposes the tissue to myositis, many practitioners will not use passive stretching to the elbow joint. Limited passive motion may be carried out or the practitioner may err on the side of caution and only use active assisted motion.

Infection (osteitis)

This often presents following an open fracture or through the pin tracks of an external fixator. The normal signs of infection appear, i.e. pain, raised temperature, swollen area with local tenderness and there may be a foul-smelling discharge or staining of POP. Bone death will occur in severe long-term cases.

Post-callus complications

These can include either nerve damage or tendon rupture. Following the normal development of callus, the soft tissue in the surrounding area may become compressed or frayed by movement over the extra bone. Thus any soft tissue near the fracture can become involved. (Note: the extensor pollicis longus tendon is very prone to rupture after Colles' fracture.)

Osteoarthrosis (OA)

Alteration in the joint articular surface, biomechanical stress changes or alteration in the bone length after fracture, all predispose the adjacent joints to increased wear and tear and early OA. OA may occur at any joint associated with the altered mechanics not just the joint involving the fracture, for instance in the contralateral knee joint following a fractured neck of femur.

Self-assessment question

- **SAQ 5.9.** Describe the immediate and more long-term complications of fracture healing and rehabilitation.

Physiotherapy cannot prevent these complications but if you are aware of them, then you will be able to recognise and treat them accordingly during the rehabilitation period.

Physiotherapy assessment and treatment

Much more caution must be exercised when assessing for the first time an inpatient with an acute fracture. By the time the patient comes to outpatient therapy, usually after bone union, a much fuller examination of the part can be made without causing damage.

The earlier the physiotherapist can start the rehabilitation phase, the greater the opportunity to influence the overall outcome through careful assessment, individual treatment and establishment of a good rapport with the patient.

There are some general principles of physiotherapy when treating fractures, which must be remembered in every case. However, the treatments themselves must be made appropriate for the individual, particularly in the duration and type of exercises given. The number of repetitions should be calculated according to the patient's ability to carry out the exercise, although many therapists start with a combination of 'fives', for instance five repetitions of the exercise held for 5 seconds, increasing either the number of repetitions or duration as possible. If a patient with an acute fracture can only manage one successful repetition then this is much more acceptable then an incorrect movement or half-hearted attempt.

Physiotherapy assessment and treatment should never be regarded as a standard recipe (see Ch. 3) as no two patients will ever be the same.

Acute unstable fractures

General points. Avoid any muscle contraction that will move the bone ends, thus inhibiting healing. It will increase pain and if vigorous may cause malalignment of the bone ends. This can occur when a strong muscle group is attached to the smaller fragment of the fracture, for instance, iliopsoas contraction on the proximal fragment of bone in a fracture of the upper shaft of femur.

If a fracture is unstable it must be supported when exercises are done distal to it. For example with a fracture of the humerus, the elbow, wrist and hand can be still exercised whilst the arm is held in the sling for support.

Joint motion. With any fracture, assisted active or passive movement is easier than active in the early stages, to increase the range of movement (ROM) and to give reassurance to the patient.

Following internal fixation try to gain as much movement as possible of the joints to be immobilised in POP, prior to its application. A good example of this is at the ankle, where often the internally fixed ankle is left in elevation without POP until the swelling in the foot and ankle goes down and the range of dorsiflexion gets to neutral (plantigrade). Gentle movements and intermittent pressure can help to reduce the swelling and allow greater movement. Continuous passive motion (CPM) machines can also assist with this in between therapy sessions (Coutts et al 1989, Davies 1991).

Swelling. Active exercise distal and proximal to the fracture will help venous return and reduction of swelling, particularly if carried out in elevation.

Weight bearing. Full or partial weight bearing must not commence until some callus formation is seen on X-ray. Touch weight bearing may be allowed in some cases where non-weight bearing is too difficult.

Walking with any walking aid at this stage must be safe, with good balance and coordination. If you are unsure whether or not the patient is safe then they must remain in hospital until they are. Non-weight bearing can be very difficult for some patients and takes quite a time to get used to, particularly in elderly patients. It is in these instances that the surgeons may agree to allow touch weight bearing, to aid mobilisation and release from hospital. (If in doubt, check first.)

Massage, especially in warm soapy water or with baby oil, will help return the nutrition to the skin, give the patient reassurance and give good sensory feedback. (Patients could do this at home.)

Function. Gentle functional movements will help the patient with any upper limb problems, but lifting of heavy objects should be avoided until the callus at the fracture site is strong enough for this.

Always use functional objectives and measurements that are particularly important to the patient.

Stable united fractures

General points. External fixators and internal fixation do not replace union of the bone; these are purely scaffolding devices to hold the bone until union takes place. Thus the bone should be treated with care, with limited weight bearing, until callus has strengthened the fracture site.

Excessive pain or fracture mobility after normal union times must be regarded as highly significant, and if there is any doubt then the patient should be referred back to the orthopaedic surgeon as soon as possible.

Joint motion. Once a fracture has been stabilised (by cast brace, external fixator or internal fixation) then the range of motion at the joints proximal and distal to the fracture can be regained. CPM machines can be used to help regain movement whilst the patient is hospitalised. Most CPM machines give support from the thigh to the knee, ensuring no abnormal strain to fractures of the shaft of the femur.

Patients can undertake some simple accessory movements themselves and these assist the return of physiological motion and may help with pain relief. Union must have occurred before these are done.

Strengthening. Do not apply excessive resistance across the fracture, either longitudinally from weight bearing or rotatory from muscle contraction, until the fracture and surrounding muscles are strong enough. For example, resistance to strengthen the rotators of the shoulder is usually given at the distal forearm; if the fracture is not well united then this rotatory force can cause a refracture of the shaft of humerus.

During strengthening exercises, do not suspend free weights distal to the fracture until after consolidation, particularly in the case of a fracture dislocation or transverse fracture near to a joint, as this causes an excessive traction force.

Suspension of weights over the unsupported joint to increase passive stretch may also be harmful with a fracture close to the joint, particularly for the knee and elbow where longer levers are involved. An example of this is when the knee is in as full extension as possible with the heel and the buttock being supported but not the femur. A physiotherapist may add either manual pressure or weights over the knee joint to assist the stretch on the posterior capsule of the knee. It can be reasoned that if there is a fracture near to a joint or an intra-articular fracture this may cause excessive stress in the anteroposterior direction thus making the fracture painful or prone to delayed union.

Muscle strength both at joints immediately proximal and distal to the fracture and at joints further away may remain weaker for quite some time (up to 2 years). Bullock-Saxton (1994) indicated that fit young men with severe lateral ligament strain of the ankle, still had proximal muscle function changes 2 years after the injury. Although this research was not undertaken on post-fracture patients, it can be assumed that the same principles apply to this category of patient. The more severe the injury the greater the risk of long-term problems, and the patient should be made aware of this.

All methods of strengthening can be introduced once the fracture has consolidated, but from union until this time the fracture site should be supported whilst resisted exercises are done.

Once good isometric strength has been achieved, endurance training with low weight but large numbers of repetitions should commence before power training (large weights, small numbers of repetitions). Isokinetic training can begin after union, again provided the fracture is supported. Torque limits can be set into the test programme then the patient cannot overwork.

Weight bearing. Weight bearing is increased as the fracture and muscle strength allow. Usually it is the patient who is reluctant to get rid of walking aids, but you must ensure that the lower limb is strong enough to take and endure the increase in weight. Limb loading with a set of bathroom scales can be undertaken to ensure:

- correct load acceptance
- level of pain on loading.

All the above points must be borne in mind when administering the treatment programme. The physiotherapist has direct control over treatment after a fracture and may influence rehabilitation for good or bad. If there is any doubt about the stability, position or overall performance then you should consult either senior physiotherapy staff or the doctors concerned.

REHABILITATION: THREE CASE HISTORIES

Rehabilitation will now be addressed using three case histories:

- A Colles' fracture, after POP fixation (Case study 5.1).
- A fractured shaft of femur, after traction/internal fixation (Case study 5.2).
- A hip fracture, after internal fixation (Case study 5.3).

Before considering any of the case histories, or indeed the rehabilitation of any patient with a fracture, five general questions must be asked about the patient and the fracture.

1. What do I know about this fracture?
2. What should I find at this stage of management if the fracture is healing normally?
3. What might go wrong with this fracture?
4. What do I know about this patient, particularly concerning his/her functional ability?
5. What are the expected overall outcomes for this patient, with this fracture?

Question 2 should be answered for both the current stage of fracture healing and for the future.

Question 4 will need to be addressed by a full subjective and objective assessment of the patient.

All questions should be answered for each of the patient's fractures. The questions can be taken in any order but all should be answered.

If all these questions can be answered then the physiotherapy treatment can be planned and any problems that might arise can be prepared for.

Rehabilitation following a Colles' fracture

Now please return to Case study 5.1, Mrs

Andrews, stage 1 (p. 82) and reread the scenario before proceeding.

Problem-solving exercise 5.2

■ Attempt to answer all the five major questions given above about Mrs Andrews and her Colles' fracture.

On reviewing the answer to the above exercise it is clear that we can only address questions 1–3 and 5 fully at this stage. Question 4 has been answered for the initial stage but a full functional assessment will depend on the results after the removal of the POP.

Case study 5.1

Mrs Andrews, removal of POP (2)
On review at 5 weeks the Colles' fracture was deemed united, and the POP was removed. Mrs Andrews was then seen by the physiotherapy consultant in the clinic and given an initial assessment.

Observation
(R) arm was held close to the body.
The skin around the hand, wrist and forearm was flaky, pale and dry.
(R) forearm was considerably thinner than the (L).
Wrist held in slight flexion and ulnar deviation.
Obvious thickening of the bone around the distal end of the radius and some soft tissue thickening around the dorsal aspect of the wrist.

Problem-solving exercise 5.3

■ Are these the normal signs of a fracture after removal of POP?
Explain why.

(See the end of the chapter if you have problems.)

Following Mrs Andrews' initial quick assessment in clinic she has been given an appointment for outpatient physiotherapy for the next day. The next stage of the normal fracture healing pathway has been reached. A full subjective and objective assessment must be undertaken to answer question 4 in full; then we can set objectives for treatment. Now return to Chapter 3 on assessment and refresh your memory.

Problem-solving exercise 5.4

■ What would you need to ask this patient to complete question 4?

Case study 5.1

Mrs Andrews, continued (3)
From what you have already been told about Mrs Andrews, some of these questions can be answered but we still need to know some details, as follows:

- Occupation: nil, retired post office manager.
- Hobbies: bowls, knitting.
- Home circumstances: widow, lives alone in a bungalow, friends have been helping out with shopping.
- Hand dominance: right.
- Main problems:
  — scared to move wrist due to pain and apprehension
  — arm feels weak and stiff
  — worried about appearance of arm
  — anxious to get back to bowls.
- What Mrs Andrews has been doing with her arm: moving the shoulder up and down, stretching the elbow, and moving the fingers. Has not been doing rotation of the shoulder and radioulnar joint, thumb also has not been moved fully.
- No other injury at the time.
- Previous medical history: nil of note, no previous fractures, operations or serious illnesses.

Self-assessment question

■ **SAQ 5.10.** What would you assess in your objective examination?

(See end of chapter, but try to come up with your own points first.)

Case study 5.1

Mrs Andrews, continued (4)
Major findings
Pain: over the dorsal and radial aspects at end of range flexion, extension and radial deviation.

ROM (right)

Wrist	Active	Passive
Extension	0–5°	0–15°
Flexion	0–45°	0–50°
Ulnar deviation	0–20°	0–25°
Radial deviation	0–5°	0–5°
Radioulnar		
Pronation	0–60°	0–65°
Supination	0–5°	0–5°

Fingers
Flexion: tip of middle finger to 5 cm from 1st palm crease.
Extension: with wrist in neutral to 20° at MCP joints.

Elbow	Active	Passive
Flexion	10–130°	10–130°
Extension	–10°	0°

Shoulder: full movement.
(L) arm: no problems.

Muscle strength: all muscles on (R) wrist isometrically contract in the neutral position. Isotonically (R) biceps, triceps, deltoid, rotator cuff, all Gd IV. Grip strength tested with a bulb grip dynamometer: records 2 kg pressure for the right hand using the large bulb.

Swelling: (R) hand 2 cm bigger than (L) at level of MCP.

Sensation: normal; (R) = (L) all tests.

Dexterity: able to grip a tennis ball, unable to pick up a 1-cm peg, hold a key, or touch thumb to little finger.

With this information we can now begin to plan Mrs Andrews' treatment, and the first step is to consider her main problems and set initial treatment objectives for them (Table 5.2).

Each time Mrs Andrews attends for physiotherapy these main problems should be

Table 5.2 Mrs Andrews' problems and treatment objectives

Patient's problems	Treatment objectives
Scared to move wrist due to pain and apprehension	Show the patient how to move without causing damage to the wrist and try to reduce pain
Arm feels weak and stiff	Encourage controlled movement of the wrist, radioulnar, elbow and shoulder joints
Worried about appearance of arm	Explain about general care of the skin
Anxious to get back to bowls, her main hobby	Explain the healing times and the need to mobilise and then strengthen the arm before returning to bowling

reassessed and any further problems which may have arisen should be noted and addressed.

Problem-solving exercise 5.5

■ Describe how you would carry out each of the objectives in Table 5.2. (Answers at the end of the chapter.)

The treatment to be carried out during outpatient sessions needs to be considered. This is based on the main problems which are clearly related to joint stiffness after immobilisation and thus are the main focus for treatment. Most of Mrs Andrews' concerns will be addressed during this consideration.

During the initial assessment it is also important for the physiotherapist to establish whether or not referral to the occupational therapist or social worker is necessary. If Mrs Andrews were having difficulties managing tasks around the house then assessment by the occupational therapist might be useful. Some basic advice, especially in the kitchen, might help considerably. If greater difficulties were encountered further assistance could also be given, such as meals on wheels, district nursing (for dressings etc.) or care assistance, but Mrs Andrews does not need these.

■ **SAQ 5.11.** How would you mobilise a stiff joint immediately after immobilisation of a Colles' fracture where union is complete? (See below.)

Answer: *If the patient is apprehensive ask her to hold just proximal to the wrist joint (i.e. across the fracture site) to gain reassurance whilst doing the exercises.*

- *Active/active assisted wrist exercises through as much range as possible especially extension and radial deviation, making sure the exercises are clearly understood and could be repeated at home.*
- *Gentle passive stretching to the long finger flexors and extensors, so stretching the soft tissues.*
- *Maitland mobilisation techniques: accessory Gd I techniques to help with pain relief or Gd II as the pain decreases, to increase range of motion. (Union must be achieved before mobilisation techniques can be done.)*
- *Functional exercises that do not involve carrying objects, e.g. opening doors with that hand, washing up dishes, getting dressed, etc.*
- *Once range has been gained then strengthening exercises should be introduced to maintain the new range.*

One of the greatest concerns of student physiotherapists is when to increase the number or type of exercises. For Mrs Andrews, there are five main pointers:

1. All ranges of motion increase, but especially extension, radial deviation and finger flexion as indicated by measurement.
2. Pain reduces at rest and does not increase with exercise.
3. Strength increases in the grip and wrist extensors and a combination of these two (functional position of the wrist).
4. Swelling decreases in the hand.
5. General hand function improves.

The patient should be aware that the wrist and hand may still become tired and ache for some time, particularly after use. As the exercises increase then the ache may return for a short time but will decrease with increased function, motion and strength.

Thus we can gradually increase first the number of exercises and then the type, that is, introduce more active motion than active assisted or passive. We would gradually bring in longer lever arms and increase resistance using small weights so endurance can be increased, until the fracture has consolidated.

Finally Mrs Andrews will be helped to return to her full function by introducing her to the techniques used for bowls. This can be started as a general exercise for the whole arm without a ball and then a small soft ball could be added. The size and weight of the ball would be increased to that of a bowls ball as Mrs Andrews became more able.

Rehabilitation following a fractured shaft of femur

These injuries can only occur when considerable force is involved, given the strength of the femur and the surrounding muscle. Thus they predominantly happen in road traffic accidents, falls, or after a violent twisting action. A fracture can also occur at the shaft of the femur immediately below the tip of the femoral component of a total or partial hip replacement. This is because the metallic component is much more rigid than the underlying bone, thus the bone takes added stress with the risk of fracture (Dandy 1993, McRae 1994).

Because there is usually considerable violence involved, it is quite common to have associated injuries, such as a fractured patella, posterior cruciate ligament rupture, posterior dislocation of the hip or skin or vascular damage.

Case study 5.2

Mr Kingston, fractured shaft of femur, post-traction and internal fixation (1)

Mr David Kingston, a 24-year-old male was admitted to hospital through A&E with a compound spiral fracture of the mid-shaft of (R) femur after being involved in a road traffic accident (RTA), where his motorbike was hit by a car late last night. He was thrown from his motorbike and landed on his (R) side.

Subjective assessment

Social history: lives with wife and two children in a house with one flight of stairs (one banister (R) going up). Bathroom and bedroom upstairs. Unemployed bricklayer (1 year); wife works and he looks after the children (aged 5 and 7 years).

Smoking: 40 cigarettes per day.

Hobbies: riding motorbike and playing Sunday league football.

Drug history: nil.

History of present complaint (HPC): on admission a Denham pin was inserted in the (R) tibia and skeletal balanced traction set up with 4 kg weight. Possibility of surgery in 3 days' time to insert an interlocking intramedullary nail. Patient cannot remember much about the accident but was not unconscious.

Painful (R) shoulder since RTA; no bony injury on X-ray.

Main patient problems:
— Pain in (R) thigh and shoulder.
— Immobilisation in hospital.
— Family (he looks after the children whilst wife works).
— Inability to move (R) leg or arm.

Objective assessment

Observation
Patient's records: temperature 35°, blood pressure 110/70, pulse 65.
   Patient: patient half lying, with skeletal traction and Thomas splint in situ suspended on overhead beam. Leg held in full knee extension and ankle in plantarflexion and inversion. Clean dressing on each side of Denham pin, and over the lateral thigh where the femur pierced the skin. Swelling mid-shaft of femur, down to and including the knee and around pin sites.
   (R) arm is held in adduction and internal rotation with elbow flexion, no support in situ. No obvious deformity, swelling or bruising. Glucose intravenous drip in (L) arm.

Leg
Palpation: lower leg feels cold (slightly blue), thigh warm. Dorsalis pedis pulse present.

ROM (R)	Active	Passive
Ankle		
Dorsiflexion	−30−(−20°)	0−10°
Plantarflexion	30−40°	0−60°
Subtalar		
Inversion	10−20°	0−60°
Eversion	−10−0°	0−30°
Small foot joints	Cannot be tested	Full (= to (L))
Toes	Full	Full (= to (L))
Knee and hip	Cannot be tested	Cannot be tested
Patella	Cannot be tested	Full (= to (L))

Muscle strength

(L) (R)	
	All groups Gd V
Dorsiflexors	Gd II, pain at pin sites
Plantarflexors	Gd III, pain at pin sites
Inversion	Gd III
Eversion	Gd III
Quadriceps	Gd I, isometric only
Hamstrings	Gd II, isometric only
Glutei	Gd III, isometric only

Neurological signs: full sensation (R) = to (L)

Vascular signs:
General fall in temperature
Pulses all present, (R) = (L)

Chest
Auscultation: (R) expansion decreased as (R) arm is held by the body. Good air entry to all lobes, slight crackles in (R) and (L) bases.

Bed mobility: not tested as patient very tired and uncomfortable.

Information about the shoulder is being withheld at the moment so as not to confuse the main facts about the leg.

Problem-solving exercise 5.6

Therefore, from Mr Kingston's assessment, can you answer the five major questions? (Answers at the end of the chapter.)

1. What do I know about this fracture?
2. What should I find at this stage of the management if the fracture is healing normally?

3. What might go wrong with this fracture?
4. What do I know about this patient, particularly his functional ability?
5. What are the expected overall outcomes for this patient, with this fracture?

The assessment of a patient with an acute fracture has to be limited to only the essential points. Any overactivity of the joints and muscles around the fracture site may cause movement of the bone ends and intense pain.

Reread Mr Kingston's assessment and compare it with that undertaken for Mrs Andrews and her more chronic state where she had been in POP for 5 weeks and the fracture was united. Bearing this in mind we need to categorise the major points from the assessment into relevant and non-relevant.

Problem-solving exercise 5.7

■ Which do you think are the most relevant points from Mr Kingston's assessment and why?

Answer:
- *Reduced bed mobility (chest and general): therefore risk of chest infection particularly if going to theatre. Also susceptible to pressure sores because of lack of general mobility.*
- *Reduced ankle movement and strength: therefore the soft tissue around the ankle may become contracted and he will not be able to walk correctly. Also loss of the venous pump means potential vascular problems (deep vein thrombosis (DVT) or pulmonary embolism (PE)).*
- *Loss of quadriceps function and immobilisation of the knee in extension: inhibition of quadriceps due to pain, swelling and bruising. Lack of control at the knee joint, and along with immobilisation of the knee in extension, this could lead to long-term loss of flexion. Knee kept in extension may also*

cause the patella to become adhered to the femur; this will have to be mobilised. Isometric quadriceps exercises and passive movements will help.
- *Potential shoulder problems: may limit the use of crutches.*

These points become the main foci for the initial physiotherapy treatment and if these are considered with the patient's problems mentioned earlier (i.e. pain in (R) thigh and shoulder, immobilisation in hospital, family problems as Mr Kingston looks after the children whilst wife works, and inability to move (R) leg and arm), then the physiotherapist and patient can work towards similar overall objectives. Of course initially the physiotherapy treatment objectives are quite specific and those of the patient more global.

In Mr Kingston's case he has indicated that he is concerned because he looks after the children whilst his wife works. This needs to be explored and if assistance is needed then the physiotherapist should check with both the nursing and medical staff to ensure that the social worker has been informed. It may not be the role of the therapist to initiate this contact, but if the patient has revealed this concern then the physiotherapist must pass it on to the appropriate people.

As mentioned earlier the treatment must be made appropriate to the individual, particularly the duration and type of exercises given. Therefore the exercise regime will incorporate the following and should be done after adequate painkillers have been administered.

- Isotonic exercise
  — ankle, dorsiflexion and plantarflexion
  — subtalar and midfoot joints, inversion and eversion
  — toe movements, flexion and extension, as often as possible.
- Passive accessory movements
  — patella, inferior and superior, medial and lateral
  — intermetatarsal joints, anteroposterior glide
  — midtarsal joints, all movements.

- Isometric exercises
  — quadriceps
  — hamstrings
  — glutei, extension and abduction of the hip.
- Encourage bed mobility: bridging, moving up and down the bed with other leg and getting up from supine to sitting.
- Respiratory: deep breathing, coughing.
- Upper limb strength: as the patient is able depending on the shoulder injury. Muscles needed for crutch walking are grip, wrist extensors, triceps, latissimus dorsi, deltoid, pectorals, trapezius.

Case study 5.2

Mr Kingston, continued (2)
After 48 hours on traction, a reassessment of the patient showed that Mr Kingston was in much less pain both at the shoulder, thigh and pin sites. The range of dorsiflexion had increased to the plantigrade position (0°) and muscle function at the ankle had increased to Gd IV, and quadriceps and hamstrings to an isometric Gd III. The shoulder joint could now be moved without severe pain.

It is quite common that once pain has been controlled and the bone ends have been stabilised that movements and muscle strength start to return. This may take up to a week depending on the patient but you would definitely expect positive change to happen in this time. There is no need to alter the exercise programme and the patient should be encouraged to do all the exercises as he/she is able.

A full examination of the shoulder can now take place.

Six days after the injury the patient went to theatre to have an interlocking intermedullary nail inserted.

Self-assessment question

- **SAQ 5.12.** What would you need to check after this type of surgery? (See below.)

  Answer:
  - *Chest function: the general anaesthetic*

slows down the normal ciliary action and more secretions can accumulate, thereby increasing the risk of infection, especially as Mr Kingston is a smoker.
- *Knee range: now measurable as the patient is out of the Thomas splint.*
- *Ankle and foot movements and power should be checked against the preoperative assessment.*

The greatest change in treatment objectives is that the knee and hip are now able to move and that Mr Kingston can get up without weight bearing. Thus to allow Mr Kingston to go home he must have muscular control of both these joints and have an adequate knee range of motion (70° of flexion and full extension).

Isometric exercises for quadriceps, hamstrings, glutei and iliopsoas can now be introduced through range, and when these are stronger, isotonic exercises can be added. Friction-free surfaces can be used to gain active hip and knee flexion and extension and CPM can be used to gain passive motion outside therapy sessions.

Prior to crutch walking, Mr Kingston's (R) shoulder needs to be reassessed and if strong enough, he may be able to transfer from bed to chair and then into standing. The intravenous drip will be in for 24 hours; therefore this will dictate the timescale for walking but does not stop transfer to a chair.

Problem-solving exercise 5.8

- What may happen and why, when a patient with a fracture of the lower limb gets up to either sit or stand for the first time?

Problem-solving exercise 5.9

- What would be the criteria for discharge for Mr. Kingston from (a) the medical, and

(b) the physiotherapy point of view? (See below.)

Answer:

(a) *All wounds have healed; fracture is stable; temperature not raised. No pain in calf or chest (indicators of deep vein thrombosis (DVT) or pulmonary embolism (PE)). Adequate support at home.*

(b) *Knee: active knee range from 0° to 70°; quadriceps strength Gd III to straighten the knee from 70° flexion to 0° extension.*

Understands exercises fully.

Function: safe non-weight bearing on crutches in standing; independent walking; sit to stand; manages stairs either with crutches or safely on his bottom.
Outpatient physiotherapy appointment made at local hospital.
Patient aware of complications especially: infection; DVT (intense calf pain with an increase in temperature); PE (chest pain, shortness of breath); persistent pain in thigh (possible loosening, refracture or infection); further or continuing loss of knee movement.
Patient knows not to weight bear until return to orthopaedic clinic, usually 6 weeks from fracture.

As Mr Kingston is returning home it may be appropriate for him to be seen by the occupational therapist to assess the home situation. This is not necessary or possible in all cases.

Mr Kingston was discharged, based on the above criteria, and is now onto the next stage of rehabilitation as an outpatient. From here on until the final stage of full functional ability, the treatment objectives will continue to progress until he can go back to his hobbies and potential work. Look back at the physiotherapy principles for a stable united fracture (p 92–93) and think how these would apply to Mr Kingston.

Problem-solving exercise 5.10

■ What would now be the treatment objectives for Mr Kingston, with realistic timescales? (See below.)

Answer:
Minimum expected timescales are shown in parentheses.

- *Maintain and increase the range of active and passive knee flexion to 0–140° (4 weeks from start of outpatient treatment).*
- *Strengthen knee flexion and extension to Gd V; can only be fully weight bearing after late union/consolidation (10–12 weeks post-fracture).*
- *Maintain and strengthen the muscles around the hips, particularly the glutei and iliopsoas on the injured side (10–12 weeks post-injury).*
- *Regain full soft tissue length particularly: quadriceps, hamstrings, iliopsoas, adductor mass, tensor fascia lata (4 weeks from start of outpatient treatment).*
- *Regain full proprioception at the knee.*
- *Return to normal gait pattern. Starts once partial weight bearing begins at 6 weeks; getting as near as possible to normal pattern with crutches and then sticks (6–8 weeks post-injury), and then with no support (10–12 weeks post-injury).*
- *Return to squats, kneeling, and step-ups on injured limb; all can commence with partial weight bearing (6–8 weeks post-injury).*
- *Able to run, jump, independent standing on one leg: needs to be fully weight bearing (10–12 weeks post-injury).*
- *Return to playing football (12–24 weeks post-injury).*

Rehabilitation following hip fracture

General information

There are two main areas containing four sites at which hip fractures occur:

1. Intracapsular (within the joint capsule) fractures may be:

- subcapital, that is, at the base of the head of femur, or
- transcervical, that is, in the middle of the neck of femur.

2. Extracapsular (outside the joint capsule) fractures may be:

- intertrochanteric, that is, at the base of the femoral neck between the trochanters, or
- pertrochanteric (through both trochanters).

Types of hip fracture are shown in Figures 5.18 and 5.19.

Displaced intracapsular fractures are the most difficult to treat and there are many surgical procedures for the surgeon to choose from. The commonest procedures include dynamic hip screw, multiple pins, hemiarthroplasty or joint replacement.

Dandy (1993) indicates that internal fixation should be considered for the younger, fitter patient with minimal bony displacement and that those who are older, unfit and with greater bone displacement require prosthetic replacement. Extracapsular fractures are usually managed with dynamic hip screws or nail-plate with a long femoral plate.

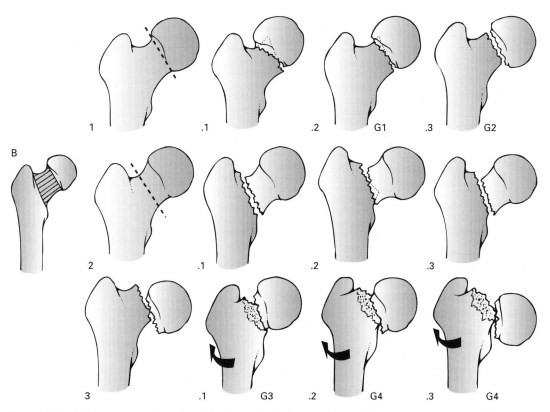

Figure 5.18 Hip fractures: neck region. B1, minimally displaced subcapital fractures: .1, impacted with 15° or more valgus; .2, impacted with less than 15° of valgus; .3, non-impacted fracture. B2, transverse fractures: .1, basal; .2, adduction pattern; .3, shear pattern. B3, displaced subcapital fractures: .1, moderate varus displacement with external rotation; .2, moderate displacement with shortening and external rotation; .3, marked displacement. (Adapted with permission from McRae 1994.)

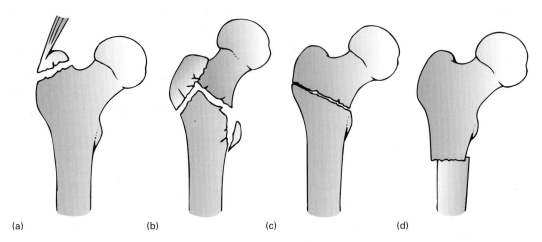

(a)   (b)   (c)   (d)

Figure 5.19 Hip fractures of the trochanteric region: (a) avulsion of the greater tuberosity; (b) pertrochanteric fracture; (c) intertrochanteric fracture between the trochanters; (d) subtrochanteric fracture. (Adapted with permission from Dandy 1993.)

Complications are common after hip fractures, many requiring revision surgery including removal of internal fixation and secondary hemiarthroplasty or joint replacement. All the early and late complications mentioned previously (SAQ 5.9) may occur with these patients, particularly related to the post-surgical condition.

Fractures of the proximal third of the femur predominantly occur in people over the age of 50 years. A report on the 300 000 hip fractures experienced in the USA during 1991 shows that 94% occurred in people over 50 years of age (US Congress Office of Technology 1994). The incidence of hip fracture, mortality and institutionalisation varies with ethnicity and geography. Recently Marottoli et al (1994) reported a hip fracture rate of 4.27% (120/2812 subjects) in Connecticut, USA. In the UK, in one English county, a discrepancy was found between the incidence of hip fracture for different ethnicities, with a 1.3:1 ratio of Asian to Caucasian hip fracture populations (Calder et al 1994).

There is a general concern that the number of hip fractures is increasing, as the population lives longer and therefore the subsequent increase in financial costs of managing these patients will be immense. Cummings et al (1990) stated that by the year 2040, 512 000 hip fractures will occur in the USA, with a management cost of $16 billion.

The prospective study of Marottoli et al (1994) from the USA established that at 6 months after fracture, 18% of their patients had died and 29% had been institutionalised. Seeman (1995) reports that a third of all hip fractures occur in men, and that they have a greater mortality rate than their female counterparts. Dandy (1993) states that, in the UK, 10% of older patients with hip fractures die within 6 weeks, 30% within 1 year and of the remaining 70%, one-third do not return to their premorbid level of activity. The mortality rate also increases with revision surgery, to 28% in the first 6 months and 36% at 1 year (Keating et al 1993). Foubister & Hughes (1989) showed that 75% of patients with hip fractures, treated in their unit in the UK, returned home following surgery but of those with complications requiring revision surgery (3.7%), only 50% returned home (Keating et al 1993). These rates vary depending on the site of the fracture, with patients with displaced subcapital fractures having a poorer return to functional independence. There is also a direct relationship between the rate of complications and functional outcome.

Thus it is not surprising to find that most acute orthopaedic, care of the elderly or rehabilitation wards have their fair share of patients with hip fractures. The demand for continuing care both at the patient's home and in care establishments has increased. Marottoli et al (1994) also indicated that the primary predictor for institutionalisation was mental status; thus care must be provided because of decreased mental as well as physical ability.

Several schemes have been implemented to try to address these issues, all aiming to return the patient to their own home or community as quickly as is feasible. In particular many accelerated rehabilitation schemes are in operation, which allow suitable patients to return home as soon as possible after the fracture, with the necessary level of care provided at home. Cameron et al (1994) studied the cost-effectiveness of this type of scheme during 1989/90 and found it to be 38% more effective than conventional hospital care, releasing resources of up to 17%. Thus the accelerated schemes are financially better, but the overall return of function may differ.

Williams et al (1994a,b) reported a prospective study on the outcomes of 120 women with hip fracture, mean age 79.9 years, who had all lived at home before the fracture and were discharged to home or nursing home care. Recovery of mobility continued during the 14 weeks post-fracture review, with the most rapid change occurring between 2 and 8 weeks. The return of mobility in patients in short-stay nursing home care (less than 1 month) was equal to that of the home discharge patients, but the longer term nursing home patients had a slower return or no change in mobility.

Those returning home showed a lower level of emotional distress such as anxiety, depression or manic behaviour than did those going to either short- or long-term nursing home care. However, in all groups the somatic mood distress was high, showing that the trauma of the fracture was highlighted more in physical terms, such as altered cardiovascular signs or functional issues.

Thus early discharge home schemes seem to assist return to function and are more cost-effective, but are dependent on good mental status and attitude and of course on adequate care at home. In this group of patients, return to independent mobility will be the main objective.

Thus the third case study is centred around this area.

Case study 5.3

Mrs Jones, fractured neck of femur (#NOF)

Present complaint
Mrs Jones, a 77-year-old lady, was admitted to hospital via casualty, after a fall at home, 2 days ago. She was discovered by her neighbour, lying on the floor, quite cold and unable to get up or walk.

Casualty report
Right leg, externally rotated and shortened; on X-ray (R) subcapital #NOF. Early signs of hypothermia and dehydration.

Initial medical care
Skin traction with 3 kg weight. For internal fixation with dynamic hip screw tomorrow, continue traction until then. Full team assessment and treatment as required.

Physiotherapy assessment

Subjective assessment

Social history: Mrs Jones lives alone in a converted first-floor flat, with 24 steps to the front door. No steps inside the self-contained flat, which Mrs Jones owns. Independent prior to fall; no social service support at all.

Mrs Jones has one son and daughter-in-law who live 35 miles away, with their two children. They visit occasionally and Mrs Jones spends a week with them twice a year.

Hobbies and interests: until 5 years ago Mrs Jones was a volunteer for the Red Cross and is still an active member of her local church. Enjoys reading, tapestry and listening to music.

Previous medical history: slight osteoarthrosis (OA) of the (L) and (R) hips and lumbar spine, for previous 10 years. (L) Colles' fracture 5 years ago, following a fall, with subsequent weakness and wrist stiffness since. Is able to use the hand functionally.

No other major illnesses or operations. Good eyesight with spectacles and good hearing.

Functional level prior to admission: functionally able about the flat but is slower in the morning than in the afternoon. Cannot easily descend stairs, particularly in the morning, because of hips, but after a walk can climb the stairs more easily. Mrs Jones can walk slowly to the local shops and church, approximately 1 mile away, and occasionally uses one stick.

Objective assessment

General posture: patient lying slouched in bed, with skin traction on the (R) leg. No pillows under either leg; patient looks uncomfortable and in some pain.

Right leg is externally rotated and adducted in the traction, and is a mottled colour and feels cold to touch.

On examination:

ROM (active)

Hips	Not tested due to patient's discomfort	
Knees	(R)	(L)
	0–40°	0–95°
	Limited due to pain and traction	No pain
Ankle	10–80°	10–80°
	No pain	No pain

Passive movement of all joints and the spine not tested.

Muscle power

	(R)	(L)
isometric only		isometric and isotonic
Gluteus maximus	1	4
Gluteus minimus/medius	1	4
Quadriceps	1	4
Hamstrings	1	4
Ankle	5	5

Neurology: no numbness or altered sensation in either leg, although Mrs Jones reports that the right leg feels as though it has cramp.
Vascular: skin dry and cold on both legs. Right leg slightly mottled and bluish in colour. Dorsalis pedis not palpable on either leg.
Respiration
Observation: decreased expansion of both bases with the main movement occurring at the apices.
Auscultation: decreased air entry to both bases with audible inspiratory wheeze.

Once again can you answer the five major questions about this patient? This time the answers will not be given separately but you can find them all in this chapter.

1. What do I know about this fracture?
2. What should I find at this stage of the management if the fracture is healing normally?
3. What might go wrong with this fracture?
4. What do I know about this patient, particularly her functional ability?
5. What are the expected overall outcomes for this patient, with this fracture?

Problem-solving exercise 5.11

■ Remembering that Mrs Jones is going to surgery the next day, what would be the physiotherapy treatment objectives at this time? (See below.)

Answer:
- *Maintain respiratory function until after surgery.*
- *Maintain venous return in the lower limbs.*
- *Teach Mrs Jones how to assist with bed mobility if possible.*
- *Try to maintain some muscle tone; it may not be practical to do this until after surgery.*
- *Try to get to know and to reassure Mrs Jones prior to surgery.*

Self-assessment question

■ **SAQ 5.13.** What are the major complications particularly associated with subcapital #NOF?

When Mr Kingston's post-surgical recovery was discussed, the main emphasis was on the return of specific muscle strength and joint motion. With Mrs Jones the primary consideration is her return to functional independence and then secondarily the return of range of motion and strength around the hip.

This change in emphasis is justified by the description of function. In Mrs Jones' case, function is mainly geared towards getting in and out of bed, rising from sitting, standing independently, independent toileting, walking and stair climbing. Mr Kingston, however, would not be classed as fully functional unless he was fit to work, to play sport, and to play with his children and so on; therefore full range of motion and strength is needed. It could be argued that physiotherapy should help Mrs Jones to gain a full range of motion and strength as well as the basic functional requirements. This of course is true, but the range of motion and strength required by Mrs Jones will be far less than that needed by Mr Kingston, and will be gained by concentrating on basic functional rehabilitation.

Now look back at the answer to SAQ 5.7 on the disadvantages of bed rest (p. 84–85). All of these points are especially significant in any elderly patient with this type of fracture but the most important is getting Mrs Jones up and out of bed to increase her general mobility. When the fracture has been stabilised then sitting out of bed can commence on postoperative day 1, and once the drips and drains are out (day 2) then walking is made easier. Assistance is obviously needed and it is advisable for two people with a walking frame to be used the first time walking is attempted. Alternatively the patient may be taken to use a set of parallel bars and, again with the assistance of two people, walking can commence. The answers to Problem-solving exercise 5.8 should be taken into consideration: any patient with a fractured neck of femur will find getting out of bed difficult. Mrs Jones' condition has been made worse by the fact that she was lying on the floor for 2 days before being found.

Whatever type of rehabilitation programme Mrs Jones might be following, several other members of the multidisciplinary team need to be involved including nursing staff, social workers, occupational therapists and the community liaison team. In a well organised rehabilitation scheme all these members of staff would already be involved in Mrs Jones' care; however, if they are not, then this will need to be instigated. An accelerated rehabilitation programme would have its own team of care staff who liaise and continue care from hospital to home environments. This team is made up of nursing staff, occupational therapists, physiotherapists and assistants as required.

On an accelerated rehabilitation programme, Mrs Jones should be ready for discharge at approximately 1 week after the operation.

Problem-solving exercise 5.12

■ What would be the criteria for Mrs Jones' discharge on the accelerated rehabilitation programme? (See below.)

Answer:
- *Support arranged at home for general day-to-day living: family, meals on wheels, community liaison team, social services, etc.*
- *Assessment and support from the accelerated rehabilitation team, i.e. physiotherapist, occupational therapists, and nursing staff.*
- *Home visit by occupational therapist and/or physiotherapist with the community liaison team.*
- *Ability to walk short distances with the use of a walking aid (probably a walking frame at this time).*
- *Some limited functional goals such as washing, toileting and dressing herself.*
- *No medical complications (see Problem-solving exercise 5.9(a)).*
- *Full cooperation of Mrs Jones and that she is happy with the arrangements.*

As mentioned previously, Williams et al (1994a,b) noted that the greatest improvement in mobility was between 2 and 8 weeks after the operation; thus it is during this time that maximum rehabilitation support is needed whatever the environment of the patient. Patients kept in hospital at this stage may be moved to care of the elderly or rehabilitation wards to free up acute orthopaedic beds. The alternative is discharge to a nursing home for either short- or long-term care. This may be confusing for patients and recovery can be delayed until patients have time to settle again.

Progression from walking with two people and a frame varies dramatically. If there are no complications then Mrs Jones might be walking with sticks in 2–3 weeks. If any of the major complications developed then this objective would obviously be delayed. Thus the physiotherapist should base mobility gains on realistic objectives which may be quite limited to start with, such as walking to the end of the bed with the assistance of two people and the walking frame.

The goals for walking will then be to reduce the number of people assisting and then to try to gain total independence with the frame. Short frequent walks are more acceptable than long walks once a day; thus cooperation of the nursing staff is essential to ensure continuity. The family can also be involved at the stage of independence with the frame, to allow them to see the progression but also to give additional encouragement when the patient is returning home. It may also be encouraging to introduce a timed walking assessment to give a truly objective outcome measurement (Macnichol et al 1980, Wade 1992).

It has been stated that function was geared towards getting in and out of bed, rising from sitting, standing independently, independent toileting, walking and stair climbing. Now that walking has been started, the other functions must be initiated. Independent toileting, for instance, involves the activities of standing independently and the movement of sitting to standing and vice versa but usually in a confined space and to a lower seat. The need to safely turn 180° is also required. Therefore this function does need to be considered separately from standing to sitting from a chair.

Each function needs to be broken down to specific components and each of these can be re-educated until the total function can be performed. For example, rising from sitting requires four basic sequences:

1. moving forward in the chair
2. moving the body weight forward over the feet (flexion)
3. lifting the bottom off the seat
4. extension of the hips, knees and spine into standing (Ada & Westwood 1992, Butler et al 1991, Kerr et al 1991, Nuzik et al 1986).

If each of these sequences is practised until the patient is proficient at them, then the overall movement will be easier. Subsequently the repeated action will help improve muscle strength and endurance, range of motion and balance.

Time must be taken to ensure that Mrs Jones is aware of each of these stages and can recognise the correct movement.

Self-assessment question

- **SAQ 5.14.** Break down the functions of independent standing, getting in and out of bed and stair climbing, into the basic sequences. (See below.)

Answers:
- *Independent standing*
  1. *Rising from sitting (as already mentioned).*
  2. *Standing holding onto a walking frame, whilst gaining balance.*
  3. *Hands off the frame, one at a time, maintain body weight equally on right and left legs.*
  4. *Reverse activities into sitting.*
- *Getting in and out of bed*
  One of two ways: either with or without rolling onto one side.
  Without rolling:
  Getting out of bed:
  1. *Move towards the edge of the bed; may be easier to go to the non-affected side, but ideally it should be the side the patient is used to getting out of bed from.*
  2. *Sit up into half-lying.*
  3. *Move feet over the side of the bed.*
  4. *Move bottom to the edge of the bed.*
  Getting into bed:
  1. *Sit on the edge of the bed.*
  2. *Shuffle the bottom back as far as possible.*
  3. *Move legs onto the bed, whilst in the sitting position.*
  4. *Lie down.*
  With rolling:
  Getting out of bed:
  1. *Move towards the edge of the bed on the non-affected side.*
  2. *With the legs together (a pillow can be placed between the legs to make this more comfortable) roll onto the side.*
  3. *Place the uppermost hand on the bed in front of the body and as the legs are being placed over the edge of the bed,*

> *push on the hand to raise the body into the sitting position.*
> *Getting into bed: Reverse the above procedure.*
>
> - **Stair climbing (no walking aids)**
>   *Ascending the stairs:*
>   1. *Holding on with one hand, body weight on the affected leg, lift the non-affected leg, flexing at the hip and knee (static standing balance needed).*
>   2. *Place the non-affected leg on the step and lean forward over the foot.*
>   3. *Extend the non-affected knee and hip, lifting the body weight up and place the affected leg on the step, beside the non-affected leg (dynamic standing balance needed whilst raising the body weight).*
>
>   *Descending the stairs:*
>   1. *In standing, flex and hitch the affected hip (with knee straight) until it clears the step.*
>   2. *Lower the affected leg and place on the step below, allowing the non-affected knee to bend in a controlled manner.*
>   3. *Shift the body weight forward and laterally onto the affected leg, whilst holding onto the banister.*
>   4. *Lower the non-affected leg onto the step below.*

Koval et al (1995) observed mobility recovery in fractured hip patients at 12–18 months postoperatively in a group of 336 community-dwelling patients who had all been ambulant prior to their fracture. Of these, 41% maintained their pre-fracture mobility, 40% remained ambulant but needed some kind of assisted device (stick or frame), 12% became independent walkers indoors but not outdoors and 8% were non-ambulant (num-

bers have been rounded so do not add up to 100%). These authors highlight a detailed scale of measurement of ambulation, which could be useful as a functional outcome measure for the physiotherapist.

The scale has seven categories:

1. independent community walker
2. community walker with a stick
3. community walker with frame/crutches
4. independent household walker
5. household walker with a stick
6. household walker with frame/crutches
7. non-functional walker.

This study highlighted the fact that 59% of their subjects did not return to their pre-fracture mobility level, incorporating 34% who dropped one level, as defined above, 7% who dropped two levels, 4% who dropped three levels and 14% who dropped four or more levels (Koval et al 1995). The premorbid mobility level was predictive for the mobility level at 12–18 months for all the patients and specifically for those in category 1. Thus the poorer the mobility level prior to hip fracture the more likely the patient was to return to that level. The other major finding of this paper is that a general health status questionnaire used (American Society of Anesthesiologists) was also a strong predictor of mobility outcome.

Therefore Mrs Jones only has a 50–50 chance of returning to full function providing that there are no complications following surgery.

The totally different emphasis and functional outcome for Mrs Jones compared with, say, Mr Kingston, means that the physiotherapist cannot work alone when the rehabilitation outcomes of a patient are more functionally based. Communication and negotiation with the patient, carers and other staff is particularly important. Thus the physiotherapist has to change his/her role depending on the short- and longer term rehabilitation outcomes of the individual patient.

Summary

This chapter has not tried to address the physiotherapy management of every fracture as this would be impossible. However, the basic principles of physiotherapy management of patients with fractures have been addressed. As you apply these to other fractures then you will be able to undertake basic problem solving to help assess and plan treatment of any patient with any fracture.

This chapter does not stand alone and there are links with those on soft tissue injury, rheumatic conditions and joint replacement. Many complications of soft tissue injury around fracture sites (e.g. of tendon, ligament, muscle or nerve) have deliberately been omitted, as these are addressed in Chapter 6 on soft tissue injury. Likewise the complications of fractures in patients with rheumatic conditions have not been covered here.

ANSWERS TO QUESTIONS AND EXERCISES

Self-assessment questions (pages 75, 78–79)

- ■ **SAQs 5.1, 5.2.** Answers follow questions in text.

Self-assessment question 5.3 (page 81)

- ■ **SAQ 5.3.** A patient has been issued with a collar and cuff immediately after a fracture of the upper third of the humeral shaft. Which joints would you advise him/her to move?

  Answer: *Move all non-painful joints, i.e. interphalangeals, metacarpophalangeals, radioulnar joints, wrist, elbow (if possible but unlikely), gentle scapulothoracic movements and neck movements.*

Self-assessment question 5.4 (page 81)

- ■ **SAQ 5.4.** How would the patient know if the POP was causing too much pressure, and what advice would be given to them?

  Answer:
  — *Vascular signs: distally the skin changes colour to a purple/blue; swelling may appear distal to the fracture or cast and will not reduce on elevation; distal segments of the limb may feel cold and clammy.*
  — *Neurological signs: altered sensation (paraesthesia) or numbness may occur in the distribution of the nerve root which is being compressed.*
  — *Pain may increase either from vascular occlusion or nerve compression.*
  — *Advice: if any of these signs occur elevate the part and return to the A&E department or general practitioner as quickly as possible.*

Self-assessment question 5.5 (page 82)

- ■ **SAQ 5.5.** Answer follows question in text.

Self-assessment question 5.6 (page 82)

■ **SAQ 5.6.** How long will this fracture take to reach union and consolidation? What do these terms mean?

Answer:
Union: 4–6 weeks. This is partial repair of the bone, when the initial callus forms around the bone ends so that there is minimal movement. The bone under pressure will still give a little and will be painful. On X-ray the fracture line will still be visible. Full bone maturity has not been reached therefore full weight bearing through the hand cannot be undertaken and some external support is usually still needed.
Consolidation: 8–12 weeks. This is full repair of the bone, where no movement takes place at the fracture site. On X-ray no fracture lines are seen and the bone trabeculae now cross where the fracture used to be. Full function can now commence without damaging the fracture.

Problem-solving exercise 5.1 (page 82)

■ What type of support will the patient be given for the arm, and what instructions should she carry out prior to review in 5 days' time?

Answer: *A high sling should be applied to support the hand and POP, in elevation.*
The patient should be instructed to:
- *Observe for any signs of POP pressure (see answer to SAQ 5.4).*
- *Keep the hand elevated to control oedema.*
- *Observe for signs of infection, e.g. staining on the POP in the presence of an offensive smell; severe cases would have a discharge from the POP.*
- *Keep the fingers mobile by putting the metacarpophalangeal and interphalangeal joints of all fingers and the thumb through as full a range of movement as possible, increasing this as the pain and oedema decrease.*
- *Remove the sling every hour, to exercise the shoulder into full elevation with full*

elbow extension and external and internal rotation.
- *Not get the POP wet.*
- *Not scratch under the POP with long-stemmed items such as rulers or knitting needles. (All of these can scratch the skin and therefore induce infection.)*
- *Take regular painkillers, if and when necessary.*

Self-assessment question 5.7 (page 84)

■ **SAQ 5.7.** Answer follows question in text.

Self-assessment question 5.8 (page 90)

■ **SAQ 5.8.** What instructions should be given to a patient with a fracture of the lower third of tibia and fibula, who is being sent home, non-weight-bearing, in a long leg POP cast from thigh to toes?

Answer:
- *Keep the limb elevated either by lying down and placing the cast on a pillow or, on sitting, support the cast on a high footstool or chair.*
- *Check that the toes do not turn a bluish colour or start to swell excessively.*
- *Observe for infection, pressure areas at top and bottom of POP and excessive ongoing pain.*
- *Keep toes moving through full range at all times.*
- *Keep tightening the quadriceps, hamstrings, and both anterior and posterior tibial muscles isometrically, in the POP.*
- *When standing up do not place weight down through the POP until medical or therapy staff indicate that this may be done.*
- *Use the crutches for sit/stand, walking, and so on, as instructed prior to leaving hospital.*

Self-assessment question 5.9 (page 91)

■ **SAQ 5.9.** Describe the immediate and more long-term complications of fracture healing and rehabilitation.

Answer:
Immediate complications

- *Infection*
- *Pressure sores*
- *Swelling\bruising distal to fracture*
- *Nerve, vascular, soft tissue damage*
- *Inability to reduce the fracture*
- *Postoperative complications:*
  — *general immobility, thus pressure sores*
  — *reduced respiratory function*
  — *reduced vascular function*
  — *electrolyte imbalance*
- *Fat embolism: not common but if undetected can result in death. Microparticles of marrow fat appear in the circulation usually a few days after fractures of the shaft of femur or the pelvis. Severe hypoxia results from pulmonary insufficiency as the fat globules block the alveoli. Changes are also seen in the brain, kidney and skin. Noticeable by change in mood of the patient, drowsiness and then unconsciousness, tachypnoea (increased rate of respiration) and petechiae (small haemorrhages under the skin) (Dandy 1993).*

Long-term complications: see text.

Problem-solving exercise 5.2 (page 94)

■ Attempt to answer all the five major questions about Mrs Andrews and her Colles' fracture.

1. What do I know about this fracture?
   Answer: We have already outlined the type of fracture, its position and expected union and consolidation times and its initial management.

2. What should I find at this stage of management if the fracture is healing normally?
   Answer: Given the case scenario at the start of treatment, then we expect to find a lady in a dorsal slab POP or a completed cast, being supported in a sling. Instruction should have been given regarding exercise, skin care and 'do's and 'don't's. Mrs Andrews will be discharged from A&E and seen in the fracture clinic in 5 days' time for review and again in approximately 5 weeks' time. The POP should be removed at 5–6 weeks when initial physiotherapy assessment and treatment would be undertaken.

3. What might go wrong with this fracture?
   Answer:
   - *Median nerve compression, carpal tunnel syndrome.*
   - *Rupture of the extensor pollicis longus (at approximately 4–8 weeks).*
   - *Potential for Sudeck's atrophy.*
   - *Mal-union: it is often very difficult to reduce the distal fragment of the radius.*
   - *Joint stiffness, predominantly at the fingers, wrist and inferior radioulnar joints, but it may occur at the shoulder and elbow (shoulder–hand syndrome).*
   - *Alteration to the healing rate.*

4. What do I know about this patient, particularly concerning functional ability?
   Answer: Mrs Andrews is a 67-year-old lady who fell onto her outstretched (R) hand. Her functional ability is limited due to her POP and a full assessment is needed once the POP can be removed.

5. What are the expected overall outcomes for this patient, with this fracture?
   Answer: If no complications arise, then in the next 4 months Mrs Andrews should have a functional wrist but may lack full movement particularly extension and supination. Depending on her hobbies, she should gain full functional use.

Problem-solving exercise 5.3 (page 94)

■ Are these the normal signs of a fracture after removal of POP? Explain why.

Answer: Yes, these are the normal signs of fracture after removal of POP.
Following reduction, the wrist is immobilised in flexion and ulnar deviation to

hold the bone ends in place, thus it would appear in this position on removal from the POP. The thickening of the radius is due to callus formation and that at the wrist is due to the periarticular and intra-articular adhesion. The skin appearance is due to altered vascularisation whilst in the POP, the skin losing its usual look and feel. The forearm is thinner because of muscle wasting on the palmar and dorsal aspects and this will emphasise the thickening at the radius and wrist. The patient will be scared to move the wrist and it will feel lighter and 'strange' immediately after POP removal; therefore it is not surprising that the patient holds the arm close to the body.

N.B. The patient may have held the arm close to the body for the last 5 weeks and therefore you need to check shoulder and elbow function.

Problem-solving exercise 5.4 (page 94)

■ What would you need to ask this patient to complete question 4?

Answer:
- *Personal details: age, occupation, hobbies, home circumstances (for instance, is there anyone to assist her, etc.), hand dominance.*
- *Main problems now, and what she has been doing with the arm since injury.*
- *History of present complaint (HPC): how the fracture occurred and how it was managed, any other injuries at the time.*
- *Previous medical history: especially history of osteoporosis, bone disease, diabetes, high blood pressure, respiratory disease, steroid use, major operations, previous fractures.*

Self-assessment question 5.10 (page 94)

■ **SAQ 5.10.** What would you assess in your objective examination?

Answer:
- *Observation: we already know the appearance of the wrist.*

- *ROM: active, passive and accessory range of motion of shoulder, elbow, radioulnar, wrist joints and joints of the hand. (Active and passive movements to be measured with a goniometer/inclinometer.)*
- *Muscle power: isometric muscle power across the fingers, wrist and radioulnar joints (this will not overstress the fracture at this stage and will not cause discomfort at the joints where isotonic strength testing will). Need to test extensor pollicis longus especially. All measured either by use of the Oxford Scale of Manual Muscle Testing or a hand-held dynamometer. Isotonic strength of the muscles around the elbow and shoulder.*
- *Sensation: light touch, hot/cold, proprioception, in the wrist and hand, especially median distribution.*
- *Dexterity of the hand, i.e. differing types of grips, general hand function. (If this is problematic then it may be necessary to refer Mrs Andrews for occupational therapist's assessment for help around the home.)*
- *Swelling: measure general swelling at the lower border of the MCP joints.*

Problem-solving exercise 5.5 (page 95)

■ Describe how you would carry out each of the objectives in Table 5.2.

Answer:
Show the patient how to move without causing damage to the wrist and try to reduce pain.

Assisted active movements using the other hand, holding the fracture whilst doing shoulder and elbow movements, thus assisting with the 'good' arm.

Gentle movement should help to reduce the pain, but Mrs Andrews can help at home by soaking the hand in contrast baths (hot then cold), or by placing ice over the dorsal aspect of the hand.

Encourage controlled movement of the wrist, radioulnar, elbow and shoulder joints.

As above but also the use of accessory

movements, e.g. rotation of the wrist joint by compressing together the palmar aspect of the pisiform and the dorsal aspect of the head of the ulna, with the index and thumb of the opposite hand. Encourage combined movements, e.g. flexion/extension of the fingers and wrist so stretching periarticular soft tissue as well as intra-articular adhesions.

Explain about general care of the skin. *Massage in warm soapy water with some baby oil in it, and then continued use of moisturiser, oil, or lanolin to help skin viability*

Explain the healing times and the need to mobilise and then strengthen the arm before return to bowling.

At this stage the fracture has united and will be consolidated in another 6 weeks' time. Then lifting of a heavy bowls ball may be attempted, provided that the strength of her right hand has reached, and slightly exceeded, that of her non-dominant left hand, and also provided that adequate range of motion has been regained. If in doubt, ask Mrs Andrews to demonstrate the bowling action using her left hand, and to weigh the ball so that you know how much she has to lift.

Self assessment question 5.11 (page 96)

■ **SAQ 5.11.** Answer follows question in text.

Problem-solving exercise 5.6 (page 97)

■ From Mr Kingston's assessment, can you answer the five major questions?

1. What do I know about this fracture?

    Answer: *It is a spiral open fracture where the bone must have pierced the skin; this is unstable and needs to be reduced. A period of traction will be needed to allow the bone ends to be realigned and to ensure that the wound is not infected; it would normally be immobilised with internal fixation, using an intramedullary interlocking nail. Union time 6 weeks, consolidation 12 weeks.*

2. What should I find at this stage of the management if the fracture is healing normally?

    Answer: *The objective assessment outlines a typical case. The patient is not able to move the limb a great deal; there is swelling and bruising of the thigh and knee. Sliding balance traction is in place, with no knee piece and 4 kg weight. The fracture is acute and still potentially unstable; there is a need to be cautious concerning over-vigorous exercise, particularly with regard to the hip flexors (iliacus and psoas major).*

3. What might go wrong with this fracture?

    Answer:
    Initially:
    — *infection (osteitis) from open wound*
    — *fat embolism*
    — *overdistraction*
    — *pressure sores from the Thomas splint*
    — *nerve damage; may occur due to pressure on the common peroneal nerve at the fibula head (unlikely)*
    — *vascular changes due to inactivity*
    — *bone position might slip if strong hip flexion action is undertaken.*
    Long term:
    — *joint stiffness at the knee (mainly flexion) and hip*
    — *reduced muscle power, quadriceps, hamstrings and anterior and posterior calf muscles*
    — *mal-union (shortening of bone)*
    — *delayed union.*

4. What do I know about this patient, particularly his functional ability?

    Answer: *Unable to function well at the moment. Reassess when initial trauma recedes, and some assistance will be needed at this moment. This limitation of movement and independence is a problem to this patient and he will need reassurance that function will return once the fracture has been internally fixed.*

Need to reassess for crutches later (after surgery).

5. What are the expected overall outcomes for this patient, with this fracture?

   Answer: *If no complications arise then Mr Kingston should regain full use of his leg, with full lower limb movement. This assumes that there are no wound or surgical problems. It will take at least 6 months and will depend on how severe the shoulder injury is. May play football once consolidation of the fracture site has occurred and full strength has been regained.*

Problem-solving exercise 5.7 (page 98)

Answer follows exercise in text.

Self-assessment question 5.12 (page 99)

■ **SAQ 5.12.** Answer follows question in text.

Problem-solving exercise 5.8 (page 99)

■ What may happen and why, when a patient with a fracture of the lower limb gets up to either sit or stand for the first time?

   Answer:
   - *The blood pressure drops dramatically due to shock, not being in the upright position, and surgery. Therefore the patient may feel faint, dizzy or nauseous. This can be prevented by having a staged approach to the vertical position, sitting the patient for longer, first with the legs up and then down.*
   - *The patient's leg may change colour to a purple/red engorged state and feel numb or tingling. This is due to the sudden gravitational increase in blood in the lower leg; the venous pump is not used to coping with this as the limb has not been dependent. The limb needs to be placed vertically, over short periods of time of increasing duration, until the signs do not occur. Isotonic exercise to the foot and*

ankle will help with venous return, and should be encouraged with the limb dependent.
   - *The leg may feel heavy. Again this is due to the increase in blood with the limb being dependent, but it is also because of lack of muscle control. Exercise will help this.*
   - *Balance, particularly in standing, may be unsafe. Again, as the patient has not been upright an adjustment of the normal balance mechanisms, that is, spatial awareness and the vestibular system, is needed. Also, of course the base of support is grossly reduced to one foot.*

     All of these factors may be greater in a patient with severe and/or multiple injuries, the elderly, or those who have been on bed rest for longer periods of time.

Self-assessment question 5.13 (page 104)

■ **SAQ 5.13.** What are the major complications particularly associated with subcapital #NOF?

   Answer:
   - *At surgery: avascular necrosis of the head of the femur, mainly due to the poor blood supply to that area. Also intracapsular fractures can disrupt the blood supply at the cartilage margins or from the circumflex femoral arteries.*
   - *Non-union, because in some cases the femoral head cannot offer adequate fixation for the pins or the dynamic hip screw.*
   - *Postoperative confusion.*
   - *Infection (either of the wound, bone around fracture or urinary tract). Johnstone et al (1995) report that 12.5% of preoperative and 42% of postoperative hip fracture patients had a urinary tract infection (UTI), and this occurred particularly in patients with subcapital fractures. Age and time delay to surgery also relate significantly to the presence of UTI.*

Self-assessment question 5.14 (page 106)

■ **SAQ 5.14.** Answer follows question in text.

Problem-solving exercises 5.9–5.12

Answers follow exercises in text.

REFERENCES

Ada L, Westwood P 1992 A kinematic analysis of recovery of the ability to stand up following stroke. Australian Journal of Physiotherapy 38(2):135–142

Bromley I 1991 Tetraplegia and paraplegia. A guide for physiotherapists. Churchill Livingstone, Edinburgh

Bullock-Saxton J 1994 Local sensation changes and altered hip muscle function following severe ankle sprain. Physical Therapy 74(1):17–31

Butler P, Nene A, Major R 1991 Biomechanics of transfer from sitting to the standing position in some neuromuscular diseases. Physiotherapy 77(8):521–525

Calder S J, Anderson G H, Harper W M, Gregg P J 1994 Ethnic variation in epidemiology and rehabilitation of hip fracture. British Medical Journal 309(6962):1124–1125

Calliet R 1975 Scoliosis, diagnosis and management. F A Davis, Philadelphia

Cameron I D, Lyle D M, Quine S 1994 Cost effectiveness of accelerated rehabilitation after proximal femoral fractures. Journal of Clinical Epidemiology 47(11):1307–1313

Clark M, Watts S 1994 The incidence of pressure sores within a National Health Service Trust Hospital during 1991. Journal of Advanced Nursing 20(1):33–36

Coutts F, Hewetson D, Matthews J 1989 Continuous passive motion of the knee joint: use at the Royal National Orthopaedic Hospital, Stanmore. Physiotherapy 75(7):427–431

Crawford Adams J, Hamblen D 1992 Outline of fractures. Churchill Livingstone, Edinburgh

Cummings S R, Rubin S M, Black D 1990 The future of hip fractures in the USA. Numbers, costs and potential effects of postmenopausal estrogen. Clinical Orthopaedics and Related Research 252:163–166

Dandy D 1993 Essential orthopaedics and trauma, 2nd edn. Churchill Livingstone, Edinburgh

Davies S 1991 Effects of continuous passive movement and plaster of paris after internal fixation of ankle fractures. Physiotherapy 77(38):516–520

Foubister G, Hughes S P F 1989 Fractures of the femoral neck: a retrospective and prospective study. Journal of the Royal College of Surgeons of Edinburgh 34:249–252

Grundy D, Russell J, Swain A 1993 ABC of spinal cord injury, 2nd edn. British Medical Journal Publications, London

Hessman M, Mattens M, Rumbaut J 1994 The unilateral external fixator (Monofixator) in acute fracture treatment – experience in 50 fractures. Acta Chirurgica Belgica 4:229–235

Johnstone D J, Morgan N H, Wilkinson M C, Chissel H R 1995 Urinary tract infection and hip fracture. Injury 26(2):89–91

Keating J F, Robinson C M, Court-Brown C M, McQueen M M, Christie J 1993 The effect of complications after hip fractures on rehabilitation. Journal of Bone and Joint Surgery 75B:976

Kerr K, White J, Mollan R, Baird H 1991 Rising from a chair: a literature review. Physiotherapy 77(1):15–19

Koval K J, Skovron M L, Aharonoff G B, Meadows S E, Zuckerman J D 1995 Ambulatory ability after hip fracture: a prospective study in geriatric patients. Clinical Orthopaedics and Related Research 310:150–159

Macnicol M F, McHardy R, Chalmers J 1980 Exercise testing before and after hip arthroplasty. Journal of Bone and Joint Surgery 62B(3):326–331

McRae R 1994 Practical fracture treatment, 3rd edn. Churchill Livingstone, Edinburgh.

Marottoli R A, Berkman L F, Leo-Summers L, Cooney L M Jr 1994 Predictors of mortality and institutionalisation after hip fractures: the New Haven EPESE cohort (established populations for epidemiologic studies of the elderly). American Journal of Public Health 84(11):1807–1812

Nuzik S, Lamb R, VanSant A, Hirt S 1986 Sit to stand movement pattern. A kinematic study. Physical Therapy 66(11):1708–1713

Pesco M, Altner P 1993 A protective orthoplast splint in the treatment of a patient with Colles' fracture by external fixation. Journal of Hand Therapy 6(1):39–41

Seeman E 1995 The dilemma of osteoporosis in men. American Journal of Medicine 98(2A):76S–88S

Tetsworth K, Paley D 1994 Mal-alignment and degenerative arthropathy. Orthopedic Clinics of North America 25(3):367–377

US Congress Office of Technology 1994 Hip fracture outcomes in people aged fifty and over. OTA-BP-H-120 US Government Printing Office, Washington, DC, USA

Wade D T 1992 Measurement in neurological rehabilitation. Oxford University Press, Oxford

Williams M A, Oberst M T, Bjorklund B C 1994a Post hospital convalescence in older women with hip fracture. Orthopaedic Nursing 13(4):55–64

Williams M A, Oberst M T, Bjorklund B C 1994b Early outcomes after hip fracture among women discharged home and to nursing homes. Research in Nursing Health 17(3):175–183

6

Soft tissue injuries

■ Soft tissues ■ Classification ■ Management ■ Complications
■ Physiotherapy management ■ Long-term outcome

CONTENTS

Objectives

By the end of this chapter you should:

1. Have an insight into and overview of the classification of soft tissue injuries, their average healing times, their different managements and common complications.
2. Understand and be able to implement the assessment of a patient with a soft tissue injury.
3. Be able to identify how to problem solve for a patient assessment and treatment of a soft tissue injury, regardless of the exact nature and site of the injury or the medical management.

Prerequisites

Make sure that you have familiarised yourself again with the physiology of soft tissue healing and the medical management of soft tissue injuries. For that you might find the following texts helpful: *Essential orthopaedics and trauma* by David J. Dandy, and *Outline of Orthopaedics* by J. Crawford Adams and D. L. Hamblen (see References).

INTRODUCTION

About the connective tissues

Connective tissues are one of the four principal tissues in the body and their general functions include (Clancy & McVicar 1995):

1. Protection for delicate organs which they surround.
2. Provision of a structural framework for the body.
3. Supporting and binding of other interconnecting tissue types within organs.
4. Transportation of substances from one region to another.
5. Internal defence mechanism against potential pathogenic invaders.
6. Storage of energy reserves.

True connective tissues have a viscous matrix and two types of cell:

- fixed cells which have either a homeostatic repair function (such as fibroblasts and fibrocytes), a homeostatic defence function (such as macrophages) or a storage function (for instance adipocytes).
- wandering cells which mostly have a defence function (such as macrophages).

They also contain three different kinds of fibre:

- Collagen fibres are long, straight, stiff and strong and give the tissue tensile strength.
- Reticular fibres, made of reticulin, are interwoven between the collagen fibres, adding flexibility to the properties provided by the collagen.
- Elastic fibres, made of elastin, are stretchable and give the tissue some elasticity (Clancy & McVicar 1995).

Having looked at the different fibres that make up connective tissues it is important to recognise that some of the latter are true connective tissues while others are specialised for different functions (Clancy & McVicar 1995).

True connective tissues (as discussed above) consist of:

- a viscous matrix

- fixed or wandering cells
- collagen, reticulin or elastin fibres.

Vascular connective tissues consist of:

- blood
  — matrix: plasma
  — cells: leucocytes, erythrocytes, thrombocytes
  — fibres
- lymph
  — matrix: lymph
  — cells: leucocytes
  — fibres: various proteinaceous materials.

Skeletal connective tissues consist of:

- blood
  — matrix: inorganic salts of calcium
  — cells: osteocytes
  — fibres: ossein
- cartilage
  — matrix: chondrin
  — cells: chondrocytes
  — fibres: elastin and collagen.

Adipose connective tissues consist of:

- blood
  — matrix: interstitial fluid with high lipid content
  — cells: adipocytes
  — fibres: collagen (rare).

As mentioned earlier, connective tissues are only one of the four principal tissues. The others are the following:

Epithelial tissues which deal mainly with:

- protection
- transport (across membranes)
- lining of internal cavities
- secretion (for instance sweat, tears).

Muscle tissue which is:

- skeletal (striped, voluntary)
- smooth (non-striped, involuntary), or
- cardiac.

Nervous tissue consisting of:

- neurons (conducting and receiving stimuli)
- neuroglia (protecting neurons).

In summary therefore one can say that there are four principal tissues which differ according to their special function and hence their location.

Self-assessment questions

■ **SAQ 6.1.** How are connective tissues classified?

■ **SAQ 6.2.** The physiological functions of collagen fibres indicate the biomechanical properties the body requires of soft tissue. What are these properties?

The soft tissues we will be dealing with are mainly ligaments, fasciae, muscles and their tendons, bursae, capsules, nerves and their sheaths. Clearly such a group of different anatomical entities has a wide variety of functions and these could be briefly summarised as follows:

- Ligaments secure joints and allow their movements.
- Muscles are responsible for movement, stability, strength.
- Bursae and capsules generally support, nourish and protect vulnerable or heavily used joint regions.
- Nerves allow for rapid communication within all parts of the body.

As with almost all other tissues and systems in the body, injury of soft tissues can occur through trauma, overuse (particularly of a repetitive kind), disease and chemical agents such as inflammatory processes. The variety of all the different functions and causes for injury puts soft tissue injury into the realm of everyday occurrences as well as, for instance, serious road traffic accidents. It also means that this kind of injury or damage happens very frequently and to most people in a variety of ways.

Stages of healing

Before the management issues can be discussed in more detail, it is necessary to look at the different stages of healing. For this the reader is referred to Evans (1980) and Clancy & McVicar (1995).

The process may be understood to involve three major stages: injury, inflammation and repair.

Dandy (1993) summarises it like this:

1. After the injury the torn fibres bleed, the space fills with clot and the surrounding vessels dilate. White blood cells invade the clot.
2. During the first 2–3 days, the wound margins fill with macrophages which remove dead tissue. Fibroblasts and capillary buds appear and the clot is replaced with granulation tissue.
3. Between 3 and 14 days, the fibroblasts form fibrous tissue, vascularity diminishes, and the scar contracts to about 80% of its original size. After 14 days the wound is healed soundly enough to withstand normal stresses, but does not regain its full strength until
3 months.
4. Between 2 weeks and 2 years, the fibrous tissue contracts further. The wound, which is a dull purplish colour at first, gradually becomes pale. Scars on the flexor aspect of joints produce tight contractures but those on the extensor aspect of joints stretch and leave ugly white scars.

From this it becomes clear therefore that a few hours, 2–3 days, 3–14 days and 2 weeks following the injury are important landmarks in the management of soft tissue injuries which will be directly related to treatment goals.

In a study of injured canine anterior cruciate ligaments, Desrosiers et al (1995) demonstrated that mechanical stimulation as provided by physiotherapy was essentially the only factor able to improve ligament healing. They found that after stimulation the scar tissue was aligned with the ligament fibres rather than being perpendicular to it. This clearly results in a more elastic and tensile ligament.

Connective tissues are unique amongst the tissues of the body in that due to their fibre make-up and distribution they are much more deformable than other tissues. Each one of the connective tissues mentioned earlier has unique mechanical properties depending on its function; for instance those structures having more elastin than collagen in their make-up are able to deform more than those with more collagen than elastin. These latter fibres being stiffer and less deformable would therefore be more prone to earlier tearing.

What happens to a ligament once it becomes stretched? The stress–strain curve will give some help in answering this question. Smith (1995) identifies the strain as the amount of force needed before collagen becomes strained and elongated. Initially, she suggests, the slack is taken up, before stress and strain become proportional to each other. In the latter situation the more force applied to the ligament the more it deforms in response to this demand. Elongation happens here and no damage is caused, meaning that the tissues can go back to neutral once the force is released. This is referred to as 'elasticity'. The ability to slowly deform under a constant load for a limited amount of time and then return to the starting point – provided the original forces decrease – is known as 'creep'.

However, if the force continues to increase microfailure starts to occur, leading to a flattening of the curve. This indicates that the fibres cannot deform any more and the 'plastic range' of the tissues has been reached. Actual break up of the tissues will occur after plasticity has been reached if the load continues. Recovery to the status quo is now no longer possible but a healing cycle involving fibrosis will take place. Smith (1995) points to the importance of connective tissue being a dynamic structure that is able to respond to applied forces with a series of plastic changes.

Fibrosis or scarring will happen in a very disorganised way with fibres pointing in any direction. In order to influence the alignment of these fibres, stresses simulating functional activities have to occur. Reynolds et al (1996) established that this remodelling process of collagen is much quicker and more effective soon after the injury, reducing massively after 2 months and being virtually nil after 1 year. This is a very important timescale for rehabilitation.

CLASSIFICATION OF SOFT TISSUE INJURIES

1. *Ligaments/tendons.* Here injuries may be cate-

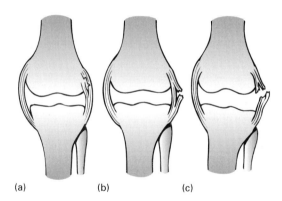

Figure 6.1 Types of ligament injury: (a) sprain; (b) partial rupture; (c) complete rupture. (Adapted with permission from Dandy 1993.)

gorised according to the loss of stability incurred (Fig. 6.1).

- Sprain: stability is not affected.
- Partial rupture: some fibres are torn and hence there is some loss of stability but some fibres are still intact as, for instance, in subluxation.
- Complete rupture: loss of stability and continuity of ligament has occurred, for instance, dislocation (Dandy 1993).

2. *Muscles.* These can be injured through:

- crushing
- laceration
- ischaemia
- ectopic ossification (Fig. 6.2).

3. *Nerves.* These can be affected by:

- division
- stretching
- crushing.

4. *Blood vessels.* These can be injured by (Fig. 6.3):

- division
- stretching
- spasm
- crushing.

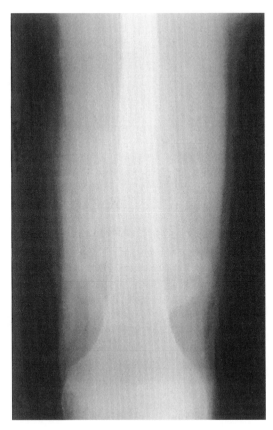

Figure 6.2 Ectopic ossification within muscle following fracture. (Reproduced with permission from Dandy 1993.)

Self-assessment question

■ **SAQ 6.3.** What is the difference between the classification of injuries in ligaments on the one hand and in blood vessels, muscles and nerves on the other?

As mentioned previously, soft tissue injuries can have a multitude of different causes, for instance road traffic accidents, sports injury, simple everyday activities like walking along the street, and so on. They can occur alone, but of course are often sustained in conjunction with other, more serious injuries. Soft tissue injuries which are associated with fractures are often classified in a different way from the above mentioned list. This classification depends on the surgical principles and on the individual prognosis for each trauma. In the Anglo–American literature these combined bony and soft tissue injuries are classified according to Gustillo as open fractures 1 to 3 with a subclassification of grade 3 lesions as A, B or C. In German-speaking countries the classification of Tscherne & Oestern is more common, using four different categories for these combined injuries (Oestern & Laque 1992). As these are not immediately relevant to the dis-

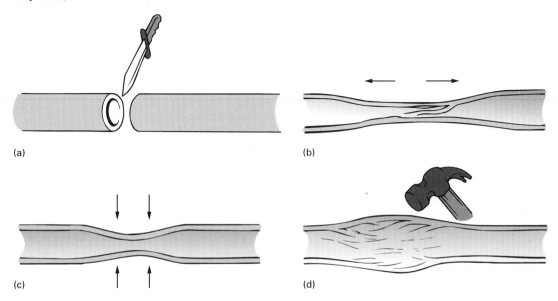

Figure 6.3 Injuries to blood vessels: (a) complete division; (b) stretching; (c) spasm; (d) soft tissue damage to the wall. (Adapted with permission from Dandy 1993.)

cussion here they will not be considered at this moment.

Injuries may not only occur as the result of a multitude of different causes but also in many different ways:

1. *Through a direct or indirect cause.* A direct cause would be, for instance, a blow to the arm resulting in a painful deltoid muscle. An indirect cause would indicate a secondary event, for instance, subluxation of a joint resulting in severe stretching of the ligamentous and capsular fibres surrounding it.
2. *Through an underlying pathology.* Several disease processes are known to involve collagen fibres, such as rheumatoid arthritis, resulting in tears of the upper cervical ligaments. It is known that age affects tendons and ligaments and makes them more prone to failure under mechanical loading (Astrom & Rausing 1995).
3. *Through stress or fatigue.* This overuse factor is often seen in sports injuries or in people who repetitively perform a particular movement such as using a keyboard. Repetitive stress injury (RSI) is a classic long-term overuse problem, though it is as yet unclear whether or not that is the whole cause of this syndrome.

How an injury is caused has a bearing, of course, on the assessment on the one hand (for instance, on whether you only assess the immediate region and investigate the mechanical nature of the injury or whether you explore lifestyle issues and take a precise medical history), and treatment management on the other.

MANAGEMENT OF SOFT TISSUE INJURIES

This is basically either conservative or surgical.

Conservative considerations include the following:

- immobilisation
- mobilisation
- rehabilitation including advice.

Surgical considerations include the following:

- For ligaments

  — repair when torn
  — replacement or reconstruction
  — shortening.
- For nerves
  — decompression
  — repair when torn
  — freeing (neurolysis)
  — grafts.
- For muscles
  — reattachment
  — transposition.
- For tendons
  — reattachment
  — transfer.
- For capsules
  — resection
  — splitting.

Immobilisation

Once the injury has occurred and bleeding is still in process any movement is going to be severely painful. Depending on the location and extent of the injury immobilisation can be either partial or complete.

It may be achieved by several different means:

1. elastic bandage (partial)
2. tubigrip (partial)
3. strapping (partial)
4. plaster of paris (complete).

Partial immobilisation
This is very specific to a particular anatomical region, for instance the ankle joint only, and will not involve the related neighbouring joint (in the case of the ankle the knee joint). With tubigrip the forefoot and the ankle up to midcalf only would be covered.

Partial immobilisation is very specific to the plane of movement involved; it will therefore assist the function of the injured structures. In the case of a twisted ankle due to an inversion injury the strapping will therefore involve the lateral and inferior aspect of the joint rather than the joint as a whole.

Tubigrip/elastic bandage
The advantage of tubigrip or an elastic band-

age is that on the whole it is affordable, and it is easily managed by the patient because its application is very general and does not require any anatomical precision. It can also be used immediately while the injured area is still swelling or while the injury is too painful to allow the detailed examination necessary for more precise techniques.

Strapping
This is mostly even cheaper and often more comfortable than tubigrip as it is less bulky. It needs to be applied very precisely to be of any use and comfortable. It can be applied once the swelling is subsiding. This method of management needs much more specialised help (and enough time to teach the patient) for it to be effective.

It is essential that strapping (in contrast to tubigrip, for example) is checked regularly for signs for skin damage caused by the sticky tape. As a matter of urgency and safety, the injury must be monitored for possibly continuing swelling.

Complete immobilisation
Plaster of paris (POP) affords complete immobilisation but in many ways its disadvantages at times outweigh the obvious advantages. Clearly, if a complete tear of a ligament (tendons tear very rarely!) has caused severe instability of a region, a POP cylinder supporting that area – especially if there has been surgical repair – might be the only option. However, it is important to remember that immobilization severely weakens soft tissue and hence makes it more liable to reinjury. In a famous study Noyes et al (1974) immobilised the knees of monkeys in POP casts for 8 weeks. The resultant weakening of the anterior cruciate ligament took 9 months to recover.

Instead of complete POP immobilisation, continuous passive motion (CPM) is currently accepted as the treatment of choice when the promotion of healing is a primary outcome. The reader is referred to Amiel et al (1995) for a more detailed discussion on the effects of CPM.

Subsequent management will obviously be dependent on the kind of immobilisation chosen initially and therefore has to be included in the goal setting as it will affect the overall outcome.

Self-assessment question

■ **SAQ 6.4**. A patient with a slight sprain of the wrist is managed with a tubigrip over the radiocarpal joint. What areas/joints would you need to include in your assessment and treatment?

LIGAMENTOUS INJURIES

Case study 6.1

John Brown (1)
John Brown is a 25-year-old man and a keen hobby footballer. Yesterday, while playing football he was tackled and fell. Although he immediately felt pain he was able to play on, but his pain got much worse once he stopped playing. He now complains of a sharp pain on the medial aspect of his right knee which increases on extension.

Self-assessment question

■ **SAQ 6.5**. What would you expect in terms of objective findings when examining his knee? (You might need to refer back to the assessment chapter.)

Answer:
Look:
This is a very new or acute injury and hence you expect to see strong reddening of the affected area (due to the dilatation of blood vessels and increased permeability of vessels). This reddening is going to be quite localized over the medial aspect of his knee.
Feel:
There is going to be a localized swelling over the injury site which feels warm to the touch.
Test:
All movements will be uncomfortable, active and passive alike, due to the inflammatory process in that area.

Flexion is full (though painful) but extension is the really aggravating movement, resulting in a very localised sharp pain on the medial aspect of the knee. This pain radiates along a narrow band of about

5 cm from the femur to the tibia (i.e. along the site of the medial collateral ligament).

Medial distraction of the knee (a valgus stress) is very painful but lateral distraction (a varus stress) is only moderately uncomfortable.

No signs of instability or locking have been elicited.

The meaning of the problem to John

John is young and a keen footballer – though clearly not as fit as he could be. It might be that his entire social life is linked to his sporting activities or that he lives up on the third floor without a lift.

Remember that the meaning of the injury to the patient is often the most important aspect to find out in an assessment.

Self-assessment question

■ **SAQ 6.6**. What kind of questions would you feel most comfortable with and which would still be probing enough for this part of the assessment to be relevant?

Case study 6.1

John Brown, continued (2)
John can only walk with a pronounced limp, leaning on an umbrella. The most likely diagnosis is going to be a medial collateral ligament sprain of the knee. Classic signs for that injury are:

● Immediate pain at injury but able to continue to play (impossible with a muscle injury), with worse pain at rest.
● Pain in the closed packed position of the knee (i.e. extension) which stretches the medial collateral ligament.
● Stable knee (hence a sprain and not a rupture).
● Localised pain (ligaments of the knee do not refer pain).

It is clear that any joint examination is never done in isolation but needs to involve related structures. In other words for the knee the other components of the closed kinetic chain must be

included, which are hip and foot. For a more detailed background on examination procedures the reader is referred to Hertling & Kessler (1990).

Management

The conservative treatment of soft tissue injuries consists of either rest or mobilisation, ice, compression and elevation (abbreviated as RICE or MICE).

Opinions in the literature are divided on the advantages of either rest or mobilisation at the start of the conservative regime. It makes sense though to be guided by the particular stage of injury or inflammation. As long as wound edges are gaping and bleeding, any increase in movement and hence tension will delay the inflammatory process and hence rest seems to be the logical advice to give. If, on the other hand, you only see the patient 3 days later, when granulation has occurred, then it seems to make sense to start some mobilisation immediately, to encourage the forming scar to be laid down in the line of stress, that is, in the way that body part needs to be used in future.

Problem-solving exercise 6.1

■ Using the examination and assessment findings, and relating them to the different stages of the inflammatory cycle, what would be the first line of John's management?

After you have worked through this exercise for yourself, compare your answerers with those in the following section.

Initial management for John Brown

1. He should be given an icepack to help minimize further haemorrhage and swelling. He should use this several times a day for short periods. (Check skin sensation as a precaution.)
2. Rest for the first 24–36 hours after the injury will help to protect the sprained ligament from further damage. This should include advice on minimising stair-climbing, sitting

in deep chairs and so on, as all of these require very strong muscle contractions which might interfere with the healing process.

3. Compression can be applied via an elastic bandage or even splint. This should extend to about 10 cm superiorly and inferiorly of the knee.

4. Elevation should be encouraged to prevent fluid stasis which would obviously prolong swelling and hence the inflammatory process.

In addition John should be given a pair of crutches for a few days (remember that he seemed to indicate problems with weight bearing by leaning on an umbrella). This will help to distribute the forces generated by walking.

With John's injury the compression element was achieved by using an elastic bandage. This aim could also be achieved by the use of tubigrip which is an elastic stocking-like tube. It is more expensive than the bandage and requires good hand and arm movement and strength to apply it. Its advantage is in the even pressure that is applied throughout.

A very important aspect of John's early management is emotional support. The suddenness and painfulness of a soft tissue lesion can knock all the confidence out of a sports person. He will need reassurance about the nature of the injury, the possible timescale and the realistically expected outcome.

Self-assessment question

■ **SAQ 6.7.** What do you base your assumptions on timescale and outcome on?

Subsequent treatment

Clearly, he is a keen sportsman who will want and need to achieve a high level of flexibility and strength as quickly as possible. This is one reason for starting his rehabilitation soon, the other being the quality of the scar. Fibrous tissues need to be laid down in the line of stress and use, which will only happen if the ligament is encouraged to simulate exactly that. John therefore needs to start moving his knee as fully as possible

as soon as the pain and swelling allow (after about 2–3 days).

He can begin with gentle autoassisted and then active exercises maintaining range of movement (don't forget the non-affected parts of his body to maintain general cardiovascular fitness), and isometric contractions first of quadriceps, later of hamstrings and hip muscles (holding the contraction to the count of 10), for the maintenance of strength. These are carried out several times a day (possibly every hour if he agrees).

You might want to try some ice and frictions at the earliest after 3 days to ensure a good quality scarring process. This is done by rubbing the fingers transversely (in a right angle across the orientation of the ligamentous fibres) and can only be tried once the internal bleeding has completely stopped.

Frictions involve enough pressure to include the patient's subcutaneous tissues in the movement. Its main action seems to be a counterirritation and hence an increase in local blood supply. Therefore it must never be done while the acute inflammatory stages have not subsided.

After a few days (3–5) John should be weight bearing, walking normally and only using his tubigrip if the swelling has not totally subsided.

After about 1 week he should be able to start gentle jogging, walking on uneven surfaces (to help proprioception), and then to commence exercising on stairs and finally to begin short 'start–stop' sprints to really load his knee and to give him the confidence that he will be alright at speed (when playing football) and at awkward angles. Remember to be sport specific with the exercises.

The management of the acute lesion therefore has the aims of (Hertling & Kessler 1990):

1. decreasing pain and swelling
2. prevention of deformity and protection of the joint
3. preventing stiffness
4. preventing muscle atrophy and tight adhesions
5. regaining strength and confidence.

Pain after medial collateral ligament strain can be felt – when stressed – for several months after the injury.

Electrotherapy

You might wish to consider several different electrotherapy modalities in John's management. The reader is referred to Low & Reed (1994) for an extensive discussion of this area and how it relates to healing times and quality of scar tissues.

Review points

John has a clearly defined simple sprain of a knee ligament, surely one of the most frequent soft tissue injuries.

Before you move on, be sure you are certain about the important aspects of this case.

1. How did it happen?
2. Did it necessitate an abrupt stop of the activity? What was the reason for this?
3. Was there any swelling, locking or giving way? Why?
4. How did the pain behave on movement and weight bearing?
5. What were the pertinent findings which helped you to identify the structure in question?
6. What pathological processes influenced the timescale of the healing?
7. What were the key aims of management, and how did these relate to the healing timescale?

Problem-solving exercise 6.2

■ How would the above principles help you with the assessment and treatment of a patient with a simple sprain in a non-weight-bearing region of the body, for instance a sprain of the interphalangeal joint (collateral ligament) of the second digit on the dominant hand?

   Include in your considerations the likely cause (?which movement) of this injury.

The following problem is equally often seen in practice.

Case study 6.2

Gemma Jackson (1)
Gemma Jackson is a 35-year-old woman who tripped on the pavement on her way to work resulting in a severe inversion sprain of her ankle. Her pain was so severe that an ambulance was called and she was seen in the accident and emergency (A&E) department. A stress X-ray (plantar flexion and inversion) demonstrated that although no fractures had been sustained a partial ligamentous rupture had occurred. This might have resulted in some instability.

Self-assessment question

■ **SAQ 6.8.** How would an X-ray demonstrate that diagnosis?

Case study 6.2

Gemma Jackson, continued (2)
When you see Gemma (coming straight from the A&E department) she complains of severe pain on the lateral aspect of her ankle.

   On examination it becomes apparent that she is unable to move the ankle in any way or bear weight on it.

Self-assessment question

■ **SAQ 6.9.** Remembering John's sprain and treatment, how would you approach Gemma's treatment?

Answer: *Gemma clearly also has a severe ligament injury and hence the initial aims are the same as John's, as the RICE regime is applied to reduce pain and swelling. Instead of just severely overstretching the ligament as John had done, she has acquired a partial rupture resulting in some instability of the ankle joint. In order to protect the joint from further damage, therefore, it is necessary to augment the stability of the joint by supplementing the injured lateral ligaments of the ankle (calcaneofibular ligament, bifurcate ligament and/or dorsal calcaneocuboid ligament). This can be achieved by strapping the ankle in slight eversion. The lower leg must be shaved and*

Friar's balsam and so on applied to the skin to protect it from the sticky tape. Then use some adhesive spray on the area, again to protect the skin as well as to increase the stickiness of the tape.

A horseshoe-shaped piece of felt of foam rubber should be used to fill in the submalleolar depressions, prior to the strapping, so that the tape will provide equal pressure and reduce the risk of a haematoma forming. The basket-weave adhesive tape strapping should always be applied from the medial aspect of the leg, passed under the heel with the foot held in eversion, and extended up the lateral aspect of the leg under slight tension in order to pull the ankle into slight eversion.

If this strapping has been properly applied, inversion, eversion and rotation of the ankle will be limited.

However the following points should be kept in mind before applying strapping:

- *Never strap before an assessment has been completed.*
- *Strapping is not a first-aid measure.*
- *Never strap if you are unsure of the injury.*
- *Check skin sensation.*
- *Never strap if there is an open wound.*

In contrast to John who needed only a locally applied bandage or tubigrip, Gemma needs to have support covering her foot and her lower leg up to the knee in order to combat swelling effectively.

Therefore, those ligamentous injuries that interfere with the stability of a joint because it is anatomically particularly reliant on the ligaments for stability, benefit from being strapped as part of the RICE regime.

Self-assessment question

■ **SAQ 6.10.** What is the rationale for the RICE regime in this case? How long would you advise the patient to persist with this approach? Are there any contraindications to this treatment?

Problem-solving exercise 6.3

■ Once the RICE regime can be progressed, what will be your treatment aims? Refer back to John's history if you need help in understanding where John and Gemma are similar and where they differ.

Progression of treatment

This will involve the following.

- Ice and frictions (be sure the bleeding has completely stopped).
- Passive movements (accessory as well as physiological) in order to maintain full ROM – think of the scar quality at all times!
- Active exercises to improve ROM and strength. Don't forget the non-affected regions.
- Gentle weight bearing, aiming at full weight bearing within a few days.
- The wobble board. Due to the force of the inversion injury, articular nerve fibres and their mechanoreceptors, which play a part in the reflex stabilisation of the ankle joint, have been separated. Thus Gemma needs much more help than John to build up her neuromuscular coordination. This can be achieved by frequent use of the wobble board, first in one movement plane then progressing to use in all possible planes. Readers are referred to Freeman & Wyke (1967) for background reading on this.
- Gentle trampolining.
- Gentle jogging.
- Any functional activity that fits in with her lifestyle. (Refer back to the subjective part of the assessment.)
- Active strengthening exercises involving the calf, ankle, and foot muscles; this is necessary for security in this area.
- Exercises involving stop/start tactics, sudden changes in direction, etc., are essential to help proprioception.

Indications for more caution would be:

- persistent pain
- swelling which reoccurs regularly.

Remember that it will take quite some time for the ligament to achieve its maximum elastic and tensile strength after an injury like this (refer back to the healing timescale if you are unsure of this). You need to caution Gemma about loading the ankle too soon in positions where it needs to rely a lot on its lateral ligaments (for instance walking on rough ground in unsupportive shoes, walking barefoot on the beach, and so on).

It is of prime importance to advise Gemma (as well as John) of the need to continue with her stretches and strengthening exercises for many weeks, if not months, in order to influence the scar as long as it still changes. This will ensure the strongest possible ligamentous repair and hence decrease the likelihood of a secondary injury due to a poor primary repair.

For more detail on the assessment techniques and the biomechanical considerations and rationale refer to Hertling & Kessler (1990).

Review of the literature on treatment of ankle soft tissue injuries

Ogilvieharris & Gilbart (1995) reviewed the English language medical literature on soft tissue injuries of the ankle published between 1966 and 1993. Altogether 84 articles were analysed, reporting the treatment results of 32 025 patients. The authors concluded from this review that non-steroidal anti-inflammatory drugs (NSAIDS) shortened the time to recovery and were associated with less pain. Active mobilisation appeared to be the treatment of choice. Ice and diapulse were also reported as being helpful while ultrasound, diathermy, aspiration and injections were not identified as being particularly helpful.

Problem-solving exercise 6.4

David is a 35-year-old architect who tripped over uneven paving stones in the street and fell onto the dorsiflexed right hand. He felt a tearing sensation in his wrist and was immediately aware of severe pain. His hand and the carpus was displaced backwards momentarily before it snapped back into place. He took himself off to the local A&E department, still in severe pain. On examination and X-ray it became clear that he

had not fractured any bones in the fall but that he had sustained a carpal subluxation. Reduction was not necessary as it had occurred spontaneously.

David is referred immediately to you. You find that the wrist and carpus are hugely swollen and painful.

- Reminding yourself of the treatment principles for John's sprained and Gemma's partially torn ligament, how would you deal with David?

Self-assessment question

- **SAQ 6.11.** What do you expect to find on examination? (Remember the internal swelling and hence the increased pressure in the carpal tunnel.)

Problem-solving exercise 6.5

- **A**. What are your treatment aims?
- **B**. How would you progress treatment? Remind yourself of the healing timetable. Refer back to both John and Gemma for details of the physical treatment.
- **C**. David is completely dependent on his hand professionally. How will you incorporate this consideration into your management?

Case study 6.3

James Low

James Low is a 46-year-old accountant who injured his ankle during a charity parachute jump. The force of his injury had been so severe that it resulted in a complete rupture of the lateral ligaments of his ankle, leading to gross instability. This diagnosis had been made by a doctor he saw in the A&E department of the local hospital.

The doctor will have arrived at this diagnosis by:

1. Grasping the calcaneus and then fully inverting the foot passively. In contrast to an ankle with an intact lateral ligament this will

result in a fairly large range of movement as the talus is now able to wobble in the mortise. As with all other ligamentous tests it is necessary to test the uninjured side in order to get a feel for the 'normal' state of the ligamentous apparatus. This is vital as it is well recognised that wide individual variations exist with regard to ligament laxity. You therefore always need to establish what is normal before you are able to discern what is abnormal.

2. A stress X-ray with the ankle in plantarflexion and inversion will have demonstrated tilting of the talus.

The best management for these injuries still seems to be under discussion. Surgical repair is regarded as second choice, and usually consists of either the repair of the ligament or the reinforcement of the lateral aspect of the ankle by transferring the tendon of peroneus brevis or by a free graft of plantaris (Dandy 1993). On examination, weight bearing is impossible due to:

- severe pain and swelling
- instability of the ankle.

Remembering Gemma's management, you know that strapping will be able to reinforce a ligament but is not strong enough to take on the role of main stabiliser by itself. Hence a plaster cast is the preferred option. This will most probably be a Litecast below-knee plaster, with the ankle in slight eversion. (Refer to Chapter 5 for more details on the different plaster materials and rules of application). Remembering the healing timetable you know that this plaster will have to be on for a minimum of 3–4 weeks in order for fibrous tissue repair to have ensued.

James will be independent in a walking plaster and might wish to use a stick for security.

After about 4 weeks the plaster will be removed and James referred to physiotherapy.

An answer is given in the following section but try to work this out for yourself first.

Problem-solving exercise 6.6

- What do you need to find out before planning your management of James'

ankle? Refer back to the healing timetable and to Gemma's and John's treatment for similarities and differences. You might also wish to reread the post-POP management concerns raised in the fracture chapter.

Further assessment of James Low

1. *Pain*

After 4 weeks in plaster this should not be a prominent feature as long as the ankle is not being moved; it might become a problem that needs addressing once weight bearing and exercises start.

2. *Swelling*

This will be a major feature as lack of movement in the plaster, and hence very reduced absorption, will have resulted in a fibrosing of the original haematoma; it will be hard and cold to touch.

3. *ROM*

This might very well turn out to be the major problem. After 4 weeks in the plaster the soft tissues (ligaments, joint capsules, membranes and so on) will have shortened in virtually all directions, but the worst will be plantarflexion and inversion. There will be very little difference between active and passive ROM.

4. *Mobility*

James has lost a lot of his neuromuscular control and strength around the ankle and therefore cannot easily weight bear through his ankle. Hence he is in danger of reinjuring the ankle. He will find himself to be more vulnerable and much less mobile than before the removal of his plaster.

5. *Social set-up*

As an accountant James is sitting at a desk most of the day but his office is on the first floor of a building without a lift. He is a widower and lives a fiercely independent life. His home is a bungalow with a small paved garden. He usually takes the bus to work. James' hobbies are mostly intellectual pursuits rather than sports.

Self-assessment question

■ **SAQ 6.12.** How would you now address the above five points in your treatment plan? After you have tried this question for yourself, check your answer against the approach described in the next section.

Physiotherapy treatment of James Low

1. *Mobility*
Clearly, he needs some help with this while his ankle is as stiff as it is at the moment. He should therefore be given a pair of crutches for a few days and taught partial weight bearing (PWB), including going up and down stairs in order for him to be able to be independent.

2. *ROM*
He needs to start with gentle active physiological movements. This is important in order to take account of the lack of elasticity in the soft tissues at the moment. (Passive movements could quickly overstretch the joint and hence result in reinjury.) He should do these for a few days to get some proprioception and movement back into the joint.

The next step will be for James to continue with his active exercises while you introduce accessory movements, particularly stressing inversion and plantarflexion (for instance Maitland grades III and IV) as far as joint irritability allows (refer back to the assessment chapter for details). It is likely that this concentrated stretching of the fibrosed scar (that is, into joint resistance) will result in some treatment soreness. This can be countered by finishing each treatment with some accessory movements of a lower grade (that is, I or II) to stimulate the mechanoreceptors and hence engender some pain relief.

The concentrated stretches will result in a low grade inflammatory reaction as some scar fibres tear. Electrotherapy might therefore be a useful pain-reducing modality at this point.

Bearing in mind the tissue-healing timetable you will remember that inflammation always goes along with some pain and definitely swelling. Hence, ice, compression (elastic bandage) and elevation after treatment will be good measures for James to use.

Can you see that he could now be treated similarly to Gemma with regard to his physical injury? What psychosocial clues have you picked up, however, that would lead you to a different treatment plan?

3. *Social set-up*
James clearly needs some advice on how to use his body. He likes doing things that require a low level of activity and hence he is quite unfit. This is compounded by his stressful and sedentary job. James must therefore be introduced to an exercise regime and be given a sound rationale for it (the biomechanics of soft tissue and their need for stretching and movement in order to remain elastic and tensile). This will allow him to be at less risk during sudden challenges to soft tissue.

Summary of important points concerning ligamentous injuries

1. You need to be aware of the anatomy and biomechanics of the injured area in order to assess it and to predict a possible outcome.
2. You need to be aware of the healing timetable of tissues in order to know whether you are dealing with an inflammatory (acute) or a repair (chronic) situation. This will direct you to the appropriate approach.
3. It is of maximum importance to take a long view and advise the patient on long-term care as the scar is going to continue to change long after the patient has been discharged from physiotherapy. Attention to the quality of the scar tissue (that is, linking the exercises and stretches to the way the area is going to be used later on) are of greatest importance.

Complications

Compartment syndrome
This can be a very serious secondary occurrence after any tissue injury. As the tissue swells up it needs space to expand. If this is not possible the tissue will become ischaemic very quickly and hence will be destroyed.

The compartments to remember are as follows (Dandy 1993):

Forearm

- The ventral compartment includes:
  — the median and ulnar nerve
  — the radial and ulnar artery.
- The dorsal compartment includes:
  — the posterior interosseous nerve, but no major vessels.

Lower limb

- The anterior tibial compartment contains:
  — the anterior tibial artery
  — the deep peroneal nerve.
- The superficial posterior compartment contains:
  — no important nerves or vessels.
- The deep posterior compartment contains:
  — the posterior tibial vessels and nerves
  — the peroneal artery.
- The peroneal compartment contains:
  — deep and superficial peroneal nerves.

It is absolutely essential to check for signs of ischaemia, that is, white colour, cold to touch, no distal pulses (if relevant) and severe pain, in patients with a history of trauma and suspected deep swelling.

Recurrent instability

If the self-treatment after discharge is not adequately executed, recurrent instability is a frequently seen complication of ligamentous sprains or ruptures. This is seen particularly often in the ankle joint but is also common in the knee or elbow. The major causes for this are cited as follows (Corrigan & Maitland 1983):

- Functional instability, due to a massive previous injury resulting in an interruption of the reflex arc and hence a loss of reflex stabilisation of the joint.
- Inadequately treated sprains, due to weakness of the surrounding muscles and shortening of the ligaments.
- Problems of the distal anatomical regions.
- Undiagnosed causes.

MUSCLES AND TENDONS

So far we have looked at ligamentous injuries only and now need to examine where muscle injuries might differ. The worked examples of the previous section are needed as a background for these.

The focus here will be particularly on:

- lateral epicondylitis of the elbow, as an example of an overuse injury
- supraspinatus tendinitis, as an example of an injury precipitated by degeneration
- hamstring strain, as an example of direct trauma.

Problem-solving exercise 6.7

Focusing on overuse or degeneration of soft tissue:

- **A.** What do you imagine the main differences to be compared with the trauma, as in the previous case studies?
- **B.** What are the hallmarks of injury and do they apply to degenerative processes and overuse?

In order to help you with these points, you might wish to reread the details on the inflammatory processes in healing and then remind yourself about the stress–strain curve and the ability to deform. You need to also remind yourself of the factors that influence (negatively or positively) these processes.

Lateral epicondylitis

Case study 6.4

Alison Hunt
Alison Hunt is a 54-year-old secretary who has developed a severe pain on the lateral aspect of her elbow over the past 2 months. It is uncomfortable most of the time but it particularly interferes with her hobby of playing tennis. Although not completely certain, she thinks that the onset was connected with her club league tournament.

She now complains of pain over the lateral aspect of the elbow, radiating distally into the forearm and into the wrist and dorsum of her hand. A diagnosis of *lateral epicondylitis* has been made.

Self-assessment questions

■ **SAQ 6.13.** Thinking about John and Gemma, what do you expect to find on observation? What will be similar and what will be different with regard to observation and with regard to testing?

Answer: Clearly you are looking for signs of inflammation because although the condition is chronic (history of 2 months), Alison is likely to reinjure her elbow by continually using it. Hence you might expect redness, swelling, tenderness and heat.

In contrast to Gemma and John there will not be internal bruising due to a sudden disruption of fibres but there might very well have been internal bleeding due to the avulsion of single tendon fibres off their insertion.

The cause of the problem is meant to be in the tendon region of a muscle. Pain therefore will not be provoked by testing the joint (that is, either the stability or the stretching of ligaments), but by contracting the affected muscles hence increasing the tension at the point of insertion to bone.

■ **SAQ 6.14.** Having established that you are dealing with a muscle tendon problem, what muscles insert into the lateral epicondyle and what tests, therefore, could you think of to test your hypothesis?

Answer: The common extensor group.
1. *Resisted extension of the wrist in order to provoke the common extensor muscle group will result in pain and might even demonstrate some weakness.*
2. *Resisted radial deviation with the fingers extended (hence the extensors stretched and therefore pulling on their insertion) will be painful.*

3. *Resisted elbow movements therefore will be unaffected.*
4. *Functional activities involving the wrist, such as shaking hands, twisting open jam jar tops and so on will all reproduce the pain.*
5. *Passive extension of the elbow will be slightly limited as well as painful due to the shortening and hardening of tendon fibres at their insertion.*

We have said that Alison's problem is most probably not due to sudden trauma but due to the painful and shortened scar resulting from overexerting or overstretching the common extensor muscle group.

Self-assessment question

■ **SAQ 6.15.** It is clearly not an acute picture as in the previous case studies but an acute incidence on top of a chronic condition. Remembering the previous case studies how would you approach Alison's treatment?
　You need to remember the tissue-healing timetable for this.
　After you have worked out your answers to this question, read the next section.

An approach to the treatment of Alison Hunt

1. *Rest*
This clearly is a problem that restarts every time the old injury pattern has occurred. Hence Alison must be advised to stop all activities that exacerbate her problem. This can be very difficult and she might need a lot of support and information in order to motivate her. Often rest is the most important factor in limiting the problem.

If Alison finds it impossible to rest the elbow enough to break the aggravating mechanical pattern, a plaster back slab can be used to enforce rest.

2. *Hydrocortisone injections*
This powerful anti-inflammatory treatment can work very quickly provided the hydrocortisone is accurately injected into the correct anatomical spot.

Unfortunately, however, a significant number of patients are not helped by this. It is as well to remember that load bearing tendons are significantly weakened by this and hence put at further risk.

3. *Ice and deep friction*
This may be followed by ultrasound.

4. *Accessory mobilisations*
These are used to gain full endrange of extension.

5. *Mills manipulation*
This manipulation of the elbow is rarely successful in the long run (Corrigan & Maitland 1983).

6. *Advice and education*
This should address the following areas:

- The cause of Alison's problems and the effect of the biomechanics on the area.
- The use of her arm, including looking at her tennis techniques.
- The need to avoid overuse of a particular area, and hence the need to 'cut up' activities of long duration and interweave them with others.
- General strengthening of the neighbouring area.
- Sensitive support while she is exploring other ways of doing her job.

Are you clear about the similarities and differences between the ligamentous injuries on the one hand and the muscle/tendon overuse on the other? If not, go back over the case studies.

Supraspinatus tendinitis

This is a very frequent complaint. The mechanism of injury seems to be overuse or trauma on top of a degenerated tendon. Due to the degenerative aspect of this condition, patients frequently describe a history of flare-ups and remissions over a long timespan, often many years.

Pain is felt over the lateral aspect of the arm, sometimes radiating into the deltoid region. The pain will rarely extend down to the elbow. Night pain is common. Look up the anatomy of the rotator cuff and remind yourself of its important function (see for instance Hertling & Kessler 1990) before continuing.

Self-assessment questions

■ **SAQ 6.16.** When a patient with supraspinatus tendinitis is examined, which movements will be particularly painful? Why are they painful and how will they need to be tested?

Answer:
1. *Active abduction is painful particularly on resistance or even during an isometric contraction. Usually pain occurs as an arc, roughly between 60 and 120° of abduction. Bringing the arm back to neutral from full abduction elicits pain in the same region, and therefore classically the patient drops the arm to a pain-free zone when starting to experience the pain (that is, the arm is dropped from about 120° to about 50°). This coincides with the tendon being compressed between the acromion superiorly and the greater tuberosity inferiorly.*
2. *External rotation is painful.*
3. *There is usually some wasting over the supraspinatus area.*
4. *The rotator cuff is very involved in the scapulohumeral rhythm and therefore a supraspinatus tendinitis is going to alter this.*

■ **SAQ 6.17.** Now that you know the signs and symptoms of this condition, come up with a reasoned plan for its management. Then compare your approach with the one presented in the following section.

Management of supraspinatus tendinitis
Treatment includes the following:

1. Rest: movements that are known to aggravate the problem must be avoided to allow the healing process to start (that is, abduction and external rotation).
2. Injection of corticosteroid around the tendon

to help with the chronically exacerbated inflammatory process.

3. Ice and deep frictions followed by ultrasound.

4. Accessory movements that move the humeral head away from the acromion (always starting from a pain-free position):
   — posteroanterior movements of the humeral head
   — longitudinal movements of the head caudally
   — quadrant position with very gentle movements.

5. Strengthening of all parts of the rotator cuff, e.g. using theraband.

Dealing with this condition is going to take a long time and a lot of patient education. Due to the degenerative nature of the underlying cause it often recurs, and therefore occasionally a surgical decompression of the tendon is needed, either by removal of the outer end of the acromion or by splitting the coracoacromial ligament. These procedures increase the subacromial space and therefore give the tendon more space in which to move around. This should result in less 'rubbing' of the tendon against the roof of this tight space and hence less scarring.

Hamstring strain

Here neither overuse nor degeneration seems to be the underlying problem but usually a direct blow to the muscles or a very forceful contraction. The patients therefore are invariably active and athletic people. A typical history might include a strenuous activity when the patient suddenly feels something give way resulting in an ache. After a few hours, though, the pain and hence loss of mobility are marked.

The diagnosis will be a partial rupture of some muscle fibres either in the muscle belly or closer to the musculotendinous junction.

Self-assessment question

■ **SAQ 6.18.** You now know the history and the signs and symptoms of this problem. You might need to look up the exact anatomy and biomechanics of the hamstrings before thinking about how you would test for the injury site and then devise a management plan. After you have done that read the following section on testing and management.

Testing hamstring injury

- Both the possible rupture sites will be aggravated by resisted knee flexion. This will only confirm the hamstring muscle as the culprit but not differentiate between the musculotendinous junction or the muscle belly.

- Straight leg raise: if this is full, you know that the insertion of the muscle into the ischial tuberosity is at fault. If it is limited you can be pretty certain that the problem lies within the muscle belly rather than near the tendon.

- Hip flexion with the knee bent takes all the tension off the hamstrings and therefore is pain-free – as long as it is done passively.

Management of hamstring injury

- *Rest.* Take weight off the injured region in order to avoid reinjury but encourage gentle active movement without weight bearing to speed up the resorption process of the haematoma for about 2–5 days.

- *Ice, frictions and ultrasound over injury site.* Remember John regarding contraindications to this treatment in the early stages of healing.

- *Strength.* After about 3–5 days start with gentle exercises through the 0–90° range, perhaps using a wall pulley. This will allow for a controlled increase in resistance. Include quadriceps in strengthening regime as the ratio of flexor and extensor strength is vital for good and safe function. Slowly include increased weight bearing in the resistance regime.

- *Control.* Devise short start–stop sprint regimes to increase the flexibility of the muscles.

- *Endurance.* Use of a bicycle, varying the height of the seat to get different parts of the muscle to work more. Also use stairs, swimming and so on.

- *Education.* This is undoubtedly the most important aspect of the rehabilitation, and the following aspects should be covered.
  - Information about the anatomy, biomechanics and mode of injury.
  - Information about the healing process, particularly the late stages, and the importance, therefore, of long-term aftercare.
  - Exploration of training style/lifestyle (that is, how does this person want to use their body).
  - Warm-up and warm-down procedures.
  - Remembering that the relationship you develop with the patient is going to be the gateway to a successful or failed rehabilitation phase. Motivation will be crucially influenced by this.

By now you should be clear about the similarities and differences between ligamentous and musculotendinous injuries. If not, please go back to the case studies and try to identify these points.

Adhesive capsulitis

In contrast to the mechanical stressors underlying the previously mentioned conditions, adhesive capsulitis of the shoulder (or 'frozen shoulder') involves an underlying inflammatory process of the glenohumeral capsule that results in thickening and contraction of the capsule. Apart from severe pain this leads to marked restriction of ROM in the shoulder.

It seems that middle-aged women are affected mainly; it has not been caused by any trauma, and the onset is more often gradual, occurring over several weeks than suddenly overnight. The underlying cause has not yet been precisely identified, but it has been noted that this condition virtually never recurs at the same site. It is as if an 'immunisation' had happened.

Self-assessment question

- **SAQ 6.19.** Remembering the capsular attachments of the glenohumeral joint, which movements would you expect to be particularly limited?

Treatment of adhesive capsulitis

As a rule of thumb, treatment (apart from pure pain-killing methods not involving movement) should not be started unless the night pain has disappeared. This can easily take 4–6 months after onset with the whole course lasting for about 18 months.

After that, treatment needs to focus on the following (Hertling & Kessler 1990):

- *Pain control*, with ice, mobilisation techniques in low grades and electrotherapy.
- *ROM*
  - accessory movements grades III and IV to increase range; caudad longitudinals in as much flexion as can be tolerated
  - posteroanterior/anteroposterior accessory movements
  - stretching, with autoassisted active exercises (using a walking stick that is grasped by both hands but guided by the non-affected side).
- *Strength*, by means of isometric exercises into flexion, abduction and adduction, internal and external rotation proprioceptive neuromuscular facilitation (PNF) patterns.

Electrotherapy is usually not helpful in the rehabilitation of this condition unless it is tried for pain relief in the early stages (for example, transcutaneous electrical nerve stimulation (TENS)).

SURGICALLY REPAIRED SOFT TISSUES

In this chapter so far we have dealt with the conservative management of soft tissue injuries; the second part will introduce some thoughts on the surgical repair of these tissues.

Surgical procedures carried out on ligaments include the following (Fig. 6.4):

1. repair when worn
2. replacement or reconstruction
3. shortening.

Surgical procedures carried out on nerves include (Fig. 6.5):

1. decompression
2. repair
3. grafting
4. freeing (neurolysis).

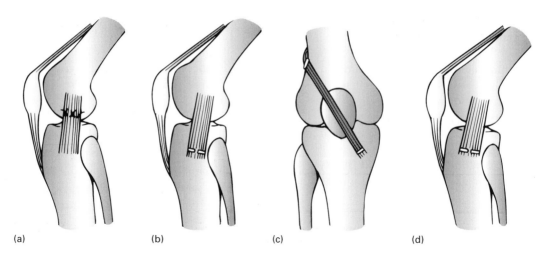

(a)   (b)   (c)   (d)

Figure 6.4 Surgery to ligaments: (a) repair; (b) reattachment; (c) replacement with tendon or prosthesis; (d) advancement of ligament attachment. (Adapted with permission from Dandy 1993.)

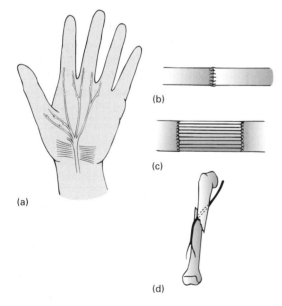

(a)

(b)

(c)

(d)

Figure 6.5 Surgery to nerves: (a) decompression; (b) repair; (c) grafting; (d) neurolysis, where tethering of the nerve to bone or other tissues is released by operation. (Adapted with permission from Dandy 1993.)

Ligament repair

Case study 6.5

Emily Jones
Emily Jones is a 21-year-old student who

dislocated her right thumb when falling on a dry ski slope. She immediately felt something 'go' and now complains of severe pain, swelling and bruising.

On examination active movements cannot be tolerated due to pain, and with passive testing of the joints her thumb appears to be unstable. Hence a complete rupture of the medial collateral ligament is suspected (which one would expect after a dislocation of a joint).

The ligament is surgically repaired and the hand placed in a splint.

Problem-solving exercise 6.8

- Identify the main difference between Emily's problem and John's or David's. What do they have in common and what are the vital differences? How should these differences influence your management approaches? How much do you need to know about the surgery itself?

Nerve decompression

Case study 6.6

Steve Morris
Steve Morris has a long history of backache

which troubles him periodically. Bed rest for a few days followed by wearing a corset until the muscle spasm had gone had always dealt with his problem. He is 40 years old and works as a computer analyst.

He and his family moved house 3 weeks ago and 2 weeks ago he developed his back pain again. Instead of being helped by his usual routine his pain got worse and started to travel down into his buttock and leg, now involving the posterior aspect of his thigh and leg and radiating into the lateral aspect of his ankle and foot.

An acute lumbar nerve root compression by an intervertebral disc is suspected.

Self-assessment question

■ **SAQ 6.20.** What would you be looking for in Steve to help clarify this diagnosis?

Answer:
Subjectively, one might expect the following:

1. *Pain worse in the morning. (As the proteoglycans in the nucleus have taken in 8.8 times their molecular weight in water throughout the night the disc is much larger and hence the prolapse is more severe.)*
2. *Standing and lying is easier than sitting.*
3. *Coughing and sneezing cause pain (increased intra-abdominal pressure).*
4. *Time lapse between back and leg pain (as the nuclear material takes some time to extrude).*

Objectively, you might find:

1. *Loss of lumbar lordosis.*
2. *Possible shift away from side of prolapse.*
3. *Flexion and side flexion to side of pain are the most painful test movements.*
4. *Passive straight leg raise is severely limited by pain (as the already stretched dura is stretched even more to between 30° to 70°).*
5. *Neurological deficit in the dermatomes and myotomes of the S1 nerve root, as shown by:*
   — *loss of sensation (lateral aspect of ankle, foot and posterior calf)*
   — *weakness (plantar flexion of ankle and toes, hip extension, knee flexion)*
   — *loss of reflex (ankle jerk).*
6. *A positive radiculogram or MRI scan.*

Steve undergoes an operation to decompress his S1 nerve root.

This is often done via microsurgery which only resects the bit of intervertebral disc that is causing the compression. On the whole this means that there is no interference with the stability of the spine as the superficial (erector spinae) and deep (multifidus) stabilising muscles of the spine have not been cut.

Self-assessment question

■ **SAQ 6.21.** Postoperative regimes obviously vary according to the differing practices of surgeons, but taking into account what you now know about wound healing and tissue healing, devise a reasoned plan for Steve's management. After you have set out your own plan, compare it with the following section.

Treatment of Steve Morris

1. *Rest*
In order to give the wound a good chance to lay down scar tissue Steve will need to stay in bed for about 2–4 days.

To help resorption of the postoperative haematoma and circulation in general, he should move his toes, ankles and knees (below about 60° of flexion so as not to move his lumbar spine too much).

2. *Mobility*
Once he is allowed out of bed Steve should walk and stand rather than sit, to put the least amount of pressure through the operation site.

3. *ROM*
Once the inflammatory process has passed and the scar tissue has begun to be laid down, it is important that Steve starts, very gently, to use his back as he wants to use it later on, that is he must

start to bend it. This will encourage the fibro-blasts to be laid down in the alignment of stress, rather than in a perpendicular fashion contracting the whole region. Extension stretches will help to protect the posterior disc wall.

Straight leg raises have to be performed regularly to prevent the nerve root from becoming stuck down in adhesions.

4. *Strength*

Isometric and isotonic back extensor exercises should be done from about the fourth day.

Abdominal exercises must be started later (after 5–6 days) as the contraction of the muscles involved increases the intra-abdominal and intradiscal pressures enormously. They need to be in good shape though, in order to contribute to the muscular corset of the trunk which will lead to greater safety later on.

5. *Education*

Again this is the most important aspect of Steve's rehabilitation and the following issues should be addressed:

- You need to be able to motivate Steve (refer back to the subjective assessment section in Ch. 3) to become involved in a back care regime for his spine.
- For this, he needs to know about his spine; the relevant anatomy and biomechanics; the effect of loading it in different positions; the contribution muscle strength can make, and the way in which strenuous tasks of long duration need to be split up.
- You need to impress on Steve that the healing process can take up to 2 years and that the quality of the healing process is in his hands once you have empowered him.

Summary

This chapter has aimed to give you an insight into some areas of soft tissue injuries. As you will have appreciated, this is a very large and complex sector of medicine where surgeons and therapists often overlap and cooperate in order to achieve the best outcome for the patient.

Use the worked example case studies in your problem solving in other settings you will be confronted with. Therefore, be clear what is characteristic for each setting and what is a general feature. It is not necessary to know every particular syndrome that can occur in this area, but it is important for you to be able to recognise the vital aspects of a person's set of problems and to identify how they are special.

ANSWERS TO QUESTIONS AND EXERCISES

Self-assessment questions (page 117)

■ **SAQ 6.1.** How are connective tissues classified?

Answer: According to their loose or dense fibre distribution and by the type of fibre they possess, that is, elastin, reticulin, collagen.

■ **SAQ 6.2.** The physiological functions of collagen fibres indicate the biomechanical properties that the body requires of soft tissues. What are these properties?

Answer: Strength, flexibility and elasticity.

Self-assessment question 6.3 (page 119)

■ **SAQ 6.3.** What is the difference between the classification of injuries in ligaments on the one hand and in blood vessels, muscles and nerves on the other?

Answer: Ligamentous injuries are classified according to the resulting interference with stability, while injuries to the other tissues mentioned are categorised according to the mechanical or chemical cause of injury.

Self-assessment question 6.4 (page 121)

■ **SAQ 6.4.** A patient with a slight sprain of the wrist is managed with a tubigrip over the radiocarpal joint. What areas/joints would you need to include in your assessment and treatment?

Answer: Inferior and superior radioulnar joints, carpal bones and intercarpal joints.

Self-assessment question 6.5 (page 121)

Answer follows question in text.

Self-assessment question 6.6 (page 122)

■ **SAQ 6.6.** What kind of questions would you feel most comfortable with and which would still be probing enough for this part of the assessment to be relevant?

Answer: If you have problems answering this question, go back to Chapter 3 on assessment to refresh your memory.

Problem-solving exercise 6.1 (page 122)

See the following section in the text.

Self-assessment question 6.7 (page 123)

See information throughout the text.

Problem-solving exercise 6.2 (page 124)

■ How would the above principles [see text] help you with the assessment and treatment of a patient with a simple sprain in a non-weight-bearing region of the body, for instance a sprain of the interphalangeal joint (collateral ligament) of the second digit of the dominant hand?

Include in your considerations the likely cause (?which movement) of this injury.

Answer: The mechanism could be, for instance, twisting something against very strong resistance, or a fall onto the distal part of the dominant hand. Non-weight bearing reduces the time of healing on the one hand, but the dominance in functional tasks lengthens the timescale and complicates the outcome. (See information in this and previous chapters, especially Chapter 3 on assessment.)

Self-assessment question 6.8 (page 124)

■ **SAQ 6.8.** How would an X-ray demonstrate that diagnosis [of partial ligamentous rupture]?

Answer: The joint surfaces of the ankle joint are gapped further than normal. (Hence the stress X-ray: a conventional anteroposterior X-ray would not demonstrate anything.)

Self-assessment question 6.9 (page 124)

Answer follows question in text.

Self-assessment question 6.10 (page 125)

See text.

Problem-solving exercise 6.3 (page 125)

See information in text.

Problem-solving exercise 6.4 (page 126)

See information in text.

Self-assessment question 6.11 (page 126)

See text.

Problem-solving exercise 6.5 (page 126)

See information in text.

Problem-solving exercise 6.6 (page 127)

See the following section in the text.

Self-assessment question 6.12 (page 128)

See the following section in the text.

Problem-solving exercise 6.7 (page 129)

See the advice following the questions in the text.

Self-assessment questions 6.13, 6.14 (page 130)

Answers follow questions in text.

Self-assessment question 6.15 (page 130)

See the following section in the text.

Self-assessment questions (page 131)

■ **SAQ 6.16.** Answer follows question in text.

■ **SAQ 6.17.** See the following section in the text.

Self-assessment question 6.18 (page 132)

See the following sections in the text.

Self-assessment question 6.19 (page 133)

■ **SAQ 6.19.** Remembering the capsular attachments of the glenohumeral joint, which movements would you expect to be particularly limited [in adhesive capsulitis]?

Answer: External rotation would be the most limited, and abduction would be the second most limited. Internal rotation and flexion should be virtually free.

Problem-solving exercise 6.8 (page 134)

See information in text.

Self-assessment question 6.20 (page 135)

Answer follows question in text.

Self-assessment question 6.21 (page 135)

See the following section in the text.

REFERENCES

Amiel D, Chiu C R, Lee J 1995 Effects of loading on metabolism and repair of tendons and ligaments. In: Gordon S L, Blair S J, Fine L J (eds) Repetitive motion disorders of the upper extremity. American Academy of Orthopaedic Surgeons, Rosemont, p 217–230

Astrom M, Rausing A 1995 Chronic Achilles tendinopathy. Clinical Orthopaedics and Related Research 316:151–164

Clancy J, McVicar A J 1995 Physiology and anatomy. A homeostatic approach. Edward Arnold, London

Corrigan B, Maitland G 1983 Practical orthopaedic medicine. Butterworth, London

Crawford Adams J, Hamblen D L 1990 Outline of orthopaedics, 11th edn. Churchill Livingstone, Edinburgh

Cyriax J 1982 Textbook of orthopaedic medicine: the diagnosis of soft tissue lesions, 8th edn. Ballière Tindall, London, vol 1

Dandy D 1993 Essential orthopaedics and trauma, 2nd edn. Churchill Livingstone, Edinburgh

Desrosiers E A, Methot S, Yahia L H, Rivard C H 1995 Response of ligamentous fibroblasts to mechanical stimulation. Annales de Chirugie 49(8):768–774

Evans P 1980 Healing at cellular level. Physiotherapy 66(6):256–259

Freeman M A R, Wyke B D 1967 Articular reflexes at the ankle joint. British Journal of Surgery 54:990

Hertling D, Kessler R 1990 Management of common musculo-skeletal disorders. Physical therapy principles and methods, 2nd edn. J B Lippincott, Philadelphia

Low J, Reed A 1994 Electrotherapy explained, 2nd edn. Butterworth Heinemann, Oxford

Noyes F R, Torvic P J, Hyde W B, DeLucas J L 1974 Biomechanics of ligament failure. 2. An analysis of immobilisation, exercise and reconditioning effects in primates. Journal of Bone and Joint Surgery 56A:1406–1418

Oestern H J, Laque K 1992 Classification of soft tissue injury. Acta Chirurgica Belgica 5:228–233

Ogilvieharris D J, Gilbart M 1995 Treatment modalities for soft tissue injuries of the ankle – a critical review. Clinical Journal of Sports Medicine 5(3):175–186

Reynolds C A, Cummings G S, Andrew P D, Tillman L J 1996 The effect of non-traumatic immobilization on ankle dorsiflexion stiffness in rats. Journal of Orthopaedic and Sports Physical Therapy 23(1):27–33

Smith N 1995 Physiotherapy practice: its relevance to healing and sports injuries. British Journal of Therapy and Rehabilitation 2(6):301–305

7

Rheumatic conditions

- Rheumatology ■ Connective tissue disorders ■ Pharmacological management
- Physiotherapy management ■ Osteoarthrosis ■ Rheumatoid arthritis
- Ankylosing spondylitis ■ Patient education ■ Function
- Biopsychosocial effects of chronic disease

CONTENTS

Objectives

By the end of this chapter you should:

1. Have an overview of rheumatic disorders.
2. Be aware of the similarities and differences between the various conditions in this group.
3. Have an overview of the assessment of patients with rheumatic disorders.
4. Recognise how to problem solve during the assessment and treatment of rheumatology patients whatever the condition or the extent of medical intervention.
5. Understand how physiotherapy management is related to pharmacological intervention.
6. Be aware of the types of physiotherapy intervention possible with a range of patients with rheumatic conditions, including patient education and a focus on a functional approach.
7. Begin to understand the implications of chronic disease for the patient including biomedical, psychological and social factors.
8. Have an overview of the roles of the members of the health care team in the management of patients with rheumatic conditions.

Prerequisites

Read the introductory chapters of the book in order to have an understanding of the background to the problem-solving approach. It is also particularly important to have read the section in Chapter 2 on the structure and function of articular cartilage. Reacquaint yourself with the features of normal synovial joints and connective tissue throughout the body (bone and cartilage are particularly important). Use any anatomy book for this, but for detailed information see, for example Williams et al *Gray's anatomy* (Williams et al 1989; see References at end of chapter). For a brief overview, see *Essential orthopaedics and trauma* (Dandy 1993), Chapter 3, pages 29–39.

Familiarise yourself with the changes that occur during inflammation and revise the cardinal signs. Make sure you understand the mechanisms involved in the development of oedema and how this can affect function.

INTRODUCTION

The approach of this chapter will be a little different from earlier ones in that it is dealing with the management of patients who have problems due to a disease process taking place in the body, rather than being due to some sort of trauma. Although the consequences of trauma can be far reaching and may involve a number of complications, with most patients it is isolated to one area of the body. But with the conditions discussed in this chapter you will discover that many patients also have to cope with wider ranging systemic problems which can affect how they react to treatment, as well as their motivation and compliance levels. For example, rheumatoid arthritis patients will find themselves extremely fatigued much of the time and this has implications for the amount and intensity of exercise that they are able to carry out. Your role as a physiotherapist often involves helping the patient to function as effectively as possible within the limits of the disease.

The range of interventions available for use in rheumatic conditions help to alleviate, but do not abolish their effects. Many patients still have to contend with pain, deformity and reduced quality of life despite extensive treatment. This would suggest that other measures such as patient education are necessary to help the patients cope with the diseases and to enable them to cooperate with the management which may be complex (Kirwan 1990). The physiotherapist is often an important link for the patient, providing much of the information necessary in this educational process.

Physiotherapists are likely to encounter patients with rheumatic disorders in all areas of practice and across all age groups. In many cases the primary problem will be arthritis, and in fact it may be the diagnosis most commonly encountered in clinical practice (Banwell & Gall 1988). At other times it may be secondary to the main problem, but it can still have a significant effect on how much the patient is able to do. Consequently it is important that all physiotherapists have a working knowledge of how to problem solve in the assessment and treatment of patients with rheumatic conditions.

Much work has been carried out in the field of rheumatology, and over the last 20 years a great deal has been discovered about the pathophysiology of the diseases as well as the mechanisms that occur during pharmacological treatment.

Treatment approaches have also developed and changed in the field of physiotherapy, especially regarding the use of exercise and the application of physical agents such as ice and electrotherapy modalities. Many of the physiotherapy treatments used in the management of patients with arthritis are in themselves quite routine. However, it is the decision making with regard to when the treatments would be most effective, combined with patient education and a focus on function that are the essential skills to learn. This also has to be closely integrated with the pharmacological management and the intervention of other members of the health care team.

THE RHEUMATIC DISORDERS

Over one hundred distinct rheumatic diseases

have been identified. The list is not static, with some problems becoming less common (e.g. acute rheumatic fever), new diseases emerging (e.g. Lyme disease and the rheumatic consequences of HIV infection), new concepts being described and some diseases being redefined in the light of further research (Christian 1992).

It is not the purpose of this chapter to try to cover all of these diseases, but rather to give a framework for physiotherapists to use in assessing and treating patients with rheumatic disorders, many of whom have very similar signs and symptoms.

The rheumatic disorders are also sometimes known as 'connective tissue syndromes'. This name indicates the more wide ranging aspects of these conditions. They are commonly thought to affect mainly the joints, hence the term 'arthritis', and many of them do have severe joint signs and symptoms. However, a large number of these conditions cause problems with connective tissue throughout the body, not just the bone and cartilage, and also have marked systemic effects. There are also some that do not affect the joints at all. In the rheumatic conditions that physiotherapists come across most commonly, the articular symptoms are often the ones that cause the most overt problems for the patient. But extra difficulties will be caused by the background symptoms such as fatigue, gastrointestinal problems, anaemia, neuropathies and so on.

Table 7.1 does not provide an exhaustive list of the rheumatic disorders, but gives an idea of the range of conditions subsumed into the field of rheumatology.

The causes of the rheumatic disorders are mainly unknown although more evidence is gradually being discovered by research. Some are much better understood than others. For example the mechanisms causing gout were described in the 1950s and 1960s, and because of this drugs have been developed that can prevent its occurrence (Gall E P 1988). However, with a disease such as rheumatoid arthritis, the aetiology is much more difficult to discover. There are thought to be several factors involved: (i) the genetic make up of the host; (ii) the immune response of that particular person, and (iii) some initiating or inciting agent (Bennett 1985). However there are so many variables it is not possible to be sure of the exact cause, and if the cause of a disease is not understood it is much more difficult to prevent its occurrence. As more is understood about the mechanisms causing these diseases, the more effective treatment will become, but in many cases at present the diseases are still chronic and incurable.

Only a few examples will be used in this chapter to represent the most common disorders that you, as a physiotherapist, are most likely to encounter. However by applying the principles you learn here to any patient with a rheumatic condition, you should be able to formulate a coherent problem list and plan of treatment.

Table 7.1 Summary classification of rheumatic disorders (adapted from Gall E P 1988)

Disorder	Examples
1. Diffuse connective tissue diseases	Rheumatoid arthritis, juvenile arthritis, systemic lupus erythematosus
2. Arthritis associated with spondylitis	Ankylosing spondylitis, psoriatic arthritis
3. Degenerative joint disease	Osteoarthrosis
4. Arthritis, tenosynovitis and bursitis associated with infectious agents	
5. Metabolic and endocrine diseases associated with rheumatic states	Gout, amyloidosis, diabetes mellitus, hypermobility syndromes
6. Neoplasms: primary or metastatic	
7. Neuropathic disorders	Charcot joints, peripheral entrapment such as carpal tunnel syndrome
8. Bone and cartilage disorders associated with articular manifestations	Osteoporosis, osteomalacia
9. Non-articular rheumatism	Tenosynovitis and/or bursitis, low back pain, myofascial pain syndromes, vasomotor disorders
10. Miscellaneous disorders	Haemophilia, internal derangement of joints

Review points

Before going on to read about the drugs used in rheumatic conditions, review the information so far. Try to think how your approach to patients with these diseases may have to be different from that used in patients with a fracture or soft tissue injury.

CATEGORIES OF DRUGS USED IN THE TREATMENT OF RHEUMATIC CONDITIONS

You will find that virtually any patient referred to you with problems due to a rheumatic condition will be taking medication. In some conditions such as rheumatoid arthritis, 'polypharmacy' is the norm, i.e. the patient with active disease will be taking a number of different drugs to combat the disease (Furst 1990, Swezey 1990a). It is not necessary for you to know every drug available, as there are many of them and new ones are being produced all the time. (If a patient mentions a drug that you are not familiar with, there should always be a reference book available to look it up in – MIMS or a British National Formulary.) But you should be aware of the categories of drugs that may be used, their effects and possible side-effects, as the patients' pharmacological management may have a bearing on their abilities to respond to your treatment and so in turn upon its efficacy.

What is expected of pharmacological therapy is alleviation of pain and swelling, reduction of inflammation and preservation of joint integrity and function (Sterling 1990, Swezey 1990a). Symptoms arising from established deformity and secondary degenerative changes will not respond (Butler 1990). Many of the drugs do cause adverse reactions due to either their pharmacological effects or patient hypersensitivity. The effects are usually mild and the patient can continue to take the drug with a dose reduction. Occasionally the effects are severe and the drug has to be stopped altogether (Brooks 1990).

Analgesics

Pain is a 'biological early warning system' which indicates tissue damage. In the case of rheumatic conditions it can arise by a number of different mechanisms which can be categorised under the headings of inflammation and mechanical derangement. It is important that the origin of the pain is pinpointed as far as possible so that the correct treatment modalities can be applied during management (Turner-Stokes 1993).

Pain is usually the symptom uppermost in the patient's mind, and sometimes analgesics will be prescribed in order to combat this or they are given as an adjunct to other drugs for symptomatic relief. Centrally acting analgesics can reduce perception of pain but have the tendency to cause constipation and drowsiness. An exception to this is paracetamol. These drugs are often prescribed but have on occasions been reported by patients to be unhelpful (Turner-Stokes 1993).

Quite often, the anti-inflammatory properties of the other varieties of drugs used in these conditions have an analgesic effect in themselves.

Non-steroidal anti-inflammatory drugs (NSAIDs)

These are generally the first agents to be employed in many rheumatic conditions. They combine pain-relieving effects with an additional action which reduces inflammation as they impede the production of inflammatory prostaglandins (Arthritis and Rheumatism Council for Research 1995, Turner-Stokes 1993).

Self-assessment question

- **SAQ 7.1.** A NSAID will suppress the classical features of inflammation (Thompson & Dunne 1995). What are these features?

These drugs are indicated where joint or soft tissue inflammation causes pain, stiffness and swelling (Table 7.2). In the acute situation a few days of treatment will usually quickly control symptoms after which the dose can be reduced or the drug stopped altogether. In chronic conditions the initial dose should be low and several drugs tried, to find the one best tolerated by the patient (Thompson & Dunne 1995).

Aspirin is often used as it is cheap and can be taken for up to a year by 60% of patients. A large

Table 7.2 Indications for the use of NSAIDs (adapted from Thompson & Dunne 1995)

Acute (short-term use)	Arthritides Gout Pseudogout Acute inflammatory flare of osteoarthrosis (Plus sports injuries, postoperative pain relief, dysmenorrhoea)
Chronic (prolonged use of drug)	Rheumatoid arthritis Ankylosing spondylitis Psoriatic arthritis Other connective tissue diseases featuring polyarthritis

dose is necessary (large that is, in relation to that taken for a headache), possibly starting with 12 tablets a day and gradually increasing (Furst 1990, Ruddy 1985). There are side-effects including tinnitus and gastrointestinal problems, but it is the least toxic of available treatments (Zurier 1990).

If the patient cannot tolerate aspirin, the next choice may be one of the other NSAIDs such as ibuprofen, diclofenac, naproxen or indomethacin (Arthritis and Rheumatism Council for Research 1995). Many patients have to try up to three of these agents before finding one that suits them, as there is individual variability in response, the reasons for which are still uncertain (Furst 1990, Thompson & Dunne 1995). They are expensive drugs and the side-effects can be more marked, such as renal function impairment, photosensitivity of the skin, bronchospasm, haematological changes, gastrointestinal problems and central effects including headache, dizziness and nausea (Brooks 1990, Thompson & Dunne 1995). Because of these problems, the long-term use of this type of drug may be contraindicated.

Disease-modifying antirheumatic drugs (DMARDs) or slow-acting antirheumatic drugs (SAARDs)

These drugs are said to be remission-inducing agents but in fact they often have unknown and probably diverse mechanisms of action, although gradually the pharmacokinetics are being eluci-dated (Brooks 1992). It is hoped that they modify the disease process. The effect of the drugs is delayed; the patient may not notice any change for 6 weeks to 3 months or longer after starting to take them (Furst 1990). As a physiotherapist, you should take this into account when assessing a patient, ensuring that you discover when a particular drug was started. This will give you a truer picture of any changes in the patient's symptoms.

Rather than just affecting the inflammation, it is thought that these agents have a more fundamental action on the disease process than NSAIDs, causing changes in laboratory test results such as erythrocyte sedimentation rate and immunoglobulin levels (Furst 1990, Ruddy 1985). It is now felt that inflammation in rheumatic diseases requires early and aggressive treatment with combinations of NSAIDs and DMARDs. As with NSAIDs there is variability in response to DMARDs and so one should be chosen that reduces symptoms and has minimal side-effects (Brooks 1992).

These drugs can be divided into two groups: weak, which are slightly less effective but less toxic, and strong. Antimalarials (chloroquine and hydroxychloroquine), often used in the treatment of rheumatoid arthritis and systemic lupus erythematosus, are weaker but have proven to be better than placebo and there is less drop out due to toxicity. There are still side-effects which include indigestion, skin rash and visual disturbances.

Sulphasalazine has been shown to be effective in the treatment of rheumatoid arthritis and the seronegative spondyloarthropathies. This drug has many toxic effects such as gastrointestinal upsets, rash, nausea, liver abnormalities and central nervous system disturbance. Here 50% of patients develop side-effects and half of these may need to stop treatment because of them (Brooks 1990, 1992, Furst 1990).

The stronger DMARDs include gold preparations (e.g. gold sodium thiomalate), d-penicillamine, azathioprine and methotrexate. Again their exact mechanisms of action are not well understood and they can have marked side-effects.

Gold has been used for the longest time (since 1935) and has also been studied extensively.

Patients on this treatment need to be monitored carefully for haematological and adverse renal effects and 10–20% have to stop taking it (Brooks 1992, Furst 1990).

D-penicillamine has side-effects similar to those of gold, but it may also cause bone marrow suppression (Brooks 1990, Ruddy 1985).

Azathioprine has anti-inflammatory and immunosuppressive effects. However, along with this there seems to be some evidence of a correlation between taking the drug and an increased incidence of malignancy, as well as other side-effects (Brooks 1992, Furst 1992).

Methotrexate is an easy drug to use in the treatment of rheumatic conditions. But again it has significant side-effects such as the possibility of liver fibrosis and cirrhosis, gastrointestinal problems, pulmonary hypersensitivity reactions or adverse central nervous system effects, including unpleasant sensations, mood alteration or memory impairment (Brooks 1992, Zurier 1990).

No single DMARD completely stops inflammation and so there is an increasing emphasis on the use of combinations of these drugs. There is also a change in when they are given in the course of the disease; the tendency is to administer them earlier in the management. If the drug prescribed is not effective then there may be repeated change to other agents, the so-called 'saw tooth strategy' (Fig. 7.1; Brooks 1992, Fries 1990).

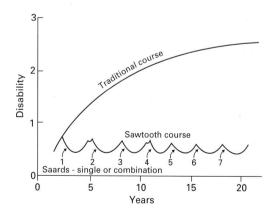

Figure 7.1 Treatment strategy for rheumatoid arthritis SAARDs, slow-acting antirheumatic drugs. (Adapted from Brooks 1992.)

Corticosteroids

These drugs play a major role in the management of inflammatory rheumatic diseases and, used carefully, can reduce symptoms and slow the destructive progression of joint disease (Brooks 1992). As with many of the drugs used in rheumatic conditions there are side-effects which in this case include water retention, osteoporosis and peptic ulceration, but at low doses these may not occur (Brooks 1992, Smith et al 1990).

Recent studies have looked into the use of intravenous 'pulses' of methylprednisolone. Results seem promising, at times giving spectacular clinical improvement, but the duration of efficacy is variable (Smith et al 1990). Pulses of prednisolone have also been shown to enhance the response of some patients to gold therapy (Brooks 1992).

Local corticosteroid injections

Steroid injections can alleviate pain and swelling. In conjunction with appropriate NSAID therapy and splinting they can help in the effective management of rheumatic conditions. The steroids are rapidly taken up by the synovium and improvement may be seen within hours and can be maintained for weeks or months. Occasionally the synovitis does not recur. The types of rheumatic condition that respond well are rheumatoid arthritis, reactive arthritis, connective tissue disorders such as systemic lupus erythematosus, psoriatic arthritis, other types of seronegative spondyloarthropathies and the inflammatory stages of osteoarthrosis. Examples of the preparations available for injection are methylprednisolone acetate, prednisolone phosphate and dexamethasone phosphate (Golding 1991).

Drug therapy: an important point

At the present time drug therapy is central in the treatment of rheumatic disorders and undoubtedly has a marked effect both on the patients' conditions and on how they respond to the other treatments available. One very important point is to remind your patients that they should not stop taking their drugs or change the dosage just because they are attending for physiotherapy. If they do this it will be impossible for you to ascertain whether it is your intervention or other factors that are responsible for causing any improvement or deterioration.

Self-assessment question

■ **SAQ 7.2.** Briefly review the types of drug used in the management of rheumatic conditions. What are the effects of each type? Try to give examples of the names of drugs in each category.

OSTEOARTHROSIS

Osteoarthrosis (OA) has been mentioned a number of times already in earlier chapters. This used to be considered a disease mainly affecting the elderly, caused by 'wear and tear'. But more recent work suggests that this is not the case and that there could be some genetic cause of the disease. Presently there are no interventions that are known to alter the long-term outcome of this condition, but there are many possible approaches that can help to alleviate the clinical problems it causes (Hutton 1995).

OA occurs with great frequency throughout the world. X-ray evidence has shown OA changes (joint space narrowing, subchondral sclerosis and osteophyte formation) in the joints of 40–60% of the population over 35 years of age. This percentage does increase with age, reaching as much as 85% in those over 75. More women show changes than men, particularly after the age of 55, but by the age of 50, X-ray changes of OA in the lumbosacral area are seen in 90% of the population (Kaufman & Sokoloff 1992). Things are not quite as grim as they sound, however, because only a small percentage of these people actually have any clinical signs such as pain, deformity and decreased joint range.

OA can affect both the axial and peripheral joints, but some joints are often involved whilst others are rarely affected (Hutton 1995). The condition is progressive and the underlying pathological processes are both destructive and productive (Gall E P 1988) so the use of the term 'degenerative joint disease' can be misleading.

Table 7.3 Classification of OA (adapted from Kaufman & Sokoloff 1992)

1. Primary (idiopathic) OA
   Can be localised or generalised
2. Secondary OA
   (a) Mechanical aberrations, e.g. meniscectomy, fracture, slipped epiphysis, avascular necrosis
   (b) Pre-existing inflammatory arthritis, e.g. rheumatoid arthritis
   (c) Occupation-related
   (d) Metabolic disease, e.g. haemophilia, gout
   (e) Neuropathic arthropathy
   (f) Immobilization
3. Endemic, i.e. only found in a certain population or in a certain region

The balance of these processes can result in either stable non-progressive and often asymptomatic disease or progression to joint destruction (Hutton 1995). There are also secondary inflammatory changes which contribute to the destructive mechanisms.

Three possible processes are postulated by which the alterations in cartilage may develop:

1. Abnormal mechanical forces which induce the failure and loss of cartilage.
2. Increased bone stiffness preceding and causing cartilage damage.
3. Chondrocyte dysfunction.

These mechanisms may be tempered by a number of factors such as age, sex hormones, obesity, physical activity, diet, heredity, structural and anatomical incongruities and metabolic disorders. This gives the range of classification seen in Table 7.3. From the available information it can be assumed that although OA is not a disease that particularly targets the elderly, its clinical effects may only become apparent and perhaps disabling in later life, meaning that many of the patients seen in physiotherapy departments with problems due to OA do tend to be older.

Self-assessment question

■ **SAQ 7.3.** What are the three main classifications of OA?

Pathological changes in OA

If you have not done so already, it would be a

good idea to read the section on articular cartilage in Chapter 2 as this will give you the 'normal' background on which to superimpose the 'abnormal' changes occurring in this disease. It is important for you to have some idea of what actually goes on inside the joints during the pathogenesis of OA.

In ageing joints, the metabolism, enzymatic modelling, collagen synthesis and the nature of the surrounding tissues remain normal (Bland 1993). But as you are already aware, changes do occur in articular cartilage with increased age. These include a decrease in water content, reduction in the tensile strength and stiffness of collagen, decrease in glycosaminoglycan chain length and fragmentation of the stabilising link glycoproteins. But these are not the same changes that occur in OA, where not just the cartilage but virtually all the tissues in and around the joint become thicker, hyperplastic and hypertrophic. This then results in increasing clinical deformity (Bland 1993, Carlstedt & Nordin 1989, Kaufman & Sokoloff 1992).

In OA there is damage to the chondrocytes and there are multiple mechanical and biological factors that can contribute to this. These cells make up about 5% of the total cartilage mass. They are responsible for synthesising and secreting the bulk of the rest of the cartilage, i.e. proteoglycans, link proteins, collagen type II and hyaluronic acid; they also regulate breakdown of the cartilage with proteolytic enzymes. Exercise, movement and force upon the joint is absolutely essential for maintenance of the cartilage (Gall E P 1988). It has been found that changes similar to OA can occur during immobilisation. However, a clinically significant finding is that the cartilage returns to normal when mechanical stimulation resumes, i.e. normal weight bearing. But if the joint is subjected to vigorous exercise at this stage the cartilage does not return to its normal state and the OA-type changes can be accelerated (Bland 1993).

Hyaline cartilage has a shock-absorbing function and its failure can be caused by either excessive loading of normal cartilage or physiological loading of abnormal cartilage (Bland 1993). Once the chondrocytes are damaged, matrix breakdown results from release of chondrocytic

enzymes and, overall, the development of OA seems to be an imbalance between synthesis and breakdown of cartilage, and attempts to repair the damage are followed by a failure in the system. The changes include an increase in water content, a reduction in the width of collagen fibrils and an overall decrease in the total proteoglycan content. Protease activity increases and the chondrocytes synthesise collagen of the Type I and III variety at the expense of the normal Type II. At the beginning of the pathological process there is considerable metabolic activity, but as the process advances the chondrocytes fail and this activity decreases. This is what causes the decrease in proteoglycans which in turn causes stiffness in the cartilage which becomes more susceptible to mechanical disruption (Gall E P 1988, Kaufman & Sokoloff 1992).

The surface of the collagen becomes roughened and particles are released which are absorbed by the synovium. There may also be crystal deposition (e.g. calcium pyrophosphate and hydroxyapatite) within the joint. Both of these factors cause an inflammatory response. But the disease is still classified as non-inflammatory because it is not a primary pathological change.

The subchondral bone is also abnormally active with an increase in bone density and in the number of cells present. New spurs of bone (osteophytes) form at the joint margins which can restrict movement (Fig. 7.2).

The bone beneath the cartilage becomes hard and dense, and there may be a change in the shape and congruity of the articular surfaces which will in turn affect where the weight passes through the joint. As the cartilage fails, the bone beneath is exposed and becomes hard and 'eburnated'. Without the articular cartilage to enhance movement, friction increases and weight transmission is uneven. Microfractures can occur which heal with callus making the bone even harder, denser and less resilient. Synovial fluid can enter cracks in the bone and form subchondral cysts (Dandy 1993).

Figure 7.3 shows exposed bone and osteophytes on the upper surface of the medial plateau of the tibia (which has been removed during an operation for total knee replacement).

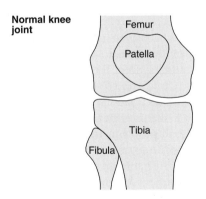

Normal knee joint

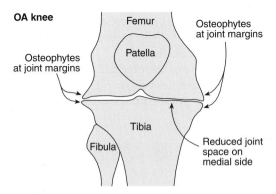

OA knee

Figure 7.2 Formation of osteophytes at joint margins.

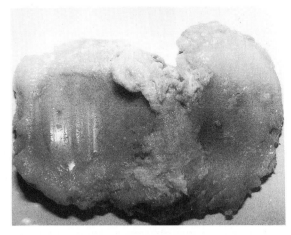

Figure 7.3 Changes on the upper surface of the medial tibial plateau in osteoarthritis (OA) (Reproduced with permission from Dandy 1993).

If the disease continues to advance, the joint becomes more and more disorganised with decreased joint space, osteophytes, instability and deformity (Fig 7.4).

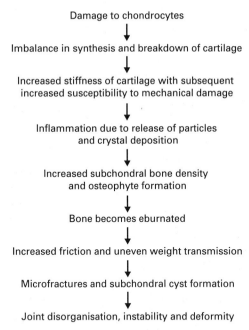

Damage to chondrocytes

↓

Imbalance in synthesis and breakdown of cartilage

↓

Increased stiffness of cartilage with subsequent increased susceptibility to mechanical damage

↓

Inflammation due to release of particles and crystal deposition

↓

Increased subchondral bone density and osteophyte formation

↓

Bone becomes eburnated

↓

Increased friction and uneven weight transmission

↓

Microfractures and subchondral cyst formation

↓

Joint disorganisation, instability and deformity

Figure 7.4 Summary of possible joint changes in OA.

Primary OA

In primary OA, that is, where the disease occurs spontaneously, the first joints to be affected are often small joints in the hand, such as the interphalangeal joints, the first carpometacarpal joint and occasionally the intercarpal joints; and the first metatarsophalangeal joint in the foot. There are also nodes that appear over the interphalangeal joints called Heberden's nodes (distal) and Bouchard's nodes (proximal); these are usually painless (Kaufman & Sokoloff 1992). The upper limb joints can be painful and range of movement may be lost, but more disabling problems tend to occur with the other areas to be affected which are the larger weight-bearing hip and knee joints and the spine (Dandy 1993).

In the elderly, OA of the knee is the most common cause of disability, with the pathological changes usually only occurring in the medial compartment. In this joint, the X-ray changes and the clinical findings parallel each other; this is unusual in OA where generally the radiographic evidence predates any clinical manifestations (Kaufman & Sokoloff 1992).

In OA of the hip the pain begins insidiously, is

usually bilateral, and leads to a limp (antalgic gait). Occasionally a patient will complain of low back pain initially, if a flexion contracture of the hip has increased the lumbar lordosis.

Within the spine the OA changes can occur both at the level of the intervertebral disc and in the synovial joints. There is little correlation between changes in the intervertebral disc and clinical signs of low back pain syndromes; however when the movable joints are affected, symptoms do occur (Kaufman & Sokoloff 1992). It is important to remember that not all of the above areas of the body will be affected in every patient with OA.

Secondary OA

A summary of the possible causes of secondary OA is shown in Table 7.3, and these are numerous. Because of this wide range of factors, not only those joints associated with primary OA will be affected; others can also be involved.

If there is an abnormality within a joint due to earlier damage, osteoarthritic changes may ensue. An example of this could be a fracture through the joint surface and consequent irregular contour due to malalignment. Soft tissue damage can also be responsible for mediating OA. For example, if a meniscus is removed from the knee because it is torn or a cruciate ligament damaged, then the biomechanics will be affected. As Wolff postulated in 1892 this tends to cause a change in the physical stimuli within the joint which in turn lead to adaptive bone formation and resorption. (This has already been mentioned in Chapter 2 on the development and growth of bone. Go back and read it again if you need to refresh your memory.) In a normal structure this remodelling would minimise the strain. But because there is already an abnormality, it tends to cause premature osteoarthritic changes. Irregularities within joints can also be due to genetic or developmental problems such as Perthes' disease, epiphyseal dysplasia or slipped epiphysis (Dandy 1993).

Inflammatory arthritis causes damage to the articular surfaces which again can predispose to premature changes of OA, and secondary OA is a common consequence of rheumatoid arthritis.

There does seem to be a correlation between OA in certain joints and specific occupations. Not all of the work has been conclusive, but for example, miners seem to develop OA in the hips, knees and shoulders; foundry workers in the elbows; fingers, elbows and knee are affected in dock workers, and occupations that involve a lot of kneeling (for instance carpenters and farmers) are associated with problems in the knee joints. These changes are thought to occur because of mechanical stresses (Kaufman & Sokoloff 1992). Conversely, as mentioned earlier, immobilisation can also adversely affect the cartilage initiating OA-type changes.

There seems to be a correlation between certain types of metabolic or endocrine disorders and osteoarthritic changes.

Age, sex, race, heredity and obesity are also implicated in the development of OA, but this may be as true for the primary disease as well as the secondary.

Self-assessment questions

- **SAQ 7.4.** Which joints are the most commonly affected in primary OA?

- **SAQ 7.5.** List the possible causes of secondary OA.

Problem-solving exercise 7.1

- With the information you have been given so far, try to work out the probable clinical features you would expect to find in a patient with OA.

If you are not sure, or wish to see if you are on on the right lines, remember you can check your ideas later in the chapter under the relevant section or at the end of the chapter.

Assessment of the patient with OA

Case study 7.1

Mrs Stamford (1)
This 70-year-old lady is attending for outpatient physiotherapy for the first time with a diagnosis

of OA knee. She has noticed increasing pain with decreased mobility in her left knee joint for the last 5 years. This has only caused her problems in the preceding 6 months and seems to be getting worse. She walks with one stick in her left hand.

Problem-solving exercise 7.2

- Decide what you need to find out during your assessment of this patient:

    1. During your subjective assessment, and
    2. during your objective examination.

- Write down a checklist of what you feel would be appropriate questions and examination techniques.

Case study 7.1

Mrs Stamford, continued (2)

On assessment the following information was obtained:

Subjective assessment

This retired teacher has had increasing problems with pain and loss of movement in her left knee for the last 5 years, but has only had functional problems in the last 6 months. These seem to be increasing in severity.

The pain is continuous but worse on movement and locomotion. It often disturbs her sleep.

The knee feels particularly stiff in the morning but loosens up quite quickly when she starts to move around. However, she generally describes the left knee as 'stiff' in comparison to the right.

She identifies her main problem as being unable to walk far enough because of pain to perform her everyday activities such as shopping, walking the dog, housework (particularly getting up and down stairs) and visiting friends. She bought the walking stick herself and finds it helps a little, but has been given no instruction in its use.

Social history: widow, living alone in a terraced

house half a mile from the nearest shops, unable to drive. Bathroom and bedroom upstairs. Four steep steps to front door. Two grown-up children living away, neighbour helps with shopping once a week.

Hobbies: walking and bowls. Unable to take part in these activities for last 6 months.

Drug history: takes aspirin as necessary for the pain. Has never taken steroids.

Previous medical history: nil of note. General health good.

Objective assessment

Observation
Patient walks with a stick, favouring left leg. Found getting up from the chair difficult after sitting for a while. Some problems removing shoe and tights from left leg. Left knee joint looks swollen and quadriceps appear decreased in bulk. Joint held in slight flexion when on plinth. Slight genu varus deformity (see Fig. 7.5). Skin colour/condition: normal.

Knee
Palpation: left knee tender on palpation medially and posteriorly. Soft effusion but no increased temperature.

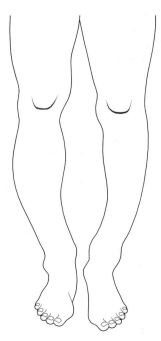

Figure 7.5 Genu varus deformity at the knee joint.

Thickening around the joint line.
Right knee: nothing abnormal discovered.

Examination
Range of movement:
Right knee active and passive: full range.
Left knee passive: extension, –5°; flexion, 90°
with discomfort at end of range.
Left knee active: extension, –5°; flexion, 80°
with pain throughout range increasing towards
maximum flexion.
Hips and ankles: full range, equal right and left,
no discomfort.

Swelling (measured at base of patella): left,
40 cm; right, 34 cm.

Muscle bulk:
5 cm above base of patella; left, 38 cm; right,
39 cm.
15 cm above base of patella; left, 38 cm; right,
42 cm.

Muscle strength: quadriceps and hamstrings on
left Gd IV; all other groups Gd V both sides.
Stability: some laxity of the joint is obvious on
testing collateral ligaments, with an increase in
pain on the medial side on varus stress.

Functional assessment
The patient has some difficulties with washing
and dressing the lower half of her body.
Walking distance is limited by pain and the
patient goes up and down steps one leg at a
time. Both ability to move from sitting to
standing and back, and bed mobility are
affected by the pain.

You now have a great deal of information
about this lady and her particular difficulties.
The next step is to sift out the main issues and
problems that you would wish to address in the
management of the patient. Before going on to
this, let's review the main areas involved in
assessment that are used to establish the initial
database. This then acts as a basis for identifying
problems, the goals of treatment in relation to the
patient's needs and designing a treatment plan in
partnership with the patient.

Assessment guidelines

The physiotherapist should be alert, listen and
respond to the questions and needs of the patient
during the assessment. It should be an interactive
session relating to the patient's goals which
change with age, lifestyle and the stage of the
disease process. The time of day that the assessment occurs and the level of patient activity just
prior to it should be taken into account (Gall V
1988).

Subjective information

*Demographic details and history of the present
condition*

1. Diagnosis.
2. Onset including symptoms, rate of
   progression and whether it is better or worse
   at present.
3. Joints affected.
4. Main problems as described by the patient,
   e.g. pain levels/behaviour, stiffness, loss of
   function. (Some of these could be assessed
   using visual analogue scales or numerical
   rating scales.)
5. Functional ability (could use some sort of
   functional scale for assessing this).
6. Systemic problems. (This will not be an issue
   for the patient with primary OA.)
7. Any previous treatment and its effect. (Not
   for the patient in this case study.)

General health and past medical history

Medication/drug history

1. Present drugs including dosage and effects.
2. Drugs taken previously with any side-effects;
   reasons for stopping. Has the patient taken
   steroids in the past?

Splints
Not relevant for this patient.

Social history

1. Occupation
2. Hobbies
3. Accommodation
4. Family/carers
5. Any help available from social services or
   voluntary organisations.

Objective information

General observation

1. Appearance
2. Gait.

A lot can be learned from observing how a patient gets up from the chair in the waiting room, walks through to the treatment area, turns to look at the physiotherapist, prepares for the physical examination, gets onto the plinth, and so on. These observations can then be used as cues to personalise the questioning during the subjective part of the assessment (Gall V 1988).

Joints involved

1. Observation of any apparent swelling/effusion, colour changes, skin condition, deformity, etc.
2. Palpation to ascertain temperature, skin condition, type of effusion, thickening, tenderness, muscle spasm and any sensory disturbances.
3. Physical examination to discover amount of swelling and muscle wasting, range of movement/stiffness, end feel, stability, muscle strength and extent/nature of any deformity.

It is important to try to differentiate where the pain is coming from. In general pain of joint origin is characterised by discomfort throughout the range whereas that from tendons or bursae can be isolated by palpation and is more likely to occur during part of the range of movement. Muscular pain can be indicated by local tenderness or by discomfort on a particular movement. It is likely to be aggravated by active contraction (Caldron 1995).

Extra-articular manifestations
Not relevant for this patient.

Functional assessment

1. Activities of daily living assessment, e.g. stairs, transfers, washing, dressing, walking, occupation, housework, hobbies, driving, and so on as appropriate.
2. Health assessment questionnaire such as the Arthritis Impact Measurement Scale (AIMS)

which also takes psychosocial and general wellbeing issues into account as well as functional problems (Hutton 1995, Rheumatic Care Association of Chartered Physiotherapists (RCACP) 1994).

This is an excellent opportunity for you to check back to the list you made in response to problem-solving exercise 7.2. See how many of the areas of the assessment you managed to come up with independently, and fill any gaps by using the information above.

This general layout will give you an overall structure to use in the assessment of most patients with rheumatic conditions in the clinical setting. Obviously assessment practices vary from centre to centre, but on the whole these are the areas that should be covered by the physiotherapist. Some departments will have their own ready-printed sheets or booklets to fill in as the patient is questioned and examined, which can be very useful as a prompt particularly for students and newly qualified staff. Part of an assessment booklet is shown in Figure 7.6.

Problem-solving exercise 7.3

■ Use the information given in the case study to try to identify this patient's major problems. Then go on to think about the goals of physiotherapy management that you could use in order to design your treatment plan.

Clinical features of OA

By now you should have a good idea of the different clinical manifestations of OA that are of relevance to the physiotherapist. This section gives a brief overview.

Clinically patients experience gradually developing joint pain with stiffness, enlargement of joint size and limitation of movement (Levine 1988).

Note here that 'stiffness' and 'limitation of movement' are used separately as if describing different concepts. Stiffness is a difficult

| ✓ *Promis* | *rheumatology assessment* |

Patient's Name		Unit No.

HISTORY PRESENT CONDITION

PREVIOUS TREATMENT/OUTCOME

PHYSIOTHERAPY TYPE (inc. HYDRO)	DATE	OUTCOME
OCCUPATIONAL THERAPY TYPE		
OTHER		

EARLY MORNING STIFFNESS	NO	YES - DURATION

RELEVANT PAST HISTORY

Course of Disease	Date onset of initial symptoms:
Therapist signature:	Date

Every entry must be signed

Figure 7.6 See also pages 155–157. A section of a ready printed assessment booklet for use with rheumatology patients. (Reproduced with kind permission of the Physiotherapy Department, Royal National Hospital for Rheumatic Diseases NHS Trust, Bath, UK.)

✓ Promis   *rheumatology assessment*

Patient's Name		Unit No.
SURGICAL INTERVENTION		DATE OF OPERATION
1		1
2		2
3		3
4		4

INVESTIGATIONS; X-RAYS

AREA	RESULT
1	1
2	2
3	3
4	4

CERVICAL SPINE; Subluxation	YES	Stable	YES	/	NO

INVESTIGATION: OTHER		RESULTS
1		1
2		2
3		3

SOCIAL HISTORY & services received

PAST	DRUG HISTORY	CURRENT

Therapist signature:	Date

NB: every entry must be signed

Fig. 7.6 *(cont'd)*

✓ *Promis*   *rheumatology assessment*

Patient's Name		Unit No.	

GENERAL HEALTH

Significant illnesses

	Cervical Spine Active range of movement		Lumbar Spine Active range of movement	
	Admission	Discharge	Admission	Discharge
Rotation Left				
Rotation Right				
Side Flexion Left				
Side Flexion Right				
Flexion				
Extension				
Therapist signature:			Date	

GLOBAL PAIN SCALE

ADMIT DATE

0   10

OTHER DATE

0   10

DISCHARGE DATE

0   10

Every entry must be signed

Fig. 7.6 *(cont'd)*

√ *Promis*				*rheumatology assessment*			
				SPECIFIC JOINT PROBLEMS			

Patient's Name				Unit No.			
	ADMISSION			DISCHARGE			
JOINT	ACTIVE R.O.M. (L) (R)	PASSIVE R.O.M. (L) (R)	MUSCLE STRENGTH (L) (R)	ACTIVE R.O.M. (L) (R)	PASSIVE R.O.M. (L) (R)	MUSCLE STRENGTH (L) (R)
Therapist signature				Date			

Every entry must be signed

Fig. 7.6 *(cont'd)*

phenomenon to define and is described in varying ways by patients. What they describe as 'stiffness' is often a collection of factors that may include some link with pain, muscle weakness and/or limitation of movement at a joint (Rhind 1987). It is a multifaceted feature of many rheumatic conditions and although patients appear able to assess its severity, they have difficulties with definition and are often ambiguous in the terms they use. The reason that this is being stressed here is that it is important for the physiotherapist to spend some time investigating the patients' perceptions of the state of their joints, i.e. the subjective aspects, as well as carrying out the objective tests. Some physiotherapy departments may use questionnaires to find out about these points, an example of which can be seen in Figure 7.7. This is particularly related to the hand but could be adapted for any stiff joint/area of the body. It utilises a series of visual analogue scales to describe the ease and quality of movement, a list of descriptors (after Rhind 1987) to ascertain which factors the patient associates with stiffness, some functional questions to ask about specific activities and also giving an opportunity to describe the main problems.

Limitation of movement, although an element of 'stiffness', is much more of an objective quantity which can be measured and recorded. But the results of both the objective and subjective tests will make up part of the initial database that the physiotherapist uses later to ascertain whether or not any changes have occurred as a consequence of intervention.

Because of the pain and limitation of movement, most often found in the weight-bearing joints, there is usually an effect on levels of function. In the later stages there may well be instability and deformity (Adler 1985, Dandy 1993). When the patient presents for assessment, the physical signs are quite variable, but may include effusion, synovitis, laxity and muscle weakness (Adler 1985). The usual symptoms that cause the patient to seek treatment are the pain and loss of function as these are the ones that have a marked effect on lifestyle.

Pain

This is usually at its worst when the joint is under load during movement or weight bearing (Dandy 1993, Hutton 1995). The pain may also continue after activity but is usually relieved by rest (Kaufman & Sokoloff 1992). There is no nerve supply to the hyaline cartilage but other periarticular structures, bone and capsule, are richly innervated and these give rise to the pain. If there is a secondary inflammatory response in a particular patient then this may also release substances that act as pain mediators, such as prostaglandins and cytokines (Hutton 1995, Kaufman & Sokoloff 1992).

The patient may describe the pain as localised or very diffuse and it can be referred to an unaffected joint, for example to the hip from the back, to the groin and knee from the hip or from the knee up the thigh and into the hip area.

Initially there will be periods when the patient is pain-free, but later on the pain will be constant and may disturb sleep.

Limitation of movement

This usually occurs slowly as the joint surfaces change shape and osteophytes form. The pain may prevent the patient moving through full range which could result in shortening of soft tissue structures so leading to further loss of movement and deformity.

If there is joint laxity, the patient may have a sense of instability and be unwilling to move fully which again, combined with the pain, will decrease mobility (Dandy 1993, Hutton 1995).

Loss or alteration of function

All of the factors mentioned so far will have a tendency to change the patients' abilities to carry out functional activities. As with the loss of movement, this process can be insidious with patients subconciously restricting their actions to those permitted by the affected joint(s). They may walk shorter distances, only go upstairs when absolutely necessary, or not work for as long or as hard without a pause. This process tends to be self-perpetuating as with decreased activity the muscle power will also decrease so causing the joint to be less stable, putting more stress on the structures so increasing pain, limitation of movement and possibly deformity. Any deformity in one joint will inevitably have an

Hand Questionnaire

This questionnaire makes up part of the assessment of your hand. The information your physiotherapist obtains from it will be used to help formulate a treatment plan tailored specifically for you. It is easy to fill in, it consists of placing a mark on several scales, choosing from a list of words and answering some simple questions. Please complete it and hand it in before you leave the department. Thank you.

1. Please place a mark on the following scales at the point you feel appropriate for the state of your hand at the moment. When you try to make a fist with your affected hand:

(a) How fully can you move it?

```
|_____|
No movement                                    Full movement
```

(b) How easily can you move it?

```
|_____|
Extremely easily                        With great difficulty
```

(c) How painful is it?

```
|_____|
Not painful at all                 The worst pain I can imagine
```

(d) How stiff does it feel?

```
|_____|
Extremely stiff                                   No stiffness
```

2. Please place a ring around any of the words below that describe the way your hand feels:

Limited movement   Painful   Tight   Rigid

Weak   Tense   Stuck   Hurts   Inflexible

Sore   Immobile   Aches   Solid

3. The following questions apply to everyday activities, please circle Yes or No as appropriate:

(a) Can you EASILY write with a pen/pencil?   Yes   No

(b) Can you EASILY turn a key in a lock?   Yes   No

(c) Can you EASILY tie the laces on a pair of shoes? Yes   No

(d) Can you EASILY button an article of clothing?   Yes   No

(e) Can you EASILY open jars of food?   Yes   No

4. What activity would YOU describe as most difficult due to your hand problem?

_____

_____

_____

_____

_____

_____

Thank you for filling in this questionnaire. Remember to hand it in BEFORE you go home today.

Figure 7.7 An example of a questionnaire that could be used to investigate hand stiffness in patients with rheumatic conditions.

effect on adjacent areas of the body and so signs and symptoms may extend over time. For example if the OA hip becomes fixed in a degree of flexion and nothing is done to prevent the consequences of this, then the level of the pelvis may drop on that side in order for the heel to reach the floor which in turn may lead to low back pain and other problems.

Much disability results from secondary weakness. If there is suitable intervention from the health care team at the appropriate time, many problems may be avoided and satisfactory functional levels maintained.

X-ray appearance

It is important for the physiotherapist to be able to recognise the common changes of OA on radiographs. The main features are:

1. narrowing of joint space
2. sclerosis (increased density) of the bone on the weight-bearing surfaces
3. formation of osteophytes at joint margins
4. possible appearance of subchondral cysts
5. changes in the shape of the bone and possibly deformity.

Many of the above features can be seen in the X-ray of an OA knee joint in Figure 7.8.

Identification of patient problems and goals of management

By now you should have the information that you need in order to identify the probable difficulties that this patient will have. This in turn should allow you to come up with physiotherapy goals which you could use in the management of this patient with OA. Go back and check on your response to problem-solving exercise 7.3 (p. 153) and compare it with the points discussed in this section.

As part of the overall process of assessment, the physiotherapist must use skill and judgement in problem solving to decide initially whether or not the patient can be helped by treatment and a self-care programme. This is probably the case with Mrs Stamford, but in some patients the disease may have progressed so far that physiotherapy intervention would be of no benefit and

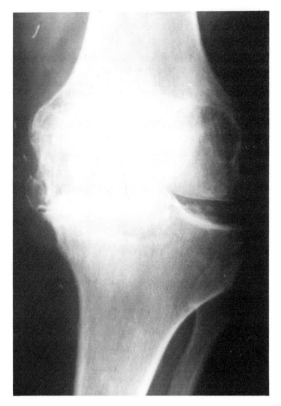

Figure 7.8 X-ray of an OA knee joint (Reproduced with permission from Dandy 1993).

surgery may be the only recourse. If this were the situation, then you may have to refer them back to the consultant/general practitioner.

For the present case study the problems that you should have identified from the information given about Mrs Stamford were:

- pain
- stiffness/limitation of movement
- muscle weakness
- functional difficulties, particularly gait problems such as walking any distance and going up and down stairs and steps.

So in the light of these identified problems, what goals might the physiotherapist decide on in partnership with the patient?

1. Reduction of pain.
2. To maintain or increase (if possible) range and ease of movement.

3. To maintain or increase (if possible) muscle strength.
4. To correct deformity or prevent any further deformity occurring.
5. To maximise functional potential and maintain or increase exercise tolerance.
6. To educate, advise and support the patient with regard to her condition.
7. To encourage the patient to take on responsibility for self-care and self-management.

Whenever necessary these goals of treatment should be formulated and carried out in liaison with other members of the health care team as appropriate, but remember that the patient is the most important facet here and the goals must take her wants and needs into consideration.

Did your list of problems and goals of treatment match these? Don't worry if you did not manage to come up with all of them. If you came up with all of those mentioned above and more — well done! But just check to ensure that they are all relevant and realistic and that you had not gone on to talk about the actual management of the patient. That's the next step.

> **Self-assessment question**
>
> ■ **SAQ 7.6.** What possible changes might you expect to see on an X-ray of a patient with OA?

GENERAL MANAGEMENT PRINCIPLES FOR PATIENTS WITH RHEUMATIC CONDITIONS

The most important issue to remember with any patient who has a rheumatic condition, is that no treatment can influence the disease progression. The principles should be the same as managing any chronic disease, with education of the patient being a key factor. It is important for health care professionals to work with patients to identify realistic expectations of intervention, and to try to help them to develop a sense of control over the disease (Hutton 1995).

When considering management in all types of rheumatic conditions you must remember several points:

1. The time course of the disease, i.e. it is a chronic condition for which (in most cases) there is no 'cure'.
2. The variability of the disease from time to time in the same patient (perhaps not quite so relevant in OA), and also from patient to patient. Many of the conditions are phasic with exacerbations and remissions. Thus it is sometimes more difficult to know whether it is the intervention that is helping or whether the patient is just entering a slightly 'better' phase. The effect that drugs may have on the condition must also be remembered and taken into account when evaluating intervention.
3. Optimal management involves the combined health care team; usually no one person can meet all of the patient's needs. Effective and comprehensive care can only be provided when the specific problems of the patient, the resources available and the patient's environment are taken into account (Banwell 1988).

In general then, management has to be geared towards the following areas:

- Minimisation of damage/destruction in the joints and other tissues.
- Maximisation of function within the boundaries of the disease.
- Matching of goals to the needs of the particular patient.

It can be seen that these aims of management relate in general terms to those already identified as aims of physiotherapy intervention.

Ruddy (1985) states that the goal of management should be the 'maintenance or restoration of the patient to a state of useful and harmonious function with her environment for the forseeable future'. In order for this to be achieved, as well as pain and functional levels, the patient's psychological status and satisfaction with treatment need to be taken into account (Wolfe 1990). This is why the physiotherapist, along with other members of the health care team, needs to take an holistic approach when planning and carrying out the management of patients with rheumatic conditions.

Review points

Use your background knowledge and the information given in this chapter to work out who might be included in the health care team responsible for the management of patients with rheumatic conditions (hint: they will not all be health care professionals).

Elements of general management

Pharmacological management

As explained earlier in the chapter, most patients with rheumatological conditions will need some sort of drug therapy as part of their management.

Rest

Although exercise has been suggested as the best form of physical treatment in the management of rheumatic conditions (Clarke 1987), it is important for many patients that this is balanced with rest periods at times throughout the day. This is especially pertinent in those conditions where fatigue may be one of the symptoms, for instance rheumatoid arthritis. Rest periods during the day have been found to improve symptoms, minimising general fatigue and local joint discomfort. But the balance between rest and exercise is essential to avoid the extra complications caused by immobility (Jarvis 1978, Swezey 1990a,b).

Occupational therapy

The occupational therapist (OT) has traditionally offered a functional approach to the management of patients with rheumatic conditions, giving practical answers to everyday problems. This may involve retraining in activities of daily living (ADL), from household and personal tasks to work and leisure activities. The OT can assist by assessing for and providing special equipment for the home and any other relevant situations (e.g. leisure, work) and teaching people how to approach problems in an active, positive way (Clarke 1987, Jeffreson 1993).

One area particularly important for those patients with rheumatic conditions is that of 'joint protection'. Both the OT and the physiotherapist may be involved with this.

Problem-solving exercise 7.4

'The destructive consequences of repetitive impulse loading [of joints] in some activities of daily living can be reduced with careful advice given to the patient' (Adler 1985).

■ With the information you have so far about the problems encountered by patients with rheumatic conditions, try to come up with a list of general points that could help a patient to protect joint surfaces and surrounding structures.

Physiotherapy

This is considered to be an important part of the management of patients with rheumatic conditions. Responsibility for physical rehabilitation falls largely to the physiotherapist at all stages, although there will be areas of overlap with other health care professionals. There are many modes of treatment that the physiotherapist can employ and, as with drug treatments, they need the same thoughtful application, monitoring and 'fine tuning' in order to fit the particular patient (Swezey 1990b). We will return to physiotherapy management later.

Patient education

This is thought to be beneficial in helping patients to cope with their disease and may also enhance compliance and cooperation with management interventions (Kirwan 1990). It might seem reasonable to assume that if a patient is being treated for a rheumatic condition, then he or she will be presented with information and will learn from that. However, this does not seem to be the case. Kay & Punchak (1988) reported relatively poor levels of knowledge in patients with a long history of arthritis who had regular contact with health professionals. Out of 100 patients, 54 felt they had received no information about the course of their disease, probable symptoms and prognosis. In general they all wanted more information. This would suggest a need for a more formalised system of patient education.

Nevertheless, before a programme of education is devised, the possibility of adverse effects must also be considered. It has been suggested that for patients with a recent onset of a chronic illness, information could cause depression, feelings of helplessness and fear (Kirwan 1990). Donovan et al (1989) also suggest that confusion can occur if the content of the programme 'does not relate to the beliefs of the group or the individual'. It must be remembered that education is an adjunct to standard care and not a substitute, and it must be adapted to the current needs of the patient.

Taking these points into account, work has been done which suggests that education for arthritis patients can be beneficial in certain aspects of management. They have shown improvements in knowledge, performance of exercises, joint protection and disability scores (Lindroth et al 1989). In some cases relaxation increased, as well as there being a decrease in pain and depression (Lorig et al 1989). However, results regarding reduction in pain have been inconsistent and therefore the aim of the programme should perhaps be to increase function within the same pain threshold (Kirwan 1990). There is evidence that more positive outcomes for health status and prognosis correlate with higher education levels and self-efficacy levels. Programmes have also been shown to positively affect knowledge levels, behaviour, attitude, disability and depression. With this evidence it is suggested that the effectiveness of current treatments for arthritis can be enhanced through education.

new information can be built onto that which already exists. It is therefore important for an agenda to be agreed by both patient and the 'educator', who could well be a physiotherapist. If this is done, it should help to enhance patient compliance, self-efficacy and coping strategies (Brattstrom 1987, Kirwan 1990).

As well as providing information and advice, the programme can also be used to reinforce any instructions from the health care team, help the patient to achieve appropriate behavioural changes and offer emotional support. It can also be used with carers (Clarke 1987, Ruddy 1985). Programmes found to be successful have the characteristics shown in Figure 7.9.

An educational programme can be arranged by a variety of people and in a variety of ways. This will probably depend more on local staffing and resources than any other factors. It could take place when a patient comes for treatment, but there is not always the time available in a busy department. Special educational sessions may be organised specifically to teach the patients about their condition. One or a number of health professionals may be involved, based at a hospital, clinic or GP practice, or the programme may be organised entirely by a self-help group run by patients and carers with input from an organisation such as the Arthritis and Rheumatism Council (ARC). This could still involve some health professionals with, for instance rheumatologists, physiotherapists or OTs perhaps being asked to come in and speak on particular areas of interest, to give demonstra-

---

Problem-solving exercise 7.5

- **A.** What subjects do you think could be usefully covered in an educational programme for patients with rheumatic disorders?

- **B.** In what ways do you think the information can be communicated to the patients?

An educational programme should be based on the needs and beliefs of the patient, so that

Characteristics of successful educational programmes
Relate to the needs and beliefs of the patient
Emphasise relief of pain and disability
Use interactive teaching methods in group settings
Develop self-management techniques, problem solving and self-efficacy
Employ exercise training

Figure 7.9 Characteristics of successful educational programmes (Kirwan 1990).

tions of equipment or run exercise sessions. For example, some National Ankylosing Spondylitis Society (NASS) groups are run on a weekly basis by physiotherapists who often work voluntarily, usually setting up exercise sessions on dry land and with hydrotherapy if a pool is available.

The meetings can be opportunities for questions and answers, group discussions, films and videos, lectures, practical exercise groups, distribution of literature and also social interaction.

The advantages of a group setting are that more people can be seen at one time, wider issues may be brought up for discussion, encouragement is often given to new members and each patient realises he or she is not the only person with the condition and the particular problems it engenders. These groups often take place outside the hospital setting and so may help patients to be less reliant on health professionals and to take more responsibility for their own management.

There are some disadvantages to the group sessions in that the information given is not tai-

lored for specific patients, and some people are discouraged by seeing others worse than themselves.

These problems are negated if it is possible to see the patients on a one-to-one basis, i.e. it is possible to make the information pertinent to each person and to ensure that they understand. But there are often difficulties with time constraints, and this method may also make the patients focus very much on their own problems.

The sort of information and advice that could be included in an educational programme for patients with rheumatic conditions can be seen in Figure 7.10. Compare this with the suggestions you came up with in response to Problem-solving exercise 7.5. This list is a basis to work from which can be added to or subtracted from as necessary to make the programme as relevant as possible to the members of the group.

Joint protection
As mentioned earlier joint protection is especial-

**Patients with Rheumatic Conditions
Educational Programme**

Nature, progression and prognosis of condition

Management

Drugs: effects and possible side-effects

Exercise/relaxation techniques

Activities of daily living (ADL) and joint protection

Surgery

Resources available, e.g. in community

Splints and orthotics

Aids and appliances

Alternative therapies

Physical problems, e.g. sexual, related to contracture/deformity

Counselling (may be available depending on local resources)

Possible variety of cognitive or behavioural strategies for coping with pain

Figure 7.10 The type of information/advice that may be included in an educational programme for patients with rheumatic conditions (Banwell 1988, Brown et al 1989, Clarke 1987, Ruddy 1985).

Principles of joint protection for patients with rheumatic conditions

1. Where possible, use the strongest and largest joints to accomplish a task.

2. Spread the load of carrying and lifting over several joints; no one joint should ever be subjected to maximum load.

3. Use each joint in its most stable and functional position.

4. Use body mechanics effectively.

5. Put less effort into accomplishing a task.

6. Maintain joint mobility and function: exercise, but where possible under low load conditions.

7. Avoid maintaining a joint in one position for prolonged periods of time (including tight grips) especially those that exacerbate a pattern of deformity.

8. Avoid excessive activity.

9. Take an equal number of rest periods as work periods.

10. Select tasks carefully.

11. Respect pain as a warning sign.

12. Avoid 'internal' as well as 'external' stresses.

Figure 7.11 Principles of joint protection for patients with rheumatic conditions (Brattstrom 1987, Clarke 1987, McKnight 1988, Swezey 1990b).

ly important for patients with rheumatic conditions. After looking at Figure 7.11, you should go back and compare the points it covers with those you came up with in response to Problem-solving exercise 7.4. Again the list of areas mentioned is general and designed to apply to patients with a range of conditions. A little later the principles will be applied more specifically to the case study you are considering.

Surgery

This is another element of the general management of many patients with rheumatic conditions. The improvement in the surgery available for these patients over recent years has probably been one of the most significant advances in treatment. It is carried out for a number of different reasons but the most common, and probably of most significance to patients, is its use in relieving pain. It can also correct deformity,

improve function, improve cosmesis and in some cases prevent further joint damage or damage to the nervous system. This is in addition to any operations performed to repair structures such as tendons (Clarke 1987, Swezey 1990a). Probably the most common operation to be carried out is arthroplasty (joint replacement) where part or all of the joint surfaces are removed and replaced with an artificial joint.

Two other common types of operation are arthrodesis (fusion) of a painful or unstable joint, and osteotomy (where a wedge of bone is taken out or inserted in order to realign the joint) which can be used to redistribute stress to a less damaged part of the joint, so relieving pain or to correct deformity.

Splinting

This may be used in the general management of patients with rheumatic conditions. Whether or not a splint is needed in the first place and then the type and purpose of it should be determined by the assessing clinician, i.e. physiotherapist, OT, splint technician, orthotist.

Splints can be used for a number of reasons:

1. To relieve pain.
2. To rest an inflamed joint.
3. To increase range of movement, e.g. serial splinting.
4. To provide support and stability, e.g. a hard collar to support the neck in a patient with an unstable atlanto-occipital joint.
5. To improve function by holding joints in a more functional position.
6. To prevent or correct deformity.
7. To aid mobility, e.g. footwear adaptations (RCACP 1994).

Self-assessment question

■ **SAQ 7.7.** What are the elements involved in the general management of patients with rheumatic conditions?

ELEMENTS OF PHYSIOTHERAPY MANAGEMENT IN PATIENTS WITH RHEUMATIC CONDITIONS

As mentioned earlier, physiotherapy is generally considered to play an important part in the management of patients with rheumatic conditions. This management includes the use of a large range of skills, techniques and concepts which can be implemented in whole or in part depending on the individual needs of each patient. Although largely related to the patient's physical rehabilitation, the physiotherapy input also impacts upon psychosocial aspects of the patient's life.

As already explained, assessment is essential, providing information on the patient's physical condition and functional levels. It also helps with overall understanding of the patient, so enabling the physiotherapist to design a treatment programme. The aims of physiotherapy management were listed earlier in relation to the case study.

Self-assessment question

■ **SAQ 7.8a.** What are the aims of physiotherapy management for patients with rheumatic conditions?

■ **SAQ 7.8b.** Why is it important that these aims are matched to the patient's needs and beliefs?

Pain relief

It is important to realise that none of the treatments in the physiotherapist's armamentarium will permanently reduce pain. They may reduce it temporarily so allowing the patient to perform more active exercise, or they could be used after exercise to soothe any 'treatment pain'. It is hoped that more permanent pain relief may occur in response to other types of intervention (see later).

The main physical modalities available to the physiotherapist for pain relief are heat, cold and some electrical techniques. But weight-relieving and supportive methods may also be included here, such as provision of walking aids and splints. Hydrotherapy is a specific method which combines heat with weight relief and ease of movement. There may also be a place for less orthodox treatments, such as acupuncture, depending on the skills of the particular physiotherapist involved.

Heat

Heat has been used for many years in different forms, varying from superficial infrared irradiation, hot packs and wax to the deeper, more penetrating short-wave diathermy and, more recently, low power laser therapy.

Many claims have been made for these methods but very few of them are supported by scientific evidence. In fact a recent study carried out by Goats et al (1996) on low intensity laser and phototherapy for rheumatoid arthritis (RA) concluded that these treatment methods have little to offer the rheumatoid patient. Swezey (1990b) states that heat 'increases molecular activity, causes vasodilatation, and increases nerve conduction, and can be used to facilitate stretching and, above all relieve pain'. Admittedly, these are very useful effects. However, he goes on to point out that it can also 'increase collagenase activity and potentially aggravate joint damage', which of course is very undesirable in patients with rheumatic conditions where joint damage is what management is aiming to minimise.

Therefore, the simpler and more superficial methods of heating are probably of most use for their short-term pain-relieving effects. They can help to reduce muscle spasm so that exercises can be carried out in more comfort. These simpler methods are also easier for the patients to duplicate at home by the use of hot water bottles, heat pads and warm baths or showers.

Cold

Cold is also used by the physiotherapist, but again for short-term pain relief. In contrast to heat, cold slows down the metabolism and reduces the speed of nerve conduction. Ice treatment should precede exercise and again patients can duplicate the method at home. Elderly patients particularly often prefer heat to cold as it is more soothing and comforting (Clarke 1987, Swezey 1990b).

Electrical techniques

There are several stimulating electrical modalities available to the physiotherapist; probably the most commonly used are interferential and transcutaneous nerve stimulation (TNS).

Claims have been made that these have longer lasting analgesic effects due to the release of endorphins by the body in response to the stimulation. Also, TNS machines are often available for patients to borrow to take home to wear over a longer time. It is also possible to buy them commercially if a patient finds this method of treatment particularly helpful. However, they have not been found to be very successful in peripheral joint pain control (Swezey 1990b).

As mentioned earlier the pain-relieving techniques available to the physiotherapist should not be used as treatments in themselves, but should always be used in conjunction with active exercise (Clarke 1987, Grahame & Cooper 1986, Haralson 1988, Ruddy 1985, Swezey 1990b).

Exercise

It has been suggested that exercise is perhaps the best form of treatment for patients with rheumatic conditions. The physiotherapist's role here is extremely important in advising on the correct levels of exercise and rest for each individual (Banwell 1988, Swezey 1990b). The necessity and reasons for exercise seem fairly well agreed upon. It helps to maintain or increase joint range, muscle strength and flexibility, as well as providing general conditioning. Traditionally patients have been excluded from vigorous activity because of their particular problems. Physicians have in fact tended to advise curtailment of exercise of this sort. However, it has been shown that people with arthritis have poor physical fitness and do have more problems due to inactivity (Ike et al 1989, Minor et al 1989).

Nordemar (1981) observed RA patients who carried out physical training for a period of 4–8 years in comparison to a control group with the same condition. The results showed significantly higher ADL capacity in the trained group, and the control group reported a more pronounced feeling of weakness and more discomfort from joints after physical strain than those in the trained group.

Ike et al (1989) report subjects with arthritis as making significant gains in aerobic capacity, functional status, muscle strength and other aspects of performance, after participating in an aerobic exercise programme. They also improved in subjective areas such as quality of life, pain tolerance, joint pain, mood and social activity.

Minor et al (1989) took RA and OA patients through a 12-week programme of exercise. They were randomised into three groups, doing aerobic walking, aerobic aquatics or non-aerobic range of motion (controls). The walking and aerobic groups showed significant improvement over the controls in aerobic capacity, 50-foot walking time, depression, anxiety and physical activity. All three groups showed improvement in scores for flexibility, number of clinically active joints, duration of morning stiffness and grip strength, indicating the importance of all types of exercise. However, the aerobic groups maintained a higher level of improvement over 1 year. They continued exercising on their own because they felt the benefit. With regard to drugs, all subjects either kept on the same dosage or reduced it; none needed an increase.

The results of these and similar studies indicate the efficacy of exercise for patients with arthritis. But all of the authors emphasise that the patients need to be well motivated and that the exercise should be supervised and of low to moderate intensity. Swezey (1990b) indicates the importance of supervision by pointing out that if exercise increases joint pain which does not subside within 2 hours, or if it causes pain and swelling which increase overnight, it is probably excessive and indicates a need for reduction in intensity.

The patient should also be encouraged to undertake leisure activities if possible, such as walking, dancing, swimming or golfing for other reasons including enjoyment and social interaction, i.e. exercise for its own sake (Banwell 1988). Even in people with no disease, physical activity has been reported as having a favourable effect on anxiety states and stress (Eide 1982), so this may be another positive factor for those with chronic disease.

In general the nature of the exercise will depend on the acuteness of joint symptoms at the time, and so treatment must be altered accordingly. This could be done for example by showing isometric methods of strengthening and reducing repetition rates during an acute period (Swezey 1990a).

Hydrotherapy

This is an ancient and popular form of treatment which, in the broadest sense, involves the external application of water for therapeutic purposes. This usually means the patients attending a warm hydrotherapy pool for exercise and relaxation.

Movement through water provides much of the resistance, and progression is achieved by working through from the easy exercise to the most difficult. The advantage here is the self-regulating nature of the exercise, in that the harder the patients work the more resistance is experienced, but this will never be more than they can manage. The water allows an almost infinite range of resistance for patients at any stage of a condition. This is a definite advantage for patients with rheumatic disease.

Buoyancy is another helpful hydrodynamic effect which reduces the amount of weight passing through the lower limbs so decreasing pain in those patients whose joints are aggravated by weight bearing. The warmth of the water also has a sedative, pain-relieving effect.

The reason that hydrotherapy is so suitable for patients with arthritis (as well as patients with other musculoskeletal/locomotor conditions) is that due to the ease of movement in water it allows exercise which may be totally impossible on dry land. This can boost morale and increase confidence. Being immersed in a pool also exercises the whole body, there is less focus on one particular area, and more of the body can be treated in less time. Large numbers of joints and muscles can be exercised in different planes with minimal change in starting position, which is an advantage for those patients who find changing position on dry land painful or difficult. Patients may learn how to swim or become confident enough in the water to then continue with exercise at their local swimming baths.

As with any treatment there are some disadvantages. It is expensive and occasionally more debilitated patients find that they are too fatigued to benefit fully from the hydrotherapy. Some people do become rather dependent on the treatment and there are a number of contraindications.

Studies have been carried out which suggest that hydrotherapy is an effective form of treatment for patients with rheumatic conditions. Reports from patients of physical, functional and psychological improvement, better quality of life and feelings of increased wellbeing, and a lack of major adverse effects would seem to support this contention (Danneskiold-Samsoe 1987, Dial & Windsor 1985, Sukenik et al 1990, Tork & Douglas 1989).

APPLICATION OF MANAGEMENT PRINCIPLES TO THE CASE STUDY

You should now have an overview of the principles that may be of use in deciding on the most appropriate type of intervention. Before going on to consider some of the other common conditions you are likely to come across, let us return to Mrs Stamford to think a little more specifically about how these principles could be applied in her case. It must be remembered that these will only be suggestions relating to a hypothetical situation, and you must use your problem-solving and decision-making skills to decide what would be the best approach for each patient you deal with.

Just as a reminder, this lady has pain and swelling in the left knee, stiffness, reduced range of movement (with some deformity), muscle wasting and weakness; all of which have led to a decrease in function. She identifies her main problem as not being able to walk far enough to carry out her usual activities.

Problem-solving exercise 7.6

■ Using the information provided earlier, jot down your suggestions for the management of this patient.

Firstly, this is not a patient whom you will see on a regular basis for a number of weeks. It is much more likely that after assessment you will give exercises and advice and then have occasional checks to see how she is progressing. If a patient is reassured and given advice, this is often sufficient as long as the opportunity is given to contact the physiotherapist if there are any problems. This means that there is not a feeling of isolation and worry. Obviously this system depends on the patient being willing to comply with the self-care type of management. If this is not the case, then it is important to agree a certain number of treatments with the patient and then to make it clear that discharge will occur after completion of the last visit.

As with many patients with OA, pain is presented as a major factor. Considering the information already given, it is unlikely that any treatment modality available to the physiotherapist will alleviate this. However, there will be ways in which the physiotherapist can help the

patient to change her behaviour which in turn may help to reduce the pain in the longer term.

It is important to explain something of the pathology of OA to the patient (if this has not been done before) and to discuss how this has affected her activities. This will mean that the patient is better able to understand the suggestions that are made regarding treatment. It will also contribute to the process of identifying realistic expectations for intervention. Many patients are reassured by being given information, particularly if it helps them to understand the low probability of a 'crippling outcome' (Hutton 1995).

We will assume that this patient has been prescribed some appropriate anti-inflammatory and/or pain-relieving drugs by her GP. This will do much to alleviate the pain and reduce swelling, but it is vital that you also teach the patient how to reduce pain as much as possible herself.

Some of the pain may be due to the fact that there is muscle weakness and deformity in and around the knee, so altering the joint biomechanics. It will be important to teach the patient exercises she can carry out at home to increase strength and to increase range of movement. In order to make this easier you can also advise her to apply superficial heat or an ice pack to the area (whichever she prefers) either before or after the exercises. Provision of an exercise sheet will act as a reminder. This could be already available in the department or you may need to make one up with specific exercises for the patient. In the case of Mrs Stamford the exercises would include work for the quadriceps, hamstrings and probably the glutei which can be taught in a variety of starting positions.

If the flexion deformity in the left knee has a bony end feel (i.e. fixed flexion deformity) then you will not be able to improve this. However, if there is a soft end feel but the joint is stiff, you may be able to mobilise it further into range. The patient must be encouraged to maintain this with her home exercises. You would not be able to improve the varus deformity, but the strengthening exercises may help to prevent further angulation. Unfortunately contractures have a tendency to recur as enthusiasm for maintenance exercises may not be long-lived, depending on the patient.

As discussed earlier, weight bearing often increases pain in OA joints. Therefore a walking aid will help to reduce the compressive forces applied to the joint surfaces and so reduce the pain. Mrs Stamford already has a stick but you should check it for height and safety and then instruct her in correct usage, i.e. particularly to use it in the right hand to deflect weight onto the unaffected leg (Hutton 1995). This can be combined with any necessary gait re-education.

Advice on the careful use of her joints will also be an important factor here and may be of considerable help in alleviating pain from over- or incorrect use. This relates back to the earlier information on joint protection. There are a number of points that may be helpful for this patient. If she is overweight there may be extra forces passing through the knee which will exacerbate her symptoms. You should encourage weight loss which will help function and reduce loading on the left knee. She should also be advised not to carry heavy weights and perhaps could use a shopping trolley, wheeled suitcases, and so on, which again reduce joint loading.

Climbing any step (for instance stairs, getting onto buses, kerbs) increases the compressive force in the knee joint to 4.25 times that of body weight (Adler 1985). You can therefore advise Mrs Stamford to lead with her unaffected leg on the way up and the affected one on the way down, so putting the stress on the non-painful limb. At home it is sensible to try to limit the number of times she goes up and down stairs each day, for example, perhaps, going up to the toilet and then performing several tasks such as making the bed, fetching clean laundry from the airing cupboard and so on, before coming downstairs again. She should also use banisters, her stick, lifts and escalators whenever available. Check her footwear and emphasise the benefits of having a cushioned sole or insole to prevent jarring.

When rising from the sitting position the forces through the knee joint are again increased. If the arms are used to help push up then the corresponding forces are much less (Ellis 1981). It is also helpful to increase the height of seats by putting blocks under the legs of the chair (and possibly the bed) or extra cushions, or newspapers under the cushions. A raised toilet seat could also be provided if necessary, probably in liaison with social services or the OT department. It may be possible to fit rails in the bathroom/toilet if this patient finds getting up from the toilet and getting in and out of the bath particularly difficult.

It would be useful to advise against standing for long periods. There may be activities that can be carried out just as easily in sitting or, possibly, perched on a high stool (e.g. ironing, preparing food, washing up). Kneeling should be discouraged and the use of long-handled tools suggested. If the patient insists on kneeling then a thick foam pad or knee pads could be used (Adler 1985).

Walking distance is a problem for this patient. She should be encouraged to continue taking walks but to plan them so that they involve calling on a friend or sitting on a seat halfway, so that she can rest before going on. Improved use of her stick will help as should the increased strength in the surrounding muscles and any decrease in pain. She should start with short distances and gradually try to increase them without aggravating her symptoms too much.

Mrs Stamford may not find all of these ideas easy to accept at first, especially if it means changing long-standing behaviour patterns. But it is hoped that by giving clear explanations and discussing the issues with her, you would be able to persuade her to try them. For some of the changes in the home it may be advisable to request the community physiotherapist to visit her if this service is available. This gives the opportunity to tailor advice very specifically to the patient's own circumstances. Carers or friends may also be present and their help could perhaps be enlisted to encourage the patient to try out the new methods of carrying out everyday tasks.

If the patient is able to comply with the management plan you have devised together, she should find that the pain does decrease and she is able to carry out her ADL more easily.

Let us return briefly to the list of goals we identified earlier in the chapter:

1. Reduction of pain.
2. To maintain or increase (if possible) range and ease of movement.
3. To maintain or increase (if possible) muscle strength.
4. To correct deformity or prevent any further deformity occurring.
5. To maximise functional potential and maintain or increase exercise tolerance.
6. To educate, advise and support the patient with regard to her condition.
7. To encourage the patient to take on responsibility for self-care and self-management.

Review points

Consider the suggested interventions for Mrs Stamford and see whether all of the above goals have been addressed.

MATCHING INTERVENTION TO GOALS

Let us assume that Mrs Stamford is a compliant patient who takes careful note of all your advice and acts upon it. The following section shows how the management plan applies to the earlier goals.

1. Pain relief:
   — drug treatment
   — application of heat or ice
   — reduced loading of the joint by careful use, walking aid, change of behaviour, improved muscle strength.
2. To maintain or increase range and ease of movement:
   — regular exercise
   — pain relief due to above factors.
3. To maintain or increase muscle strength:
   — regular exercise
   — gradual increase in activity level.
4. To correct deformity or prevent further deformity occurring:
   — as for point 3, especially the mobilising exercises to correct deformity, and the strengthening to prevent further deformity occurring.
5. To maximise functional potential and maintain or increase exercise tolerance:

— ability to do more as pain decreases and strength/mobility increases
   — changes in methods of carrying out ADI
   — aids provided
   — improved use of stick, gait re-education.
6. To educate, advise and support the patient with regard to her condition:
   — information about OA and how it has affected the patient's abilities
   — advice on exercise and ADL
   — availability of physiotherapist over the telephone for further support if necessary
   — follow up appointment for reassessment
   — provision of literature from department and possibly leaflets and videos from ARC as an adjunct to treatment.
7. To encourage the patient to take on responsibility for self-care and management:
   — overall approach to management of patient but with contact when necessary to prevent patient feeling isolated or unsupported.

The interaction of these goals and interventions may vary from patient to patient, depending on their attitude to health, the home environment and the severity of the condition, but this gives an example from which you can extrapolate. You may need to use all or only some of the ideas suggested, and once you are more used to dealing with this type of patient, you will develop your own approach.

Remember, your problem-solving abilities in any particular area improve with experience but you also need to have a good knowledge base from which to work. In this way you move from being a novice towards the expert end of the continuum.

Before moving on to rheumatoid arthritis, you will be presented with a more complex case study of a second OA patient. Use the information you have gained so far to think about which aspects of your physiotherapeutic intervention would be similar and which different to those of Mrs Stamford.

Case study 7.2

Mr Nicholls
This gentleman is 70 years old with a 20-year

history of OA. He is a retired carpenter (retired at 60 due to problems with knees, hips and right shoulder). He had a right hip replacement 4 years ago, but over the last year the pain in the right knee has increased markedly and his mobility is severely limited. He has been admitted to the orthopaedic ward for a right knee replacement.

He lives with his wife in a terraced house with steep stairs. His bed was moved downstairs 6 months ago; there is a downstairs toilet.

On observation he is rather overweight and moves with difficulty, complaining of pain both at rest and on movement. Right knee is swollen, with decreased muscle bulk, fixed flexion deformity (15°) with marked osteophyte formation and joint thickening felt on palpation. (These findings are mirrored on the left side but with no flexion deformity.) Range of movement is decreased and there is marked tenderness medially and posteriorly.

His cervical spine is stiff with some discomfort on movement, the right shoulder, left knee and left hip have reduced range and he has pain in them.

Functionally he can get up from the chair if the seat is high and there are arms. Needs help getting in and out of bed and it is difficult to turn over. He sleeps with a pillow under the right knee and reports that he has not had an unbroken night's sleep in the last 3 months due to the pain.

He can walk a short distance with two sticks. He is now unable to drive (his wife cannot drive).

He cannot get into the bath; there is a separate shower at home but it is upstairs and so difficult to get to. There is a high seat for the toilet and grab rails already fitted.

Problem-solving exercise 7.7

- **A.** Try to work out a realistic set of goals of treatment for this gentleman and suggest possible interventions which you think may be of use in this case.

- **B.** Which other members of the health care team may be involved?

The approach to Mr Nicholl's physiotherapy treatment is discussed in the following section, but it is important that you should first try to work it out for yourself.

Physiotherapy treatment for Mr Nicholls
Mr Nicholls has a lot more problems to deal with than the previous case study, Mrs Stamford. However your approach with regard to physiotherapy input may be very similar. It is also important to keep in mind which other members of the health care team may be involved and how and when you need to communicate with them as appropriate. Another essential point to remember is the patient's viewpoint – what needs does he perceive that he has?

This patient has been admitted for a total knee replacement, and thus your intervention is likely to be affected by a number of factors:

1. Orthopaedic surgeons often have specific postoperative regimes for their patients. In the ideal situation the physiotherapist will have been involved in the initial design of this regime.
2. In some hospitals there are systems whereby the physiotherapist is involved throughout the management of the patients, that is, seeing them in the orthopaedic clinic before admission, then whilst in hospital and finally through to the home visits and occasionally post-discharge. In other situations you will only see the patients while they are on the ward.

Hopefully you can see how these points would affect both the amount and type of your intervention.

For issues specific to dealing with Mr Nicholls after his operation, please read the appropriate sections of the chapter on joint replacement.

A. *Goals of treatment*
This gentleman has a long history of OA and is quite disabled. He will probably have had physiotherapy before. Your goals of treatment may involve the following:

1. Reduction of pain.

2. To maintain or increase range of movement in the joints not involved in the operation.
3. To work on range of movement in the new right knee joint – hopefully to reach 90° for good function.
4. To maintain muscle strength or increase it if possible.
5. To maximise function within the limits of the patient's abilities.
6. Education/advice/support as necessary for both patient and carer, encouraging self-care and management.

These goals would need to be tailored specifically for Mr Nicholls and related to his environment and abilities.

Possible interventions

- Much of the pain will be relieved by the knee replacement itself (once the soreness of the wound has gone).

  He is used to using two sticks; you may change his walking aid if you and the patient feel it would be helpful. For example, elbow crutches or a walking frame may be useful, at least initially, to relieve weight and in turn reduce pain. This can then be changed as he improves.

  It is unlikely that you would carry out any local pain-relieving techniques.
- For increase of range in the operated knee there is often use of a continuous passive motion machine, plus a set of exercises as appropriate.
- Increase in range, muscle power and function are usually addressed by some sort of exercise regime, starting with bed exercises and then becoming more active as the patient mobilises. Exercise sheets are sometimes used; these can be standardised or, if the appropriate computer software is available, one could be designed specifically for Mr Nicholls.
- Hydrotherapy may be indicated if a pool is available on site. This type of treatment can reduce pain due to warmth and weight reduction. It is useful for general exercise which would be important for a patient like Mr Nicholls who has widespread problems.

It is also useful for increasing exercise tolerance.

- Education, advice and support resources will vary from place to place. This element could be on a one-to-one basis with the therapist talking to Mr Nicholls and to his wife, or there may be a group setting. Some hospitals have information available in written and/or audiovisual forms. Occasionally this support is continued at home by community services especially if there is a 'fast track' discharge system in operation.

  Possible advice for Mr Nicholls may include:
  — 'do's and 'don't's after joint replacement
  — information on joint protection
  — advice on home exercise and amounts of general activity
  — dietary information (as he is overweight)
  — available aids and appliances
  — services available in the local area and how to access them
  — benefits he may be entitled to
  — useful addresses.

  It is also important to encourage the patient and his wife to ask questions, particularly if anything is worrying them.

B. *Other members of the health care team*
The other members of the health care team who may be involved include:

- Mr Nicholls and his wife (plus any other family or friends who may help out)
- Orthopaedic surgeon
- Nursing staff
- OT
- Social worker/social services
- Dietician
- Community staff, e.g. physiotherapist, OT, nurse, home help
- General practitioner
- Self-help groups (if available in the locality)
- Volunteer helpers.

This list may be longer or shorter for each patient you come into contact with.

RHEUMATOID ARTHRITIS

Rheumatoid arthritis (RA) is a chronic, inflammatory condition mainly affecting the joints. It is manifested by a destructive, symmetrical polyarthritis but it also has many systemic effects. It is almost 200 years since RA was first described, and it is still not known whether it is a 'disease of antiquity' (Bellamy 1991), that is, some sort of inherent weakness in the human make-up, or whether it is a disease of only the last two centuries due to some infection or combination of environmental factors. It is possible that RA is a recent entity, not seen in Europe until the end of the 18th century, but there is also some evidence that it may have been a condition described by Hippocrates and other early writers. The latter possibility is very difficult to substantiate however. There is little help from palaeontologists as the soft tissue pathological changes of the condition are not well preserved in fossil specimens, in contrast to other diseases where there are bony changes, such as ankylosing spondylitis and osteoarthrosis (Harris 1985a).

RA was not clearly defined until 1958 and there are still differences of opinion regarding its classification (Gall E P 1988). There is even clinical and serological evidence to suggest that the disease commonly known as RA may not be a single entity, but could represent a collection of several diseases with similar features (Bhardwaj & Paget 1992).

RA is one of mankind's most significant diseases due to its relatively high incidence throughout the world. The onset often occurs in early life at a critical time for the patient in terms of career, family and activities. It is also notable because of its chronicity and potentially disabling effects (Anderson 1985).

Data on incidence (that is the number of new cases of a disease occurring in a defined population within a defined period) and prevalence (that is the frequency of a disease in a defined population) of RA do vary somewhat. This may be due to problems encountered in the classification and therefore the diagnosis of the condition. But using the American Rheumatism Association 1987 revised criteria for the classification of RA

Table 7.4 The American Rheumatism Association 1987 revised criteria for the classification of rheumatoid arthritis (Arnett et al 1988)

Criterion	Definition
1. Morning stiffness	Morning stiffness in and around the joints, lasting at least an hour before maximal improvement
2. Arthritis of three or more joint areas	At least three joint areas simultaneously have had soft tissue swelling or fluid (not bony overgrowth alone) observed by a physician. The 14 possible areas are right or left proximal interphalangeal (PIP), metacarpophalangeal (MCP), wrist, elbow, knee, ankle and metatarsophalangeal (MTP) joints
3. Arthritis of hand joints	At least one area swollen (as defined above) in a wrist, MCP or PIP joint
4. Symmetric arthritis	Simultaneous involvement of the same joint areas (as defined in 2) on both sides of the body. (Bilateral involvement of PIPs, MCPs or MTPs is acceptable without absolute symmetry)
5. Rheumatoid nodules	Subcutaneous nodules over bony prominences or extensor surfaces or in juxta-articular regions, observed by a physician
6. Serum rheumatoid factor	Demonstration of abnormal amounts of serum rheumatoid factor by any method for which the result has been positive in <5% of normal control subjects
7. Radiographic changes	Radiographic changes typical of rheumatoid arthritis on posteroanterior hand and wrist radiographs, which must include erosions or unequivocal bony decalcification, localised in or most marked adjacent to the involved joints (OA changes alone do not qualify)

Criteria 1 to 4 must have been present for at least 6 weeks. RA is defined by the presence of four or more criteria, and no further qualifications (classic, definite, probable) or list of exclusions are required. These criteria demonstrated 91–94% sensitivity and 89% specificity for RA when compared with non-RA rheumatic disease control subjects.

(Table 7.4) the prevalence is consistently between 1 and 2% of the adult population in every part of the world (Bhardwaj & Paget 1992). Variation from this is very rare and tends to occur only in certain populations that appear to have a predisposition for the disease, for example urban South African blacks have a prevalence rate of 3.3% (Harris 1985a). In the United States, however, there is no difference between black and white populations. Unfortunately there are no data available for ethnic groups in the UK, but prevalence is fairly constant in white populations (Hazes & Silman 1990). There is also an increase in prevalence with increase in age in both males and females, possibly exceeding 10% in persons aged 65 years and over. The incidence of RA ranges from a high of 2.9 to a low of 0.097 per 1000 population with an increase for each decade of life (Bhardwaj & Paget 1992).

There is a marked sex difference overall and it is generally agreed that women are affected up to three times more frequently than men. This female predominance may become less prominent in patients over 65 (Anderson 1985, Bhardwaj & Paget 1992, Harris 1985a, Hazes & Silman 1990). It has been postulated that there may be some hormonal influence in the pathogenesis and course of certain rheumatic and autoimmune diseases, one of which is RA. This would seem to be supported by the beneficial effects that many women with RA report during pregnancy. (A completely opposite effect is found in women with systemic lupus erythematosus who find that pregnancy causes an increase in symptoms.) Work is going on to investigate whether or not hormonal therapy could be used to prevent or treat RA (Yaron 1995).

The onset of the condition is usually between the ages of 25 and 55 but it can affect those both younger and older. Epidemiological studies suggest that RA is 30 times more common in the identical twin of an affected individual than in the general population and some familial clustering has been noted (Sterling 1990). It is also possible that some socioeconomic factors are related to RA. There seems to be a decreased prevalence in men with higher education, but a twofold increase in those in the lowest income bracket. The overall prognosis appears to be worse, as does functional outcome, in poorer, less educated patients (Bhardwaj & Paget 1992).

There is some evidence to suggest that there may be a declining trend in incidence, especially in the female population, and an indication that the severity of the condition could be decreasing. But the latter may only be due to better prevention of joint damage and abnormalities by early treatment and rehabilitation (Hazes & Silman 1990).

Aetiology

A great deal of work has been carried out on RA, and although the clinical features and treatment are now better defined, the specific cause is still unknown and there is much to be learned regarding the pathogenesis of the disease (Anderson 1985, Bhardwaj & Paget 1992).

As mentioned at the beginning of this chapter, there seem to be several interacting factors which are responsible for the onset of RA. Research has shown that immunological mechanisms are of crucial importance both in the initiation and perpetuation of the disease. These are linked with some genetic predisposition and an inciting agent. In the 1970s advances were made in relating histocompatibility markers located on the 6th chromosome to the epidemiology of certain diseases. These major histocompatibility complexes (MHCs) control the surface antigens which are specific glycoproteins in the surface membranes of cells in the blood and tissues throughout the body. In RA the primary association appears to be with the DR4 locus, at least in certain populations. Over 70% of white patients with RA will have the DR4 haplotype as opposed to less than 30% of controls. In comparison 46% of black patients with RA have DR4 present in contrast to 14% of the normal population. This does seem to be an indication of susceptibility to the disease and there also appears to be a link between more aggressive disease states and the presence of DR4. It must be remembered however that there are 30% of patients with RA who are not DR4-positive as well as there being people who do not have RA but do have the DR4 haplotype. Other genes involved in the development of RA may soon be identified which would make it easier to predict susceptibility with more accuracy (Banwell & Gall 1988, Bennett 1985, Bhardwaj & Paget 1992, Harris 1990).

As to the initiating factors, the stimuli that can activate the immune response in a susceptible host are probably multiple and ubiquitous and so difficult to detect and prevent. There is evidence pointing to infectious agents, i.e. a virus or bacterium, as aetiological pathogens of RA. The Epstein–Barr virus which belongs to the herpes family of DNA viruses has been implicated in the pathogenesis of RA for a number of years, but the actual relationship has still to be determined. Lentiviruses, parvoviruses, the rubella virus and mycobacteria are also suspected, but again the specific link is unclear. Other research has identified endogenous substances such as connective tissue proteins (collagen, proteoglycans) or altered immunoglobulins which could act as immunogens in a genetically susceptible host (Bhardwaj & Paget 1992, Harris 1990).

It is hoped that with more work in both cell biology and genetics, it will eventually be possible to fully understand how all of the factors interlink to trigger the pathogenesis of RA.

Self-assessment question

■ **SAQ 7.9.** Briefly review the factors involved in the pathogenesis of RA.

Course and prognosis

There is a slow, insidious onset in 55–70% of patients and the initial symptoms can be either systemic or articular. In some there is fatigue or diffuse musculoskeletal pain followed later by joint involvement, but morning stiffness may be the first symptom.

In 8–15% of patients onset is acute, tending to begin in the joints with severe muscle pain. This group is the most troublesome to classify as there are many possible differential diagnoses.

Lastly 15–20% of patients exhibit an intermediate onset where symptoms develop over days or weeks and the systemic effects are the most noticeable. Generally the small joints in the hands and feet are affected before the large ones. In the majority of cases depression, anxiety and fear for the future can accentuate the symptoms (Harris 1985b).

The course of RA is variable. Remission is the most hoped-for outcome leaving little or no abnormality. The more classic course is intermittent, with relapse followed by complete or partial remission, with a slow but steady progression of damage to articular and periarticular structures and gradual increase in disability. The third possibility is a relentless progression, either rapid or slow, with no remission and many complications (Anderson 1985, Harris 1985b, Rasker & Cosh 1989).

Generally the prognosis in RA is not good, but it is a dynamic process when placed within the settings of patient response, changing therapy and alteration in the natural course of the disease. There does appear to be a direct correlation between RA and decreased life expectancy. In a long-term study over 25 years Rasker & Cosh (1989) found that on average patients died 15 years earlier if the death was directly attributable to RA, 10 years earlier if RA was a contributory factor and 5 years earlier even when death was totally unrelated to RA. It has also been found that patients with RA are more likely to develop other chronic disorders which may be a contributory factor in decreased life expectancy (Bellamy 1991). Onset and death appear to occur earlier in men than women and their overall mortality is higher. However, in those men who survive, the expression of the disease is less severe. In general, women tend to have more chronic and disabling disease than men (Bhardwaj & Paget 1992, Rasker & Cosh 1989).

RA certainly has an effect on how long patients can continue to work. Those performing light work fare the best and are still often able to continue for 10 years after diagnosis, whereas the person carrying out a job involving heavy labour is often work-disabled. Work type and the physical demands are related to the patient's ability to continue. The problems encountered by 'homemakers' are more difficult to quantify as there is no control group. However, as you would expect they do report reduced ability to carry out usual activities (Wolfe 1990). People with RA will have a reduced income leading to a toll on livelihood and quality of life, indicating not just physical problems but defining the impact of RA in terms of significant financial, social and psychological costs.

The worse a patient's condition at 1 year after diagnosis, the worse the prognosis. A poorer prognosis also seems linked with the presence of rheumatoid factor in the blood, X-ray evidence of erosions, insidious onset, delay in treatment and poor initial response to treatment (Bellamy 1991, Bhardwaj & Paget 1992).

There seem to be varying opinions on whether or not treatment is effective in altering prognosis. Harris (1990) states that there is little evidence that present treatment alters outcome although he concentrates mainly on drug therapy, whereas Wolfe (1990) is of the opinion that outcome can be improved by treatment. He looks at a wider spectrum of management including orthopaedic surgery, disease-modifying drugs, patient education and self-management as well as other types of therapy including occupational and physiotherapy. Bhardwaj & Paget (1992) state that outcome appears to be more favourable if there is a good initial response to treatment.

Self-assessment questions

■ **SAQ 7.10.** The course of RA will differ from person to person. What are the three possible courses that it can take?

■ **SAQ 7.11.** What factors may have an effect on the prognosis of RA?

Pathological changes in RA

Stage 1

Antigen-presenting cells (macrophages or dendritic cells in synovial membrane) are the first to be involved in the human immune response. They ingest, process and present foreign protein antigens to T-lymphocytes. The processed antigen binds to glycoproteins and is then recognised by helper T-cell receptors. A cellular immune response is then initiated where B-lymphocytes differentiate into plasma cells which secrete immunoglobulins that act as antibodies to the autoantigenic components of IgG. This is the early stage of RA where no symptoms occur.

Stages 2 and 3

These are similar to stage 1, the main difference being in severity of the reactions. Antibody–antigen complexes activate the cascade of reactions known as the complement system and this causes substances to be released into the synovial fluid that influence the behaviour of certain cells. The inflammatory reaction begins with the induction of vascular exudation by vasoactive substances leading to congestion and oedema of the synovial lining, followed by effusion into the joint space (Anderson 1985, Bhardwaj & Paget 1992). Cytokines such as interleukins-2, -3, and -4 and interferon-gamma, produced by immunocytes, macrophages and fibroblasts, amplify and perpetuate the inflammation which becomes self-sustaining (Harris 1990). They also cause proliferation in the cells of the synovium within the joints and tendon sheaths. The hypertrophied synovium is sustained by increased capillary growth (angiogenesis).

Clotting cascades are activated which cause fibrin to be deposited on the synovial membrane and articular cartilage. Lysosomal enzymes are released which begin to degrade cartilage, any menisci present and ligaments.

These stages become gradually symptomatic and the products of inflammation then drive the proliferative response into stage 4 of the disease (Anderson 1985, Harris 1990).

Stage 4

In this stage, irreversible destruction of cartilage occurs. There is an enormous increase in synovial surface area due to the formation of villi. It organises and becomes an invasive front (pannus). Proteinases are released that are capable of destroying almost all proteins making up the matrix of articular cartilage and bone. Pannus actually replaces bone at the joint margins and erosions appear. Prostaglandins are released which increase osteoclast activity, minerals are resorbed from the underlying bone (osteolysis) which is then further degraded by collagenases and proteinases. Pseudocysts may form (Anderson 1985, Bhardwaj & Paget 1992, Harris 1990).

The articular cartilage is also replaced by the pannus which is subsequently transformed into fibrous tissue. This can go on to cause decreased movement in the joint and in some cases leads eventually to fibrous ankylosis.

Very little gross destruction of cartilage is necessary before normal function is reduced to the point that progressive disintegration occurs in response to everyday activities involving the weight-bearing joints (Harris 1990). In fact, much damage can take place before any joint space narrowing shows up on X-ray.

Proliferation and destruction also occur in the capsule, ligaments and tendons. This can cause an altered use pattern and the structures may become very lax or rupture and this will affect the stability of the joint (Anderson 1985, Harris 1990).

Stage 5

This is a continuation of the irreversible destructive changes in the joint. There may be subluxation of the joint surfaces in addition to muscle atrophy and fibrosis, leading to a significant decrease in functional ability. There may also be secondary OA changes by this time (Anderson 1985).

Table 7.5 presents a summary of the stages of RA.

Table 7.5 A summary of the stages of rheumatoid arthritis, including radiographic changes (Harris 1990)

Stage	Pathological process	Symptoms	Physical signs	Radiographic changes
1	Presentation of antigen to T-cells	Probably none	—	—
2	T-cell proliferation, B-cell proliferation, angiogenesis in synovial membrane	Malaise, mild joint stiffness and swelling	Swelling of small joints of the hands or wrists, or pain in hands, wrists, knees and feet	—
3	Accumulation of neutrophils in synovial fluid. Synovial cell proliferation without invasion of cartilage	Pain, swelling, morning stiffness, malaise and weakness	Warm, swollen joints, excess synovial fluid, soft tissue proliferation within joints, pain and limitation of motion and rheumatoid nodules	Soft tissue swelling
4	Synovitis polarised into invasive pannus. Activation of chondrocytes. Initiation of enzyme degradation of cartilage	Same as stage 3	Same as stage 3 but swelling more pronounced	Magnetic resonance imaging (MRI) reveals proliferative pannus, radiographic evidence of periarticular osteopenia
5	Erosion of subchondral bone. Invasion of cartilage by pannus. Chondrocyte proliferation. Stretched ligaments around joints	Same as stage 3 plus some loss of function and early deformity (e.g. ulnar deviation at metacarpophalangeal joints	Same as stage 3 plus instability of joints, flexion contractures, decreased range of motion and extra-articular complications	Early erosions and narrowing of joint spaces

Try the following problem-solving exercise before you go on to read the next section.

Problem-solving exercise 7.8

Using the information given so far, try to work out:

■ **A.** The possible symptoms that a patient with RA would describe to you.

■ **B.** The clinical signs you would expect to find on examination.

Clinical features of RA

You are already aware that RA affects all parts of the body and not just the joints (i.e. it is an autoimmune disease affecting connective tissue which is present in all areas), and as such it has a very broad spectrum of clinical presentations.

Case study 7.3

Mrs White (1)

This 60-year-old lady has been admitted for bilateral total hip replacements. She was diagnosed with RA 6 years ago. Within 12 months the disease had affected her neck, shoulders, elbows and small joints of the hands. Later on the hips and knees started to give problems, the knees getting worse as the hips deteriorated. On the whole her feet and ankles have been fine but are now starting to be affected and to cause more functional difficulty. At present her hands are sore but the hips are giving the most problems. She has deteriorated quite rapidly over the last 6 months.

She lives at home with her husband and son, sleeping downstairs (and has done for the last 3 years). There is a shower and toilet downstairs. Her husband is self-employed and helps with most things. She was able to get around with a walking frame until about 2 months ago.

She worked as a dispenser in a chemist but had to give up work 5 years ago.

Problem-solving exercise 7.9

■ **A.** Review your answers to the previous exercise and now briefly relate them to this case study. Do you think that all of the symptoms and clinical signs you came up with would be relevant to this lady?

■ **B.** Make a list of headings that you would use when assessing this patient.

The headings you might use are discussed in the following section but, as ever, it is important that you try this for yourself first.

Approach to the assessment of Mrs White

Make a note of the time of day you make your assessment; this could be very important for your reassessment, that is, many RA patients have variation in symptoms during the day.

Subjective assessment

1. *Demographic details and history of present condition*

For Mrs White you would be particularly interested in time since diagnosis, how quickly the disease has progressed and how she is at present (whether her symptoms are better or worse). You also need to know which joints are affected apart from the hips which are to be replaced, her main problems as she perceives them and what she has most difficulties with functionally.

Morning stiffness: how long does it last?

It will also be relevant to investigate any systemic problems that could impact upon your intervention. For example has the RA affected her heart or does she fatigue very easily?

Lastly in this section, has she had any physiotherapy before and how did she respond?

2. *General health and past medical history*

It is important to get an overall picture of her pattern of health and wellbeing as it could affect your intervention. There are some questionnaires that can be used to investigate this area.

3. *Present medication and drug history*

Again this is important as it could affect your intervention. You would also need to know if her drug treatment changes during the period she is receiving physiotherapy as it could give false impressions of the effectiveness of treatment.

4. *Splints*

Does she have any? Does she wear them regularly? Has she had them in the past and if so have they been helpful? Which joints?

5. *Social history*

Particularly her living conditions, who (if anyone) is available to help at home, leisure activities (present or those she has had to give up recently).

Objective assessment

1. *General observation*

For example: appearance and gait; how does she get in and out of chairs, on and off the bed? How well does she manage getting dressed/undressed?

2. *Joints involved*

Observe, palpate, examine.

In each case is there pain, swelling, tenderness, decreased range, decreased power in muscles around the joint, instability, deformity? Is there spasm in the muscles? Are tendons affected? Can you get access to any X-rays?

3. *Extra-articular manifestations*

Has she any nodules? What is the condition of her skin: thin/papery, any ulcers? Does she have any areas of reduced or altered sensation?

(You may need access to medical notes for results of tests such as ESR, presence of rheumatoid factors or anaemia.)

4. *Functional assessment*

This would need to be tailored particularly to Mrs White in the light of her specific problems.

Now we will continue with more information about this patient.

Case study 7.3

Mrs White, continued (2)
Subjective assessment
You already have information on diagnosis, onset, rate of progression, the present state of her condition and the joints affected, as well as her social situation.

The main problems are pain, stiffness and loss of function in all the affected joints, particularly over the last 6 months. She describes herself as having good and bad days. At present there is no pain at rest but it is induced by any movement or staying in one position too long. It is eased by painkillers (every 4 hours). She wakes 2–3 times every night and has marked morning stiffness (1.5 hours).

Functionally she is able to do less, needing help with all activities of daily living, and she can no longer walk with her ordinary walking frame.

She is anaemic but this is being treated. Fatigue is a problem particularly in the evening. Apart from this her general health is satisfactory.

Concerning drugs, she is taking penicillamine, a non-steroidal anti-inflammatory drug (naproxen), paracetamol/codidramol as necessary, and asilone and vitamin B_{12} supplement. She has never taken steroids.

Previous treatment has involved hydrotherapy and land-based physiotherapy which helped her to retain function for a longer period.

Objective assessment
Generally this lady looks very thin and quite pale. She has great difficulty moving about the bed and is unable to walk more than a few steps around the bed.

Muscle strength is reduced in all groups: Gd III+ to IV.

Joints: all affected joints have a reduced range of movement; both hip and knee flexion is limited by pain, particularly on the left side. She was unable to lie in supine and so the tests had to be done in long sitting. It was not possible to test hip extension as she was unable to get into position. The knees and shoulders were warmer to the touch than the other joints. Swelling was obvious in the knees, elbows, wrists and fingers.

Areas of pain and tenderness were as shown on the body charts in Figure 7.12.

Self-assessment question

■ **SAQ 7.12.** Briefly review the five stages in the pathogenesis of RA with particular reference to the changes occurring in the joint and whether these are symptomatic or not.

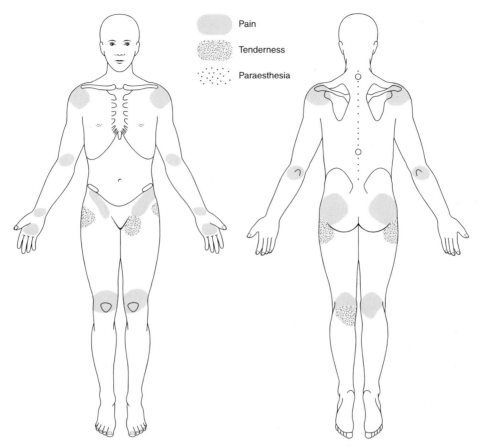

Pain

Tenderness

Paraesthesia

Figure 7.12 Body charts showing areas of pain and tenderness in the patient Mrs White.

Review of clinical features seen in RA

Characteristically the patient is a woman aged between 20 and 50 years with a symmetrical poly-arthritis, usually involving the small joints of hands and feet. She will complain of fatigue and morning stiffness. Blood tests will show an elevation in ESR (erythrocyte sedimentation rate), anaemia and the presence of rheumatoid factor. However there are many other ways in which this disease can present (Bhardwaj & Paget 1992).

Early in the course of the disease, symptoms can be either articular or systemic. There may only be prodromal symptoms at first, that is fatigue, weight loss, and diffuse musculoskeletal pain with low grade fever. The fatigue is often accompanied by morning stiffness which is very characteristic of inflammatory joint disease and diagnostically significant if it lasts for more than

half an hour. The onset of joint disease varies; this has already been covered in the section on course and prognosis.

Joint symptoms are usually symmetrical and, as mentioned earlier, often begin in the small joints of hands and feet. Hips and ankles are rarely affected in the early stages. When the pathological changes are confined to the synovial membrane, capsule and tendon sheaths, the patient complains of pain, swelling, tenderness and stiffness of a number of joints. Initially there will be pain on movement but with increasing disease activity there is pain at rest. Movement is guarded and there is a subjective feeling of stiffness and decreased range of movement.

In the finger joints the swelling produces a spindle shape, they may be warm and tender and feel 'boggy' and difficult to move. Effusions are commonly found in the knees, and swelling of bursae and tendons occurs especially related to the wrists and dorsa of hands and feet. There may be swelling at the hip joint but this is very difficult to assess due to the large muscle mass in the area. If swelling is visible, it is seen in the groin or femoral triangle. There can be trochanteric bursitis with tenderness directly over the greater trochanter.

As the joints become more painful and stiff there will be atrophy of muscle tissue due to altered use patterns. As well as this, there is often muscle tenderness and decreased strength. These factors lead to an overall reduction in functional activity. In the case of the lower limbs mobility will be inhibited, and because of the changes occurring at each joint there will be altered gait patterns. A knowledge of the normal biomechanics of the joints, the changes due to the disease process and the requirements for normal mobility is necessary in order to design an appropriate rehabilitation programme.

Morning stiffness remains a prominent symptom throughout and can be used as a guide to the activity of the disease and to gauge responses to therapy.

Joint deformities are not usually present early on and X-ray will only show soft tissue swelling and osteoporosis around the joints with no erosions.

The outstanding complaints are of joint pain, stiffness and loss of function.

In the later stages of the disease, with cartilage destruction, necrosis and fibrosis of synovial membrane, contracture or stretching of the joint capsule and ligaments, and granulation tissue invading tendons and sheaths, there tends to be increasing and irreversible impairment of function. There may be limitation of movement in some joints but there also may be subluxation and instability.

There are some characteristic deformities associated with RA. Ulnar deviation at the metacarpophalangeal joints is common but causes surprisingly little functional disability. Deformities of the fingers may be more problematic. 'Swan neck' deformity (Fig. 7.13) is hyperextension of the proximal interphalangeal (IP) joints and fixed flexion of the distal

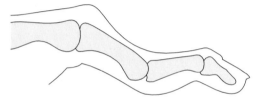

Figure 7.13 'Swan neck' deformity.

IP joints. This stops the patient making a fist. The 'boutonnière' (or button hole) deformity (Fig. 7.14) is due to protrusion of the proximal IP joint through the extensor expansion producing fixed flexion, with extension of the distal IP joint. This again will markedly affect grip.

Of the 20% of patients whose initial joint involvement is in the foot, for 80% of these it will begin in the forefoot. Common deformities are hallux valgus, dropped metatarsal heads and possibly hammer and claw toes. With hindfoot involvement there will be excessive pronation subjecting the foot to extreme stress on weight bearing.

At the knees there may be fixed flexion deformity and valgus or less commonly varus. The typical RA knee deformity has been described as one of flexion, subluxation, valgus and external rotation. The valgus deformity is often combined with an eversion deformity at the subtalar joint with increased pronation of the forefoot. There may be deformities at other joints, depending on the amount of destruction, bony erosion and the effects of the disease on the capsule and other soft tissue structures that normally play a supporting role.

The following clinical manifestations also occur to varying degrees in RA patients

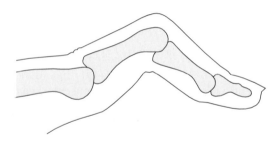

Figure 7.14 'Boutonnière' or 'button hole' deformity.

(Anderson 1985, Barnes 1980, Bhardwaj & Paget 1992, Harris 1985b, Levine 1988, Sterling 1990):

1. Subcutaneous rheumatoid nodules over pressure points in 20% of patients. Nodules can also be found in the lungs, pleura, heart, pericardium and the eye.
2. Vasculitis with all layers of the vessel wall infiltrated by lymphocytes, proliferation of the intima and possible disruption of the elastic lamina. This can lead to occlusion, ulceration or occasionally thrombosis.
3. The skin becomes atrophic, thin and papery.
4. Peripheral neuropathy may occur and, if there is subluxation of the cervical spine, cord compression.
5. The lymph nodes and the spleen may be affected with marked splenomegaly, leucopenia and reduced resistance.
6. Amyloidosis can occur rarely in the spleen, liver or kidneys.
7. Some degree of anaemia almost invariably accompanies RA.
8. X-rays show soft tissue swelling, osteoporosis, narrowing or loss of joint space, erosions and any deformities.
9. On laboratory tests many RA patients have a raised ESR. However, a normal ESR does not preclude the presence of active disease.
10. In approximately 80% of patients rheumatoid factors are found in the serum. This is a standard test in the diagnosis of the condition and if they are present it indicates a less favourable prognosis.

Problem-solving exercise 7.10

Using the information from earlier in the chapter on management of patients with rheumatic disorders and the findings from the assessment of Mrs White, formulate:

■ **A.** a problem list

■ **B.** goals of treatment, and

■ **C.** a treatment plan for this lady.

Take into account her physical, social and psychological wellbeing. (Keep in mind that she has been admitted for hip replacements, but don't spend too much time on immediate postoperative management as this is covered in the chapter on joint replacement. Also make the assumption that her drug regimen is adequate.)

After you have done this, you can check your ideas in the following section.

An approach to the physiotherapy treatment of Mrs White

This section will give some possible problems, goals and treatment ideas for Mrs White. However, it is important for you to remember that these will differ for each patient that you see; there will need to be additions and/or subtractions depending on the particular circumstances. This is not a 'recipe' for you to follow but a template for you to adapt and build on.

A. *Problem list*

- Pain in all joints affected especially hips and knees.
- Reduced range of movement in all joints affected.
- Reduced muscle strength.
- Reduced mobility both in bed and during locomotion (no longer able to get around with walking frame).
- Reduced function.

The above problems will impact upon her everyday activities and probably the amount of interaction she has with others. This could cause her to feel despondent. This is turn may reduce her willingness to socialise. So it is possible to get into a descending spiral where pain and other physical problems cause difficulties in the social and psychological areas of a patient's life. If this increases negative feelings it could magnify the pain even further by causing the patient to focus on the physical problems. Much of this will of course depend on your patient's outlook and the support she gets from family and friends.

Obviously you are not a psychiatrist or psychologist and so are not expected to be able to examine the patient's mental state. However, during your assessment you should be able to get an idea of how the patient is feeling and how motivated she is to help herself.

B. *Goals of treatment*

- To reduce pain. This may or may not be a goal for the physiotherapist involved with RA patients. As with Mr Nicholls and his knee, the pain from Mrs White's hips will be reduced by the surgery once the operative soreness fades. But her other joints will continue to be painful.
- To maintain or increase range of movement in affected joints within the limits of the disease and the patient's tolerance level.
- To maintain or increase muscle strength in affected muscle groups (with the same proviso as above).
- To improve bed mobility if possible whilst the patient is on bed rest, and then to help the patient to mobilise after the hip replacements.
- To help the patient with functional activities particularly locomotion (and any others in discussion with Mrs White and other appropriate members of the health care team).

C. *Treatment plan*

This could be dictated to a certain extent by the regime within the particular hospital. But it could include the following:

- Pre- and postoperative care as necessary, e.g. regarding respiratory function and bed exercises.
- Pain relief. If one or possibly two of the non-operated joints is/are particularly problematic you may use ice or superficial heat for temporary pain relief before giving exercises. Most of the pain relief should be taken care of by the drug therapy. Due to her widespread problems, this patient would appear to be an ideal candidate for hydrotherapy which does have a pain-relieving aspect – but again this would be temporary, acting only whilst Mrs White is in the pool. You would have to ensure that the treatment did not increase her fatigue to a debilitating level. Pain relief may also be achieved by the use of appliances such as splints and walking aids.
- Range of movement and muscle strengthening will be addressed by an exercise regime. This could include passive or active assisted movements to begin with, moving on to active and then resisted work as appropriate. Static muscle work could be used to begin with if movement was particularly difficult. Bed mobility could be addressed at the same time (as it is something the patient has problems with).
- Mobility once out of bed usually involves the use of a walking aid; perhaps a gutter frame would be helpful with Mrs White so taking the strain off hands and wrists. Her gait and the distance walked each time should be worked on, and you may change the walking aid as it becomes appropriate, for example, you might progress onto gutter crutches. The rate of progression may be dictated by the surgeon (that is, it may be a set number of days before she is allowed out of bed), or it may depend on the patient's own abilities.

It would be usual to check Mrs White's safety on the stairs (this sometimes needs more practice) before she could go home.

- Advice/education. This should be an integral part of your treatment. Mrs White will definitely need information about do's and don't's after hip replacement; this could be verbal, written or a combination. As for advice about other issues, this will vary from patient to patient. Mrs White has a 6-year history of RA and so she may know a lot about the condition and the possible self-help strategies such as joint protection. However, this is not always the case and you may need to spend some time with her and her husband going over important points. This should be done in conjunction with other relevant members of the health care team.

Review points

If you look back at the answer to the problem-solving exercise regarding Mr Nicholls (p. 172), you should see lots of similarities between that and Mrs White's management. This should help to reinforce the fact that although patients may have different conditions, often the problems they have and the possible interventions are very similar. Obviously, this book cannot cover all eventualities, but at least you should now be getting the idea that as long as you keep the principles in mind, you can apply them to a wide range of situations. The important point for you is to really look at your patients and investigate their problems during the assessment period. Then decide on your intervention and tailor it to the particular patient in each instance.

Additional treatment modalities

Some patients have reported finding relief from symptoms when trying out alternative therapies. These include modalities such as homeopathy, acupuncture, aromatherapy and reflex therapy.

There is also the suggestion of some connection between RA and hypersensitivity to environmental toxins, especially food and food-related products. However it has been proven that no food has anything to do with causing arthritis and no food is effective in treating or curing it. But some observations suggest that for selected patients, dietary manipulation may be beneficial, although there is no proof of this. If a patient has found a strong relationship between the eating of a certain food and a flare, then it would seem sensible to avoid that food. It has been found that cow's milk may induce or exacerbate symptoms in some patients and a controlled fast can help to alleviate this. There is some new evidence to suggest that dietary fish oil supplements could help to alleviate the symptoms of RA; however it should be noted that this oil can prolong bleeding time and inhibit platelet aggregation. This could be dangerous if the patient was taking another anticoagulant such as aspirin (Bhardwaj & Paget 1992).

Conclusion

Around 70% of patients with RA will experience chronic disability with remission and exacerbation. Total clinical remission is a very rare event and therefore most patients will require intervention from the health care team.

Drug therapy is essential and at present is the only way in which the disease can be retarded, and this is usually only a temporary reduction in the rate of progression.

The physiotherapist's role is one of attempting to enhance the patient's functional abilities within the limits of the disease. This is done by active treatment, advice, education, splinting and provision of or advice about aids and appliances. (The latter is done is consultation with the OT.)

At present, the overall functional status of the patient is maintained by medication, physiotherapy, education, emotional support, and surgery where indicated. This is really the limit of medical intervention until the aetiology and pathogenesis of the disease is understood more clearly.

ANKYLOSING SPONDYLITIS

The last example of a common rheumatic disorder to be considered in this chapter is ankylosing spondylitis (AS). As the condition is presented to you, try to think about the similarities and differences between this disease and the two you have already learned about.

AS belongs to a group of disorders known as the seronegative spondyloarthropathies. This term means conditions where there is no rheumatoid factor found in the serum and which predominantly affect the joints of the spine. They share a number of characteristic clinical features which are listed in Table 7.6.

Ankylosis means bony fusion and spondylitis is inflammation of the spine. AS is a chronic, progressive inflammatory arthritis, predominantly affecting the axial skeleton, but peripheral joint involvement is often a significant feature, most commonly the hips and shoulders (Bhardwaj & Paget 1992). It affects both synovial and cartilaginous joints as well as the sites of insertion of both tendons and ligaments (enthesopathy). The inflammation is followed by fusion (partial or complete) of the joints mentioned above.

It is a significant cause of disability in young men (0.4% in men; 0.05% in women). It is more common in males than females, but this sex-linked ratio becomes less marked as the age of onset increases (for onset at less than 16 years the male: female ratio is 6:1, and for onset at 30 years,

Table 7.6 Characteristic clinical features of the seronegative spondyloarthropathies. (Adapted from (Caldron 1995, Inman 1992, and Rai & Struthers 1994)

1. Sacroiliitis
2. Peripheral arthritis; often asymmetrical and in the lower limbs
3. Absence of rheumatoid factor
4. Absence of extra-articular features of RA
5. Presence of other extra-articular features characteristic of the group, e.g. iritis, ulcerative colitis and cardiac involvement
6. Enthesitis: inflammation at the site of tendon and ligament insertions
7. Significant familial incidence
8. Association with the HLA-B27 genetic marker
9. Male predominance

it is 2:1). It is estimated that there are approximately 70 000 cases of AS in the UK but there are probably large numbers of subclinical, undiagnosed cases within the population. Many of these may well be female as this still tends to be thought of as a predominantly male condition.

As with RA there also seems to be some difference in the prevalence of AS with different races.

Aetiology

There is a marked familial incidence, but other factors probably determine onset in predisposed individuals. Of the spondyloarthropathies the association with HLA-B27 is greatest in AS; it is present in over 95% of patients (Rai & Struthers 1994). But it must be remembered that not everyone with the HLA-B27 genetic marker will develop AS: out of 8% of the American white population with HLA-B27, only one in five has any signs of the disease (Caldron 1995). As with other rheumatic conditions, there seems to be some environmental trigger, possibly a virus, which causes the development of the disease.

The risk of a patient who is HLA-B27-positive transmitting the same antigen to his or her child is 1 in 2. The risk of an HLA-B27 relative developing AS is about 1 in 3. Hence the overall risk for the children to develop the condition is 1 in 6. Because of these factors, part of the management for these patients may involve genetic counselling (Rai & Struthers 1994).

Course and prognosis

The onset and course of the disease are variable but it usually occurs in a young adult (15–30 years) who complains of gradually increasing back pain and stiffness. It is not unusual for there to be a delayed diagnosis as it can present as chronic, mechanical low back pain (Gall E P 1988, Rai & Struthers 1994).

The disease runs a progressive cyclical course with each exacerbation leaving an increase in the amount of residual damage and disability. The eventual outcome may be total fusion of joints particularly in the spine and thorax with consequent reduction in functional ability. However, many patients never reach this stage and still retain some movement. It used to be believed that AS would burn out when the patient reached the fifth decade; however more recent work does not indicate this. It seems that progression and severity depend on the disease activity when it is initially diagnosed; the more severe it is the worse the prognosis. There is also a correlation with age: the older the patient, the more severe the disease activity (Kennedy et al 1993).

AS does not in itself cause a reduction in life expectancy, but there may be associated problems. These would usually be due to the extra-articular manifestations affecting the heart and/or lungs. There can also be secondary amyloidosis which can cause premature death (Viitanen & Suni 1995). If the thorax is so fused as to seriously reduce chest expansion there may also be some extra risks involved in surgery, particularly for those patients with marked deformity.

However, in the majority of cases, with treatment and advice including family education and awareness of the condition, a good prognosis can be achieved (Rai & Struthers 1994).

Pathological changes in AS

As mentioned earlier, AS is an inflammatory arthritis that affects the synovium, capsule and ligaments around the joints, as well as the insertions of tendons into bone. This inflammation is known as an enthesopathy and is particularly obvious around the spine and pelvis. During this process the adjacent bone is destroyed and eroded. A healing process then occurs where there is increased bone production, causing a protuberance which gets larger with each episode. As this continues it can eventually cause bridging between the bones involved. In the spine the inflammation occurs where the annulus fibrosus joins the margin of the vertebral body, and the bony overgrowth which results is referred to as a syndesmophyte. The posterior and anterior longitudinal ligaments are also affected. When the syndesmophytes of adjacent vertebrae join, the spine takes on a particular appearance on X-ray and is referred to as a 'bamboo spine' (Fig. 7.15). Obviously, by this time the spine is fused as are the sacroiliac joints. Similar ankylosis occurs in the symphysis pubis, costovertebral and manubriosternal joints.

Up to 50% of AS patients have clinically significant hip involvement which is often bilateral. In severe cases, findings here can include protrusion deformities and/or completely ankylosed hips. Osteoporosis is also seen (Ranawat et al 1992).

The ESR is sometimes raised early on or during a period of active disease but conversely there is sometimes a normal ESR during this time (Rai & Struthers 1994).

The earliest X-ray changes are seen in the sacroiliac joints.

Problem-solving exercise 7.11

- Using your experiences so far and the information you have been given, see how many of the possible clinical features of AS you can come up with before reading the next section.

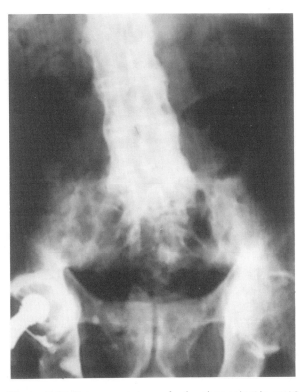

Figure 7.15 X-ray appearance of a 'bamboo spine' in an AS patient (Caldron 1995).

Self-assessment question

■ **SAQ 7.13.** Jot down as many of the characteristic clinical features of the seronegative spondyloarthropathies as you can remember. (Clue: there are nine.)

Clinical features of AS

The onset of AS is insidious in most cases and as mentioned earlier, it often begins with low back pain and stiffness. Patients are generally seen after several months of symptoms for which an inciting event cannot be recalled. The pain which is usually described as severe aching, can also radiate to the buttock and posterior aspect of the thigh or knee and it can be uni- or bilateral. At first the pain and stiffness are episodic and worse after immobility. The patient may also complain of fatigue due to the chronic discomfort which disturbs normal sleep patterns. There may also be weight loss and low grade pyrexia. Commonly there is morning stiffness, but this can be variable.

As the disease affects more joints, the pain will spread to encompass these: it may include the thoracic and cervical spine, the manubriosternal and costochondral joints, the hips, knees, shoulders and heels. The latter is due to enthesopathy at the tendocalcaneus (with pain at the back of the heel) and possibly the plantar ligaments (pain on weight bearing in the morning, from plantar fasciitis). Some patients also complain of pleuritic-type chest pain due to the disease affecting the insertions of the intercostal muscles. Muscle spasm may accompany the pain in any of the above areas.

Later in the course of AS the patient will complain of more constant pain and stiffness. This is still worse after immobility and improves with exercise. There will also be a noticeable decrease in spinal mobility and chest expansion. The patient may complain of tenderness, particularly in the axial joints: spine, sacroiliac, manubriosternal, costovertebral and symphysis pubis.

In progressive disease the patient will have noticeable deformities which often include the following:

- increased thoracic kyphosis

- poking chin
(If the above deformities are severe, they can cause problems with intubation during surgery.)
- flattened lumbar lordosis with posterior pelvic tilt
- slightly flexed hips and knees (which can become fixed with habitual change in posture).

The above postural changes are often grouped together and called the 'question mark' deformity, as this can be the appearance of the patient when viewed from the side (Fig 7.16). The characteristic stooping posture and stiff spine lead to muscle shortening and further loss of movement.

There will also be abnormal loading in and around the joints which can lead to secondary problems including degenerative changes. Loss of muscle strength is common and this may be due to reduced activity levels, limited movement or some structural change in the muscle cells (Viitanen & Suni 1995).

Self-assessment question

■ **SAQ 7.14.** Using your knowledge of anatomy, work out which muscle groups may become shortened and tight due to the changes in posture which occur in AS.

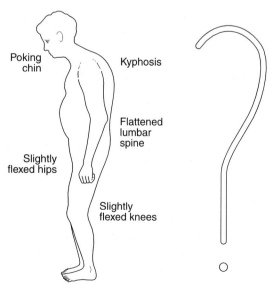

Figure 7.16 'Question mark' deformity.

The extra-articular features which some patients experience are:

- recurrent iritis
- aortic incompetence
- Crohn's disease
- ulcerative colitis
- (sometimes associated with psoriasis).

All of the above may need treatment in their own right; for example iritis will need treatment with topical corticosteroids and the patient often needs to wear sunglasses due to acute light sensitivity which causes pain.

The distinguishing clinical features for recognising inflammatory back pain (as opposed to mechanical) include (Caldron 1995, Chartered Society of Physiotherapy (CSP) 1993, Rai & Struthers 1994, Viitanen & Suni 1995):

- Pain and stiffness which are worse in the morning and improve with activity.
- Insidious onset with no inciting incident.
- Pain present for more than 3 months.
- Onset of symptoms usually well below the age of 40.

Case study 7.4

Mr Smith
This gentleman is attending the outpatient department with a suspected diagnosis of AS. He is a 29-year-old carpenter, married with two young children, living in a sixth-floor flat. He has been unable to work for the last 2 weeks and has spent most of that time on bedrest. His symptoms have improved somewhat after starting on NSAIDs and this is his first visit to a physiotherapy department.

Problem-solving exercise 7.12

■ Decide how you would assess this patient. If you wish, go back to the earlier section about OA to refresh your memory about assessment, but keep in mind how this patient differs from the scenarios you have dealt with so far.

Assessment

It is not intended that this section repeat all of the information given earlier in the chapter. By this time it should be fairly clear that you can use very similar questioning and examination techniques for all of the patients who have been presented. The overall structure is the same, but you need to make sure that the structure you choose to adopt is flexible enough to be personalised for each patient you see. Decide which sections you need to keep and which can be left out or looked at in less detail. As mentioned in the last problem-solving exercise, for general assessment guidelines go back to the section on OA.

As an autonomous practitioner you need to carry out a thorough enough examination to satisfy yourself that the diagnosis the patient comes with matches your findings. You are now aware that AS can sometimes present as chronic low back pain, so answer the following SAQ to make sure you have remembered how to tell the difference.

Self-assessment question

■ **SAQ 7.15.** What are the clinical features you can use for distinguishing inflammatory back pain from mechanical back pain?

There are a number of issues that you should have addressed during your assessment of this patient which are different from those you dealt with earlier in the chapter. These are particularly related to his functional and psychosocial status. Perhaps some of the following questions would be useful:

- At the time of assessment what is his function like?
- Does he feel that he is getting better, worse or staying the same?
- Is he able to manage his ADL?
- Can he get up all six flights of stairs to his flat? If not, why not? Is it too painful, does he get tired or breathless?
- How long does it take him to work off his morning stiffness?
- Can he drive? (if this question is relevant)
- Is he the main breadwinner for the family?

- How will the disease affect his ability to carry out his job?
- Exactly what activities does his job involve?
- What are the other activities he normally carries out, e.g. work at home or hobbies and so on? Can he do them now?

The above questions need to be asked along with the usual ones about pain behaviour, stiffness, and so on. This patient is much younger than the others you have considered and has a very different set of circumstances. You need to look at these issues in relation to the findings of your physical examination.

You already know a lot about how to assess a patient with a rheumatic condition, but there are certain measurements taken with an AS patient that are a little different due to the specific problems experienced.

Until recently it has been the norm to take a large number of measurements of range of movement in all joints, vital capacity and height and posture, on a regular basis, to assess both the disease progression and the effects of exercise. However, recent work at the Royal National Hospital for Rheumatic Diseases in Bath, UK, has streamlined this approach to a smaller number of measures which appear to give the same information about disease activity. Of the 20 measurements, five were found to most closely coincide

with the X-rays and laboratory results that are used to indicate disease status (Mallorie et al 1995). The five measures are:

1. cervical rotation
2. tragus to wall distance (Fig. 7.17)
3. lateral flexion
4. modified Schober's test of lumbar flexion (Fig. 7.18)
5. intermalleolar distance.

This makes for a much speedier assessment and gives a baseline from which to measure any changes in the patient's condition. However, if you found your patient had a problem with a particular joint or area not included here, you could of course use any measures you felt appropriate. Other possible measurements can be seen in Table 7.7.

Remember that these measures are just sug-

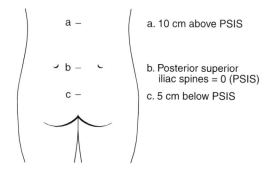

a – 　　　a. 10 cm above PSIS

b – 　　　b. Posterior superior iliac spines = 0 (PSIS)

c – 　　　c. 5 cm below PSIS

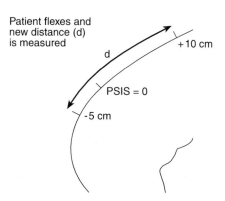

Patient flexes and new distance (d) is measured

d

+10 cm

PSIS = 0

-5 cm

Figure 7.18 Modified Schober's test of lumbar flexion.

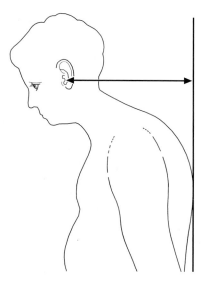

Figure 7.17 Measurement of tragus to wall.

Table 7.7 Possible physical measurements for use with ankylosing spondylitis (AS) patients (CSP 1993, Helliwell et al 1996, Rai & Struthers 1994, Viitanen & Suni 1995)

Height
Cervical spine: all movements
Thoracic spine: flexion/extension
Chest expansion at xiphisternum
Lumbar spine: flexion/extension/side flexion
Finger to floor distance (unreliable by itself for lumbar flexion as it includes hip flexion)
Hip: all movements (with goniometer), Thomas' test
Knee: check for flexion deformity
Shoulder: particularly flexion
Exercise tolerance
FEV₁ (forced expiratory volume in 1 second)
Vital capacity

gestions and it would not be necessary to use them all for every AS patient.

Management

Apart from the patient in this case study being much younger, there is one key point concerning the management of the AS patient. Any ideas?

The main thing to be aware of is that the pain and stiffness improve with exercise. This is extremely important and the patient must be helped to understand that activity is a major part of the management of the condition. Although exercise plays a large part in the treatment of many rheumatic conditions, in AS it is a major consideration.

Drug treatment usually consists of analgesics and NSAIDs which are taken to reduce inflammation. This in turn reduces pain and stiffness allowing the patient to be generally more active and to undertake an exercise programme.

Self-assessment question

■ **SAQ 7.16.** What are the five main objective measures that can be used to record the progress of an AS patient?

Problem-solving exercise 7.13

Assume that during your assessment you have found that Mr Smith has low back pain referring into his buttocks and posterior thigh region. Movements of the whole spine are restricted and painful but there is no fixed deformity at this time. He also has discomfort and reduced range of movement in both hips and shoulders (especially flexion and abduction). He feels stiff in the morning and this decreases if he gets up and about a little during the day. Generally he feels rather fatigued and gets breathless on light exercise.

■ Devise a plan of physiotherapy treatment for this patient. Include any advice you might give him regarding ADL. Note any points where input from other members of the health care team may be useful.

You can look at the following section for some ideas on this – but try it yourself first.

A plan of treatment for Mr Smith

The plan of physiotherapy for Mr Smith will mainly involve exercise and stretches for the following reasons:

- To maintain muscle strength (and improve it if necessary), generally, but also to target specific muscle groups that are in danger of becoming weak, for instance back extensors, shoulder and hip abductors.
- To maintain or improve muscle length and joint range of movement (especially in the spine, hips and shoulders).
- To improve exercise tolerance.

Both hydrotherapy and land-based regimes are used regularly in AS.

Advice on ADL

The plan should also include advice on ADL.

Overall the patient needs to take on responsibility for his own management: looking after his health and posture. This includes not allowing himself to become overtired or taking on too many commitments.

If the AS is very active then rest may be indicated (which could involve time away from work or even in hospital), but rest does not mean immobility as this could increase the stiffness in the spine. It is important that the person continues to exercise and to practise good posture.

It is good to encourage prone lying even if the patient needs a pillow under his chest at the beginning. Twenty minutes is an acceptable period but the patient may have to work up to this. It will help prevent the hips and back from becoming too flexed.

The bed should be firm without sagging. This will again help to keep a good posture.

A high chair with a firm seat and upright back is often found to be better for the posture but may not be as comfortable as an easy chair. Sitting in low, soft chairs will result in bad posture and increased pain. Also the patient should keep his head against the back of the chair (or a small cushion if necessary); this will reduce the chance of developing a poking chin.

If the patient travels by car it is important to get out periodically to stretch, as pain and stiffness can distract attention.

It is important to remain physically active. Contact sports can be risky as damage to the joints can occur. Swimming is excellent as it exercises the whole body without jarring and includes cardiovascular and respiratory factors (respiratory exercises are very important for some patients with thoracic cage joint involvement: it helps to maintain vital capacity). Some other possible activities are cycling, badminton, squash, netball, basketball and running (preferably not on roads, but on grass if possible to reduce jarring).

The patient should also be given the following advice about ADL:

- Do not use a revolving chair if you work at a desk: this will stop you rotating the spine. This lack of turning will lead to you being unable to turn.
- Get up to change the channel on the TV, don't use the remote control!
- A hot bath may help to ease aches and pains. You could do some exercises in or after the bath.
- Avoid working at a flat-topped desk or table as this means you are bending your head forward. Try to arrange some sort of inclined surface.

- When working in a standing position, try to raise the task up so you are not bending forward.
- Check posture regularly and correct it as much as possible. You can use a wall to stand against; try to get the back of your head, hips and heels touching it.

Some specific exercises, advice and activities can be found in *Stretch, relax and a little bit more … Exercises for ankylosing spondylitis* (Barefoot 1993).

Other members of the health care team
The members of the health care team involved with this patient may vary depending on his specific needs. The GP will certainly be involved and the OT may have an input. Mr Smith may wish to attend the local National Ankylosing Spondylitis Society group if there is one available.

As patients with AS tend to be less disabled than those with severe RA or OA, they may not need intervention from a large health care team. But if you do come across any patients who are severely affected (that is, those who are having problems with ADL due to marked deformity, weakness and reduced exercise tolerance), then more members of the team would be involved.

Conclusion

Work has been done which shows definite improvement in AS patients when they have drug therapy plus an exercise regime. Different approaches have been investigated, for example 2–3 weeks as an inpatient with daily land-based exercise and hydrotherapy, out-patient treatment with land-based and/or hydrotherapy and home exercises, or home exercises alone. Other patients attend groups run by the National Ankylosing Spondylitis Society (NASS) which is more of a self-help group with input from health professionals.

Improvement has even been found in patients who have had the condition for many years with decrease in range of movement and marked deformity. Often this improvement is not great in terms of degrees of increased movement and so on but it is usually of functional significance to the patient.

It is not easy to get an overview of the available research regarding exercise and AS, due to the differences and shortcomings of the methodologies. But the main message that comes through from virtually all the studies is that patients must maintain the exercise level themselves, incorporating it into their lifestyle, otherwise any improvement seen with treatment (whatever approach is used) is not maintained. The exercise should also be as intensive as the patients can tolerate in order to keep any improvement to a maximum (Helliwell et al 1996, Viitanen & Suni 1995).

You should keep this in mind whenever you are treating patients with AS. It may be your input that helps to motivate them to continue with their exercises. You could even become involved in running sessions in the pool and on dry land at a NASS group.

As with all the rheumatic diseases, the patients must be encouraged to take on the responsibility for their own management, with support and input from the health professionals when necessary.

A NOTE ON THE IMPACT OF CHRONIC PROGRESSIVE DISEASE

When you are involved in the management of patients with chronic progressive disease, it is imperative that you take the psychological and social implications into account alongside the purely physical effects. Inevitably when a patient presents with an illness, both the health professional and the patient have to 'make sense' of the disease. However the meanings that the disease has for each will be very different. For the health professional the diagnosis, symptoms and treatment are often the initial considerations, but for the patient the main focus may not be on the disease but on the impact it has on his or her life. Awareness of this difference in approach is important when devising a treatment plan and when deciding what may need to be covered in a patient education programme. Overall it should help to improve communication between the patient and health professionals as well as improving compliance with treatment.

Responses to treatment depend on the patient.

Different people have different coping mechanisms, motivational levels and values regarding aspects of life which are important. There can also be variation in one patient at different times, considering the phasic nature of many of the rheumatic disorders. Patients therefore have to be flexible if they are to cope with variation in pain, functional ability and possibly progressive deformity.

Major problems can occur if patients perceive that the disease is controlling their lives instead of them controlling it. Stress and anxiety levels increase and it is difficult to know whether this is a cause or effect of the condition. Patients make attributions for their overall disease and may even make separate attributions for flares and remissions. It has been found that the presence of psychological stress is most often cited as the reason for a flare in RA patients. The second most popular reason for a flare was given as excessive physical activity, but patients who gave this as a reason felt less helpless. This may be because activity levels can be altered easily by the patients themselves, so enabling them to believe that they may have some control over the disease (Selley 1990).

Points to consider

Self-concept
This relates to the way we perceive ourselves and our relationship to/with the environment. Patients with a chronic progressive disease will revise their own self-concept and it is axiomatic that this will have an effect on how well they cope and their response to treatment. But interestingly it has been shown that people will only seek as much help as is compatible with maintaining their self-concept (Skevington 1990).

Self image
This is made up of several facets. Firstly, there is the physical image which may be positive or negative. The media are constantly reinforcing so-called 'acceptable' images and many people feel they should conform to these. This will of course be affected when a person has a chronic progressive disease, particularly if there is reduction in functional ability or any deformity.

Secondly there is the public image of people with arthritis, particularly related to altered appearance. These two areas of self-image may cause isolation or withdrawal.

Closely connected to this is the third facet of self-image which concerns sexual identity. A person with arthritis may feel that it is more difficult or even impossible to form relationships, or the consequences of the disease could even affect established relationships.

Disease process

The possibility of eventual deformities is very important to patients. These may be difficult to conceal if they affect the gait or, particularly, the hands, which are used for expression and non-verbal communication. Perceptions also differ, with one patient's 'mild' deformity being perceived as 'severe' by another patient who has the same degree of change. This relates to the patient's coping strategies (Newman 1990).

Because of the disease process, patients may have to rely on others for selecting clothes, putting on make-up and doing their hair. This can cause problems especially if the carer has different ideas.

Treatments given to combat the disease process can also affect appearance, for example water retention due to steroids. There could be scarring from surgery and some patients may be required to wear obtrusive splints or orthoses.

Perceptions

People with chronic progressive disease also have to deal with common public perceptions. Some people expect that someone with arthritis will be 'old, gnarled and twisted' and may be surprised when they meet a person with a rheumatic condition who is none of those, whereas others will not expect any change in appearance. Some will perceive those with rheumatic conditions to be disabled and some will not.

There seems to be a general need to appear 'normal', whatever that is. But many people with arthritis get to a stage where they also need to acknowledge that they do require help, which can be difficult.

Role changes

Chronic progressive disease does force role changes, both within society and with other people which can be very far reaching.

1. *Employment*

Someone with arthritis may have to get up extremely early to get over morning stiffness before going to work. In conditions where fatigue is often an issue, this will only compound the problem. Generally the person has decreased energy and needs more time to do things. Because of these problems, the evenings and weekends are used for rest which means that there is a decreased social life.

A variable condition (that is with flares and remissions) will mean variable performance, possibly with time away from work and, depending on the situation, fear of dismissal. If the person is unemployed it is probably more difficult to get a job and career opportunities will be reduced.

With less work or the loss of a job, financial resources will be decreased, there will be less purpose and structure to the person's life and decreased independence. If the patient is a housewife there may be problems managing the home.

2. *Family*

If an individual develops a rheumatic condition it can affect the whole family. Employment issues may impinge here, especially if the patient is the main breadwinner.

Partners may begin to feel isolated if they have to sleep in separate rooms or beds because of the patient's pain and/or sleeplessness. The person with the disease may have less energy and be unable or unwilling to go out very much. There could also be decreased physical contact, mainly because it hurts.

Individual and family plans will be affected. People may feel guilty and stress levels may rise, making it difficult to talk. This is important in its own right, but even more so if we take into account the evidence regarding the link between stress and possible exacerbation of the disease.

3. *Community*

Because of the disease process and consequent possible changes in employment and family situations, the person will also perceive a change in role in the wider community setting. This will involve a narrower social environment.

There are also issues concerning the different concepts of 'disability' in varying cultural settings.

4. *Stages of life*

The disease process will have different effects depending on when it starts in the person's life. Think back to the case studies earlier in the chapter and consider the differences due to age at onset.

Review points

Suppose a patient with a rheumatic condition came to you for help and advice. Try to imagine how the above issues could affect your approach and the patient's response.

For more detailed coverage of these important issues you can refer to *Arthritis and the psyche* (Selley & Kirwan 1990).

Summary

This chapter has given you an overview of the issues involved in the management of rheumatic conditions, including background information on a number of common conditions, assessment, identification of problems and treatment planning. It has also addressed pharmacological management, the roles of the health care team and the implications of chronic progressive disease for the physiotherapist and the patient.

As stated at the beginning of the chapter, the physiotherapy interventions used with patients with rheumatic conditions are often quite routine – but it is the decision-making process of when and where to use them that is the most important. Obviously it is impossible to cover every eventuality, but it is hoped that if you now come across patients with any rheumatic condition, you would feel more confident in your ability to deal with them appropriately. Remember that one of the most important points is that there is no cure for these diseases and the patients are not going to 'get better'. Your role is to help them to cope and function more effectively within the limits of the condition, using a whole gamut of knowledge and techniques in partnership with other members of the health care team.

On reading this summary, do you feel you have grasped the above points? If not, perhaps you should go back and re-read any appropriate parts of the chapter before moving on.

ANSWERS TO QUESTIONS AND EXERCISES

Self-assessment question 7.1 (page 144)

■ **SAQ 7.1.** An NSAID will suppress the classical features of inflammation (Thompson & Dunne 1995). What are those features?

Answer: The classical features of inflammation are: redness, heat, swelling, pain and loss of function.

Self-assessment questions 7.2–7.5

See information in text.

Problem-solving exercise 7.1 (page 150)

■ With the information you have been given so far, try to work out the probable clinical features you would expect to find in a patient with OA.

Answer:
— *Joint pain*
— *Stiffness*
— *Enlargement of joint size*
— *Limitation of movement*
— *Loss of function.*

Problem-solving exercises 7.2 and 7.3

Refer to text.

Self-assessment question 7.6 (page 161)

See information in text.

Problem-solving exercises 7.4 and 7.5

Refer to text.

Self-assessment question 7.7 (page 166)

See information in text.

Self-assessment question 7.8 (page 166)

■ **SAQ 7.8a.** What are the aims of physiotherapy management for patients with rheumatic conditions?

See information in text.

■ **SAQ 7.8b.** Why is it important that these aims are matched to the patient's needs and beliefs?

Answer: If patients do not perceive that the aims of physiotherapy treatment are relevant to their particular situation and environment, then they may be less willing to participate and less compliant. This is particularly important when we are expecting patients to take on responsibility for their own management. Your success in dealing with patients will depend to a certain extent on how effectively you identify their problems (related to assessment and your modification of it as necessary) and then on how appropriately you intervene.

Problem-solving exercise 7.6 (page 169)

Refer to text.

Problem-solving exercise 7.7 (page 172)

See following section in text.

Self-assessment questions 7.9–7.11

See information in text.

Problem-solving exercise 7.8 (page 179)

See information in text.

Problem-solving exercise 7.9 (page 179)

A. Compare with your response to problem-solving exercise 7.8.

B. See the following section in the text.

Self-assessment question 7.12 (page 180)

See information in text.

Problem-solving exercise 7.10 (page 183)

See the following section in the text.

Problem-solving exercise 7.11 (page 187)

See information in text.

Self-assessment question 7.13 (page 188)

See information in text.

Self-assessment question 7.14 (page 188)

■ **SAQ 7.14.** Using your knowledge of anatomy, work out which muscle groups may become shortened and tight due to the changes in posture which occur in AS.

Answer: Because of the overall flexed position of the typical AS patient, it is the flexor groups of muscles which become shortened and tight because of changes in posture (and possibly due to physiological changes in the muscle itself). This means that physiotherapy intervention often involves a large element of stretching exercises as well as strengthening of the antagonists. The patient needs to be given advice and to be reminded about positioning and posture.

Although the flexor groups are the obvious muscles to stretch, the exercise regime always includes more general stretching (often of adductor and rotator groups) to combat reduced range of movement.

Problem-solving exercise 7.12 (page 189)

See information in text.

Self-assessment questions 7.15 and 7.16

See information in text.

Problem-solving exercise 7.13 (page 191)

See following section in text.

REFERENCES

Adler S 1985 Self care in the management of the degenerative knee joint. Physiotherapy 71(2):58–60

Anderson J R (ed) 1985 Muir's textbook of pathology, 12th edn. Edward Arnold, London

Arnett F C, Edworthy S M, Bloch D A et al 1988 The American Rheumatism Association 1987 revised criteria for the classification of rheumatoid arthritis. Arthritis and Rheumatism 31(3):315–324

Arthritis and Rheumatism Council for Research 1995 Pain and arthritis: a booklet for patients. Arthritis and Rheumatism Council for Research, Chesterfield

Banwell B F 1988 Comprehensive care. In: Banwell B F, Gall V (eds) Physical therapy management of arthritis. Churchill Livingstone, New York, ch 2

Banwell B F, Gall V (eds) 1988 Physical therapy management of arthritis. Churchill Livingstone, New York, p ix

Barefoot J 1993 Stretch, relax and a little bit more … Exercises for ankylosing spondylitis, 3rd edn. Georgian Music Desktop Publishing, Bath

Barnes C G 1980 Rheumatoid arthritis. In: Currey H L F (ed) Mason and Currey's clinical rheumatology. Pitman, London, p 30–62

Bellamy N 1991 Prognosis in rheumatoid arthritis. Journal of Rheumatology 18(9):1277–1279

Bennett J C 1985 The etiology of rheumatoid arthritis. In: Kelley W N, Harris E D, Ruddy S, Sledge C B (eds) Textbook of rheumatology, 2nd edn. W B Saunders, Philadelphia, p 879–885

Bhardwaj N, Paget S A 1992 Rheumatoid arthritis. In: Paget S A, Fields T R (eds) Rheumatic disorders. Butterworth Heinemann, Boston, ch 3

Bland J H 1993 Mechanisms of adaptation in the joint. In: Crosbie J, McConnell J (eds) Key issues in musculoskeletal physiotherapy. Butterworth Heinemann, Oxford, ch 4

Brattstrom M 1987 Joint protection and rehabilitation in chronic rheumatic disorders. Wolfe Medical, London

Brooks P 1990 Monitoring drug therapy in rheumatoid arthritis: toxicity. Reports on rheumatic diseases (Series 2) No. 16. Arthritis and Rheumatism Council, London

Brooks P M 1992 Medical management of rheumatoid arthritis. Rheumatology Review 1(3):137–145

Brown G K, Nicassio P M, Wallston K A 1989 Pain coping strategies and depression in rheumatoid arthritis. Journal of Consulting and Clinical Psychology 57(5):652–657

Butler R 1990 Monitoring drug therapy in rheumatoid arthritis: efficacy. Reports on rheumatic diseases (Series 2) No. 15. Arthritis and Rheumatism Council, London

Caldron P H 1995 Screening for rheumatic disease. In: Boissonnault W G (ed) Examination in physical therapy practice – screening for medical disease, 2nd edn. Churchill Livingstone, New York, ch 11

Carlstedt C, Nordin M 1989 Biomechanics of tendons and ligaments. In: Nordin M, Frankel V H (eds) Basic biomechanics of the musculoskeletal system. Lea and Febiger, Philadelphia, ch 3

Chartered Society of Physiotherapy (CSP) 1993 Standards of physiotherapy practice for the management of people with ankylosing spondylitis. Chartered Society of Physiotherapy, London

Christian C L 1992 Introduction and differential diagnosis of rheumatic disorders. In: Paget S A, Fields T R (eds) Rheumatic disorders. Butterworth Heinemann, Boston, ch 1

Clarke A K 1987 Rehabilitation techniques in rheumatology. Williams and Wilkins, London

Dandy D J 1993 Essential orthopaedics and trauma, 2nd edn. Churchill Livingstone, Edinburgh, ch 16

Danneskiold-Samsoe B 1987 The effect of water exercise therapy given to patients with rheumatoid arthritis. Scandinavian Journal of Rehabilitation Medicine 19:31–35

Dial C, Windsor R A 1985 A formative evaluation of a health education water exercise programme for class II and III adult rheumatoid arthritis patients. Patient Education and Counselling 7:33–42

Donovan J L, Blake D R, Fleming W G 1989 The patient is not a blank sheet: lay beliefs and their relevance to patient education. British Journal of Rheumatology 28:58–61

Eide R 1982 The effect of physical activity on emotional reactions, stress reactions and related psychological reactions. Scandinavian Journal of Social Medicine 29(suppl):103–107

Ellis M 1981 Knee joint forces whilst rising from a chair. Leeds newsletter – Demonstration centres in rehabilitation. January 20–23

Fries J F 1990 Re-evaluating the therapeutic approach to rheumatoid arthritis: the 'sawtooth strategy'. Journal of Rheumatology 22(17)(suppl):12–15

Furst D E 1990 Rheumatoid arthritis – practical use of medications. Postgraduate Medicine 87(3):79–92

Gall E P 1988 Pathophysiology of rheumatic disease. In: Banwell B F, Gall V (eds) Physical therapy management of arthritis. Churchill Livingstone, New York, ch 1

Gall V 1988 Patient evaluation. In: Banwell B F, Gall V (eds) Physical therapy management of arthritis. Churchill Livingstone, New York, ch 4

Goats G C, Hunter J A, Flett E, Stirling A 1996 Low intensity laser and phototherapy for rheumatoid arthritis. Physiotherapy 82(5):311–320

Golding D N 1991 Local corticosteroid injections. Reports on rheumatic diseases (Series 2) No. 19. Arthritis and Rheumatism Council, London

Grahame R, Cooper R 1986 What can physiotherapy offer? Reports on rheumatic diseases (Series 2) No 3. Arthritis and Rheumatism Council, London

Haralson K 1988 Physical modalities. In: Banwell B F, Gall V (eds) Physical therapy management of arthritis. Churchill Livingstone, New York, ch 6

Harris E D 1985a Pathogenesis of rheumatoid arthritis. In: Kelley W N, Harris E D, Ruddy S, Sledge C B (eds) Textbook of rheumatology, 2nd edn. W B Saunders, Philadelphia, vol 1, p 886–914

Harris E D 1985b Rheumatoid arthritis: the clinical spectrum. In: Kelley W N, Harris E D, Ruddy S, Sledge C B (eds) Textbook of rheumatology, 2nd edn. W B Saunders, Philadelphia, vol 1, p 915–949

Harris E D 1990 Rheumatoid arthritis – pathophysiology and implications for therapy. New England Journal of Medicine 322(18):1277–1289

Hazes J M W, Silman A J 1990 Review of UK data on the rheumatic diseases 2, rheumatoid arthritis. British Journal of Rheumatology 29:310–312

Helliwell P S, Abbott C A, Chamberlain M A 1996 A randomised trial of three different physiotherapy regimes in ankylosing spondylitis. Physiotherapy 82(2):85–90

Hutton C W 1995 Osteoarthritis – clinical features and management. Reports on rheumatic diseases (Series 3) No 5. Arthritis and Rheumatism Council for Research, Chesterfield

Ike R W, Lampman R M, Castor C W 1989 Arthritis and aerobic exercise: a review. Physician and Sports Medicine 17(2):128–137

Inman R D 1992 Reiter's syndrome and reactive arthritis.

In: Paget S A, Fields T R (eds) Rheumatic disorders. Butterworth Heinemann, Boston, ch 6

Jarvis R E 1978 Physiotherapy for children and young adults with arthritis. Physiotherapy 64(5):143–145

Jeffreson P 1993 What can occupational therapy offer the patient with rheumatic disease? Reports on rheumatic diseases (Series 2) No. 25. Arthritis and Rheumatism Council for Research, Chesterfield

Kaufman L D, Sokoloff L 1992 Osteoarthritis. In: Paget S A, Fields T R (eds) Rheumatic disorders. Butterworth Heinemann, Boston, ch 5

Kay E A, Punchak S S 1988 Patient understanding of the causes and medical treatment of rheumatoid arthritis. British Journal of Rheumatology 27:396–398

Kennedy G, Edmunds L, Calin A 1993 The natural history of ankylosing spondylitis. Does it burn out? Journal of Rheumatology 20(4):688–692

Kirwan J R 1990 Patient education in rheumatoid arthritis. Current Opinion in Rheumatology 2:336–339

Levine P 1988 Gait and mobility. In: Banwell B F, Gall V (eds) Physical therapy management of arthritis. Churchill Livingstone, New York, ch 7

Lindroth Y, Bauman A, Barnes C et al 1989 A controlled evaluation of arthritis education. British Journal of Rheumatology 78:7–12

Lorig K, Seleznick M, Lubeck D et al 1989 The beneficial outcomes of the arthritis self-management course are not adequately explained by behaviour change. Arthritis and Rheumatism 32:91–95

McKnight P T 1988 Splinting and joint protection. In: Banwell B F, Gall V (eds) 1988 Physical therapy management of arthritis. Churchill Livingstone, New York, ch 8

Mallorie P A, Whitelock H C, Garret S L et al 1995 Defining spinal mobility in ankylosing spondylitis (AS): the Bath AS Metrology Index (BASMI). Procedings of the 12th International Congress of the World Confederation for Physical Therapy. American Physical Therapy Association paper PL-RR-0886-T

Minor M A, Hewett J E, Webel R R et al 1989 Efficacy of physical conditioning exercise in patients with rheumatoid arthritis and osteoarthritis. Arthritis and Rheumatism 32(11):1396–1405

Newman S 1990 Coping with rheumatoid arthritis. In: Selley S, Kirwan J (eds) ARC Conference Proceedings No. 9 'Arthritis and the psyche'. Arthritis and Rheumatism Council, London

Nordemar R 1981 Physical training in rheumatoid arthritis: a controlled long term study. II. Functional capacity and general attitudes. Scandinavian Journal of Rheumatology 10:25–30

Rai A, Struthers G R 1994 Ankylosing spondylitis. Reports on rheumatic diseases (Series 3) No. 3. Arthritis and Rheumatism Council for Research, Chesterfield

Ranawat C S, Maynard M J, Flynn W F 1992 Total hip replacement arthroplasty in patients with inflammatory arthritis. In: Paget S A, Fields T R (eds) Rheumatic disorders. Butterworth Heinemann, Boston, ch 14

Rasker J J, Cosh J A 1989 Course and prognosis of early rheumatoid arthritis. Scandinavian Journal of Rheumatology 79(suppl):45–56

Rheumatic Care Association of Chartered

Physiotherapists (RCACP) 1994 Guidelines of good practice for the management of people with rheumatic diseases. Chartered Society of Physiotherapy, London

Rhind V M 1987 Assessment of stiffness in rheumatology: the use of rating scales. British Journal of Rheumatology 26:126–130

Ruddy S 1985 The management of rheumatoid arthritis. In: Kelley W N, Harris E D, Ruddy S, Sledge C B (eds) Textbook of rheumatology, 2nd edn. W B Saunders, Philadelphia, p 979–992

Selley S 1990 Patients' views on the causes of arthritis. In: Selley S, Kirwan J (eds) ARC Conference Proceedings No. 9 'Arthritis and the psyche'. Arthritis and Rheumatism Council, London

Selley S, Kirwan J (eds) 1990 ARC Conference Proceedings No. 9 'Arthritis and the psyche'. Arthritis and Rheumatism Council, London

Skevington S 1990 Psychological consequences of chronic pain. In: Selley S, Kirwan J (eds) ARC Conference Proceedings No. 9 'Arthritis and the psyche'. Arthritis and Rheumatism Council, London

Smith M D, Ahern M J, Roberts-Thompson P J 1990 Pulse methylprednisolone therapy in rheumatoid arthritis: unproved therapy, unjustified therapy or effective adjunctive treatment? Annals of the Rheumatic Diseases 49:265–267

Sterling L P 1990 Rheumatoid arthritis: current concepts and management, part 1. American Pharmacy 30(8):47–52

Sukenik S, Buskila D, Neumann L et al 1990 Sulphur bath and mud pack treatment for rheumatoid arthritis at the Dead Sea area. Annals of the Rheumatic Diseases 49:99–102

Swezey R L 1990a Rehabilitation in arthritis and allied conditions. In: Kottke F J, Lehmann J F (eds) Krusken's handbook of physical medicine and rehabilitation. 4th edn. W B Saunders, Philadelphia, p 679–716

Swezey R L 1990b Rheumatoid arthritis: the role of the kinder and gentler therapies. Journal of Rheumatology 17(suppl):8–13

Thompson P W, Dunne C 1995 Non steroidal anti-inflammatory drugs: use and abuse. Reports on rheumatic diseases (Series 3) No. 4. Arthritis and Rheumatism Council for Research, Chesterfield

Tork S C, Douglas V 1989 Arthritis water exercise program evaluation – a self assessment survey. Arthritis Care and Research 2(1):28–30

Turner-Stokes L 1993 Treatment and control of chronic arthritic and back pain. Reports on rheumatic diseases (Series 2) No. 23. Arthritis and Rheumatism Council for Research, Chesterfield

Viitanen J V, Suni J 1995 Management principles of physiotherapy in ankylosing spondylitis – which treatments are effective? Physiotherapy 81(6):322–329

Williams P L, Warwick R, Dyson M, Bannister L H 1989 Gray's anatomy, 37th edn. Churchill Livingstone, Edinburgh

Wolfe F 1990 50 years of antirheumatic therapy: the prognosis of rheumatoid arthritis. Journal of Rheumatology 17(suppl):24–32

Yaron M 1995 Hormonal problems and rheumatic diseases. Reports on rheumatic diseases (Series 3) No. 6. Arthritis and Rheumatism Council for Research, Chesterfield

Zurier R B 1990 Conventional drug therapies and complications, novel therapies and non-drug treatments. Current Opinion in Rheumatology 2:463–468

8

Joint replacements of the lower limb

■ Joint replacement ■ Classification ■ Management ■ Complications
■ Physiotherapy management

CONTENTS

Objectives

By the end of this chapter you should:

1. Have an overview of the type of joint replacements for the lower limb and when they are used.
2. Understand the assessment of a patient before and after joint replacement.
3. Recognise how to problem solve for patient treatment and assessment, whatever the type of joint replacement in situ.

Prerequisites

Re-read the chapters on assessment (Ch. 3) and fractures (Ch. 5), and *Essential orthopaedics and trauma* (Dandy 1993), Chapter 24 and Chapter 6 (p 78–82).

INTRODUCTION: OVERVIEW OF JOINT REPLACEMENTS FOR THE LOWER LIMB

Joint replacements are now a very common surgical event and many are undertaken each year in the UK. The first completely successful joint replacement in a human subject took place in 1959, although many previous attempts had succeeded for varying lengths of time. The hip was the first joint to be successfully replaced, and internal prosthetics for the metacarpophalangeal (MCP), wrist, elbow, shoulder, knee and ankle joints were all developed after this.

A full joint replacement, or total arthroplasty, replaces both sides of the joint, that is, the acetabulum and the head of the femur. Partial joint replacement (hemiathroplasty) restores the aspect of the joint that is damaged; the surfaces most commonly replaced are the head of the femur and the femur and tibia in the medial compartment of the knee. All partial replacements may be upgraded to a full replacement at a future date if necessary.

A joint replacement can be further classified according to whether it is constrained, semiconstrained or unconstrained. In a constrained joint there is a link between the two components and all anatomical movements of the artificial joint are restricted to a greater or lesser extent. In a semiconstrained joint some movement, although restricted, is allowed in all planes, and an unconstrained joint permits free movement in all anatomical planes. Examples of these will be discussed with reference to particular types of joint.

Commonly, the replacement prosthetic parts are made out of inert metals, such as stainless steel or chrome–cobalt–molybdenum alloys, and high density polyethylene. These components have been shown to produce low friction motion at the joint so decreasing the chance of abrasion or damage (wear) to the internal joint surfaces, aiding longevity of the joint.

The overriding issue through the years has been the survival of the replacement, that is, the length of time the patient may expect the joint to last with 'normal' use. Loosening, deep infection, fracture and dislocation remain the main complications of joint replacement surgery (Rothman &

Hozack 1988). The successful survival of a joint replacement relies on all members of the team understanding the underlying biomechanical principles of the 'normal' joint and its replacement, the limitations of the materials used, and the surgical procedure undertaken. More importantly the patient must understand why these things matter, so that the rehabilitation programme can be modified to protect the joint.

It is the advancement of the understanding of these issues that has lengthened the average survival of a replacement hip joint to 25 years and that of a knee joint to 15 years. However not all joints will last this length of time, because of poor insertion, loosening, dislocation or fracture.

This chapter will explore the issues outlined above and discuss the rehabilitation programmes for patients who have undergone hip and knee replacements. Ankle replacements will not be discussed, as they are not routine surgical events.

First the indications for a joint replacement and its complications will be discussed.

INDICATIONS FOR JOINT REPLACEMENT

The commonest reasons for a patient to undergo a joint replacement are pain and loss of function (Stanic et al 1993). It is therefore not surprising that the major weight-bearing joints (hip and knee) are the joints most commonly replaced. The repetitive high loads and torsional stresses being taken across these joints predispose them to wear and tear (osteoarthrosis) and the signs and symptoms outlined in Chapter 2. In patients with multiple joint pathology, such as rheumatoid arthritis, replacement of damaged joints may include the MCPs, elbow, and/or shoulders as well as the more routine hips and knees, providing pain-free movement after surgery, with some improvement in function. The functional gains following surgery are not as good as those where there is single joint involvement but, as a result, joint survival is usually longer because the demands made on the new joints are far less.

Pettine et al (1991) compared the outcome of total hip replacements between an over-80-year-old group and a more normally representative group aged 64–67 years. The outcomes did not differ significantly, and the authors advocated that elective hip replacement surgery should be offered to the over-80-year-olds. A similar study has not been undertaken for total knee replacements.

Post-traumatic joint stiffness or avascular necrosis (see Ch. 5) would also predispose the patient to pain and loss of function at specific joints. A partial or total joint replacement may be indicated, even in the younger patient, if the joint destruction was irreversible. The commonest example of the use of a hemiarthroplasty is the replacement of the head of the femur following a subcapital fracture. If the blood supply to the head of the femur has been traumatically interrupted then avascular necrosis will ensue and internal fixation of the fracture alone will not prevent bone death. Hence a hemiarthroplasty of the head of femur may be undertaken if the acetabulum is free of obvious signs of degeneration. Austin–Moore or Thompson hemiarthroplasties are the commonest types used in the UK. The Austin–Moore type does not have to be cemented in place (Fig. 8.1).

An alternative example would be a hip replacement performed several years after a hip

arthrodesis (surgical fusion of the hip joint). Arthrodesis is often performed in the younger patient if the hip has been severely damaged and joint destruction is irreparable. The patient is left with no hip movement and uses compensatory lumbar spine and knee motion. Over time the excessive use can cause trauma and pain to these joints and therefore a hip replacement can be an option in later years.

The outcome of the two above examples would be very different for obvious reasons. Chapter 5 outlines the rehabilitation of a patient following a subcapital fracture. The functional achievements following an arthroplasty for post-traumatic joint stiffness depend on the range of motion gained by surgery and the length of time since, and extent of, the initial damage.

In the younger patient a total hip replacement can be prescribed if there is joint destruction following congenital dislocation of the hip (see Ch. 9). Again, the outcome will not be the same as for conventional total hip arthroplasty because there is likely to be severe weakness of the abductors.

IMPORTANT ASPECTS OF JOINT REPLACEMENT

Fixation

The incidence of loosening of the prosthetic components is dependent on the skill of the surgical technique and the type of fixation to the underlying bone. Originally all joint replacements were inserted with a bond of polymethylmethacrylate cement (PMMA) which held the prosthetic component tightly to the bone.

Acrylic cement can sustain compressive stress well but cannot control shear or torsional stress, so that repeated rotational movement across the bone–cement interface will result in a splitting of the cement and release of cement particles. These particles may then cause bone destruction, and along with the initial damage to the cement, loosening of the prosthetic component will occur. Care during the operative procedure to clean and dry the prepared bone surface before application of cement will reduce the incidence of loosening, but biomechanically, loosening is inevitable at

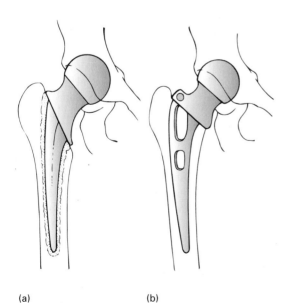

(a)   (b)

Figure 8.1 Hip prosthesis for fracture of femoral neck. (a) Thompson prosthesis secured with cement; (b) Austin–Moore prosthesis with no cement. (Adapted with permission from Dandy 1993.)

some stage because cement is stiffer than bone. Thus the bone–cement and cement–prosthesis interfaces become the weakest points under the excessive loads. The more obese or active the patient the greater the loads and risk of loosening. Also a greater surface area of cement will create more problems; this is of particular significance in long-stem femoral implants.

An alternative to cementing the prosthesis in place is bio-ingrowth: the natural growth of bone around or through the prosthetic implant. No cement is used and attachment is achieved by new bone growth at the bone–prosthesis interface. Bone growth is enhanced by the tightness of the 'press fit' of the component, where the resulting trauma and compression to the bone stimulate new growth (Rothman & Hozack 1988). Alternatively a coating of hydroxyapatite on the prosthetic component may stimulate bone growth. The surface of the prosthetic component is often shaped with bumps, grooves or holes to allow easier attachment of the new bone. A non-cement technique necessitates a period of non-, or partial weight bearing to allow stabilisation of the component. The length of time of reduced weight bearing depends on the type of joint being replaced, the expectations of the patient and the rate of bone growth.

More and more joints are being replaced using a cementless technique and this is often the preferred choice in 'younger' (under 65 years) patients undergoing arthroplasty. In some cases only one component of a total joint replacement may be cemented in. For example, only the acetabular component of a total hip replacement may be cemented in, allowing the femoral component, with its greater surface area and higher rotational forces, to attach via new bone growth, hopefully reducing the risk of loosening.

If loosening has occurred an uncemented joint can be revised to a cemented joint (Rothman & Hozack 1988).

Rehabilitation issues

A prosthetic replacement will normally ensure relief of pain and return of function following surgery, but this is dependent on the range of motion before surgery, the strength of surrounding musculature and the laxity of the joint.

The replacement is guaranteed to remove the bony destruction caused by the underlying pathology, and the release of tight soft tissues or the repair of damaged ones will help to realign the new joint. However it is only the rehabilitation programme, that will help the patient to achieve full return of function, strength and stability to the joint (Fernandez-Galinski et al 1996). This point is often forgotten when the patient awakes pain-free and more mobile.

At the moment there is little evidence to show whether lack of a rehabilitation programme is detrimental to the biomechanical aspects of joint replacement, particularly loosening. There is research evidence to show that patients do have problems for quite a while after surgery (Zavadak et al 1995).

Assessment

The importance of assessment in joint replacement surgery, both pre- and postoperatively, cannot be forgotten. Specific issues will be mentioned in the following sections, but it is important to remember that a full clinical examination is not necessary for a preoperative assessment of a total joint replacement, because joint stability, range of motion, muscle power and proprioception will all change postoperatively. Thus the therapist should concentrate on respiratory function, range of motion in the particular joint, muscle power and general functional ability, such as walking (distance travelled and aid used), sitting to standing, stair climbing, bending forward and dressing tasks.

Acknowledging and recording the altered patterns used preoperatively to perform or compensate for these functions will help the therapist to build a postoperative rehabilitation programme appropriate to the specific needs of the patient. If a patient has been overusing the lumbar spine to gain sufficient forward flexion to put on shoes or socks, then back pain may be a problem. There will need to be a specific strengthening programme for the hip flexors and extensors to achieve the hip motion required to reduce the compensatory spinal movements; otherwise the patient will continue with the 'learned' pattern.

Patients are individuals, and how they compensate for loss of motion/strength/proprioception will be different, although the overall loss of function may be the same.

Leg length discrepancies are not uncommon prior to joint replacement, particularly of the hip, because of bone erosion and pathology. Measurement of leg length discrepancy preoperatively will help the physiotherapist to evaluate the change in biomechanics which may occur following surgery. Hopefully the discrepancy will be corrected at the time of surgery although muscle weakness will continue and may mask leg length equality.

Self-assessment question

■ **SAQ 8.1.** How would you measure apparent and true leg length discrepancies?

Unsure of the answer? Read pages 151–153, Chapter 10, of *Clinical orthopaedic examination* (McRae 1990), then see the end of the chapter.

General rehabilitation

Hydrotherapy is an excellent treatment for a patient following joint replacement surgery, once the wound is healed and there are no signs of

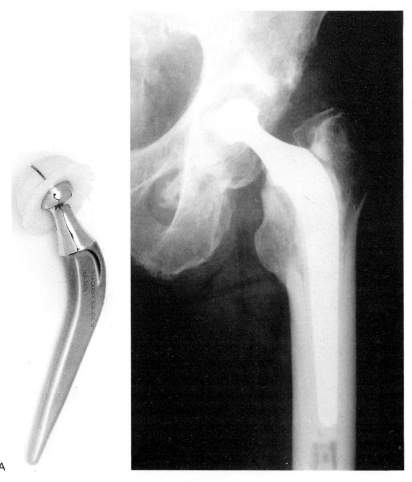

A   B

Figure 8.2 A Charnley total hip replacement. (a) The prosthesis; (b) appearance on X-ray. (Taken with permission from Dandy 1993.)

infection. Some hospitals may allow patients in the pool at an earlier stage as long as the wound is covered. Use of a gymnastic ball in supine lying and sitting will encourage control around the new joint and can help to promote proprioceptive feedback.

HIP JOINT

Types of hip joint

The commonest type of hip replacement in the UK today is the Charnley low friction arthroplasty (Hasheminejad et al 1994) which was first used in the 1960s. The femoral component is structured from stainless steel and the acetabular cup from high density polyethylene (Fig. 8.2).

At the same time McKee was developing a completely stainless steel hip joint but the cup's wear capacity was not as good as that of the high density polyethylene. The modern hip arthroplasties still use a combination of chrome–cobalt–molybdenum alloys, or stainless steel femoral shafts with a high density polyethylene acetabular cup. The acetabular cup may have a metal back in some cases. Fixation of both components may be with or without cement. If no cement is used, fixation of the femoral component depends on a tight 'press fit', whereas the acetabular cup is fixed with either screws or pegs (Goldie 1992).

There is a huge variety of prosthetic hip replacements available to the surgeon and these are usually of the unconstrained type. Semiconstrained hip joints are available but they are not very common. The normal hip joint has the greatest range of motion of any of the lower limb joints. Thus, following surgery an unconstrained joint will allow the hip to return to its preoperative range of motion or greater. The disadvantage of this free movement with no prosthetic constraint is that the joint will be prone to dislocation. The greatest risk of dislocation is immediately after surgery and it is common up to 6 weeks postoperatively. By then a new capsule should have grown around the hip joint. It is only when this has occurred that the patient should be advised to aim for full movement of the hip joint.

Incision sites

The incision site for a total hip replacement may be:

- Anterolateral: between the tensor fascia lata and the glutei.
- Posterolateral: through the posterior capsule.
- True lateral: with the Charnley approach the greater trochanter is excised and reattached with wire fixation (Fig. 8.3). If this is done then rehabilitation is slower and should be more representative of an uncemented arthroplasty. The 'Liverpool' approach is an alternative lateral approach, which does not remove the greater trochanter.

Each surgeon will have their own preference but it is very important that the therapist knows which incision has been used, and any specific requirements that should be met. Whatever the type of prosthesis or incision used, a suction drain will be in situ for up to 48 hours postoperatively. The surgeon and/or nursing staff will also dictate management of the wound and all physiotherapy staff should be informed about this.

Complications

Dislocation

The positions leading to dislocation depend very much on the incision site used for the operation:

- Anterolateral and true lateral: the hip will dislocate if placed in excessive extension, external rotation and adduction, or a combination of all three.
- Posterolateral: the hip will dislocate in excessive flexion, internal rotation and adduction, or a combination of all three.

Thus for at least 6 weeks and preferably up to 12, the patient's hip should not be placed in these positions.

The patient must be aware of the possibility of dislocation and this knowledge should be reinforced, especially immediately following surgery. To assist in the prevention of dislocation, the patient should sleep with an abduction pillow between the legs when supine, or may lie on their

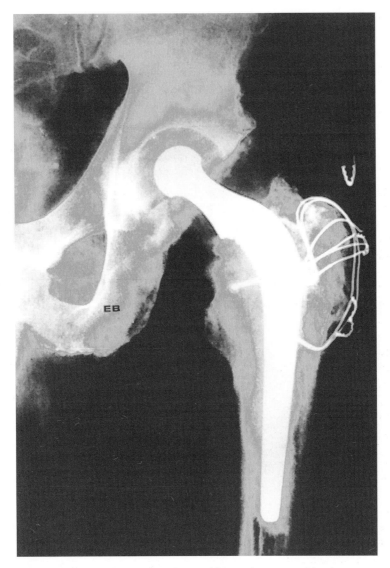

Figure 8.3 X-ray showing Charnley total hip replacement with wire fixation of the greater trochanter. (Taken with permission from Rothman & Hozack 1988.)

operated side once the drain is out. Whilst in bed it is recommended that the patient's locker be placed on the operated side, so that if the patient leans over then the leg would not roll into internal rotation and adduction (Goldie 1992)

Dislocation of the hip is easily recognisable because the leg is shorter, externally rotated and in extension if it has dislocated anteriorly, or shorter, flexed and internally rotated if dislocated in the posterior direction. An X-ray of the hip will clearly show the dislocation (Fig. 8.4). Treatment then will be relocation of the hip under general anaesthetic, followed by a period of bed rest with traction for up to 6 weeks (Dandy 1993, Goldie 1992). If the hip is unstable in flexion then plaster of paris (POP) may be applied to keep the leg in extension.

Wear

Any material will develop signs of wear, that is

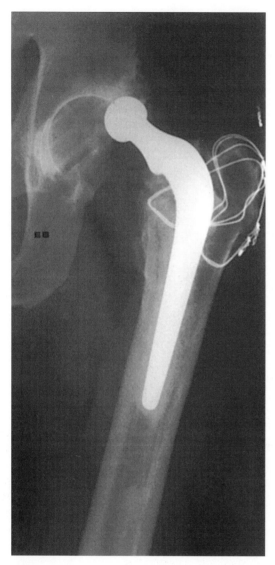

Figure 8.4 X-ray showing dislocation of total hip replacement. (Taken with permission from Rothman & Hozack 1988).

pits and holes in the material or fragments of debris flaking from the material, with repeated loading to its surface. This is true of the high density polyethylene of the acetabular cup or the tibial plateau. Failure of a total hip joint will occur if the prosthetic material cannot sustain the forces on it and it starts to flake or crumble. Revision of the cup is essential if signs of debris occur, as the opposing surface will eventually become pitted as well.

Other complications

Other complications are those common to any surgical procedure. SAQ 5.7 in Chapter 5 on fractures highlights the main complications for people on bed rest, and these are very similar to the complications following an operative procedure.

Problem-solving exercise 8.1

■ To which of the common surgical complications mentioned SAQ 5.7 do you think patients are most prone following total hip replacement?

If there is any reason why a patient cannot have a general anaesthetic, such as severe respiratory disease, then the procedure could be done under an epidural anaesthetic. Brinker et al (1997) reported equally good results when using epidural compared to general anaesthesia with regard to 'length of hospitalisation, non-surgical operating room time, intraoperative blood transfusions, intraoperative femur fractures, deep vein thrombosis, deep infections, death, or the prevalence of postoperative urinary tract infections'. Significant differences were found for estimated intraoperative blood loss, surgical time and the drain output, with the epidural group having the 'best' results in unilateral hip replacement surgery.

Venous thrombi

Prophylactic medication for the prevention of deep vein thrombosis and pulmonary embolus, both before and after total hip replacement, is routine in most surgical units, although the need for its use has been questioned (McGrath et al 1996). In most cases a programme of prophylactic warfarin or aspirin will be given to reduce the risk of a venous clot (Hull et al 1997). An alternative to this would be intermittent pneumatic compression (IPC) of the lower limbs both during and after surgery (Woolson & Watt 1991). These authors have shown that there is no significant difference between treatment with war-

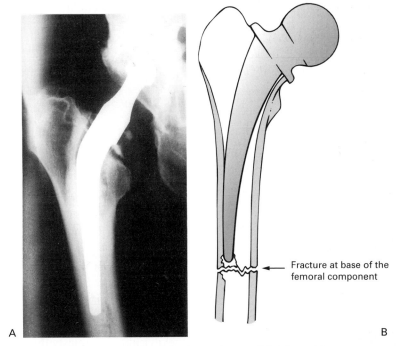

A   B

Figure 8.5 Fractures around the femoral stem. ((a) Taken with permission from Dandy 1993; (b) adapted with permission from McRae 1994.)

Fracture at base of the femoral component

farin, aspirin and IPC, with a mean occurrence of thrombosis being 10%.

It is also common practice, whatever type of prophylactic treatment is used, for the patient to wear an elasticated antiembolus stocking on the operated limb, or possibly on both limbs (Woolson & Watt 1991).

Fracture

Femoral fractures particularly around the stem of the femoral component of the hip can occur either at the time of surgery or at a later date. The femur can fracture either just distal to the tip of the stem of the prosthesis or the lower tip of the stem can protrude through the lateral wall of the femur (Fig. 8.5). It is common to see bone erosion at the site of the fracture, which may indicate excessive loading at that point (McRae 1994). It may be possible to fix these fractures without revision of the femoral stem but this is highly unlikely.

Longitudinal fractures around the stem can be repaired successfully with internal fixation with wires or screw and plate. The femoral prosthesis can fracture transversally mid-stem and this may cause an associated fracture of the femur at this point. If the fracture occurs at a late stage postoperatively then signs of loosening often accompany the fracture. It would be normal practice to revise the stem of the prosthesis when this fracture occurs (Fig. 8.5) (Dandy 1993).

Postoperative thigh pain

Pain can arise in both cemented and uncemented hip procedures but for very different reasons.

Thigh pain immediately following an uncemented hip replacement is quite usual and will diminish once new bone growth has occurred and the implant becomes secure, at any time up to 6 months (Engh et al 1987). Occasionally patients can complain of pain at a point equivalent to the end of the femoral stem after activity. The repetitive compressive loading on the bone distal to the femoral stem may cause the end pain but this has not been confirmed (Maihafer 1990).

If a patient has thigh pain following a cemented prosthesis, this is not normal, and signifies loosening of the femoral component. Any signs of unresolving thigh pain should be reported to the consultant surgeon for review. The patient should be reminded of this on discharge, as the loosening pain may not arise until many months or years after the operation.

Failure

Total hip arthroplasties fail in approximately 0.5–1% of all the hip joint replacements undertaken (Dandy 1993). If failure occurs then revision arthroplasty may be a possibility.

The main reasons for this are loosening or deep infection. As discussed previously biomechanical loosening between the bone and the cement is inevitable at some stage but the aim is to delay this for as long as possible. This is particularly prevalent around the stem of the femoral component and the patient will complain of pain and discomfort down the thigh and loss of function. On X-ray a dark line occurs between the cement–prosthesis interface, indicating a gap between the surfaces (Fig. 8.6). Loosening of the acetabular component can also occur but the

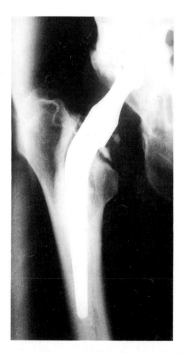

Figure 8.6 X-ray showing loosening of the femoral stem. (Taken with permission from Dandy 1993.)

patient now complains of pain in the groin and loss of function (Dandy 1993).

Infection

Infection can occur at any time following surgery although the surgeon takes great care to prevent this happening. As with any infection the patient will have a raised temperature and complain of pain around the groin or thigh. Infections rising after the initial operation period may be secondary to infections elsewhere in the body, such as the urinary tract or teeth. There is also a direct relationship between mouth infections that are present preoperatively and late onset infection of total hip replacements (Bartzokas et al 1994).

Patients must be advised of the possibility of infection and the need to seek medical help if this should arise.

If infection persists following management with antibiotics, the only option for the surgeon is to undertake a revision arthroplasty. Prior to the revision arthroplasty the infected arthroplasty would be removed (excision arthroplasty) and the remaining hole would be filled with antibiotic beads. The patient would then be kept on bed rest and traction for up to 6 weeks or until the infection subsided. Only then would the revision be undertaken.

Rehabilitation

Once the hip joint is altered by disease pathology or trauma, it will develop fixed contractures in flexion, adduction and external rotation. These contractures have to be resolved either preoperatively, in the operating theatre, or in the postoperative rehabilitation phase, for the operation to be classed as a complete success. If the hip is left in the contracted position then full range of extension, abduction and rotation will remain lost thus maintaining the altered biomechanics of the pre-surgery joint.

A flexion contracture tends to emphasise an adduction contracture and will severely exaggerate a discrepancy in apparent leg length and may add to any true discrepancy after surgery.

Therefore after surgery the therapist must measure the length of the legs on a regular basis. If a true leg length discrepancy is present then a temporary shoe raise can be given. If the discrepancy is over 1 inch (2.4 cm) then only provide half of this height until the hip and lumbar spine adapt to the change of alignment. If there is only an apparent leg length discrepancy, then do not give a shoe raise until any contracture or muscle weakness has been resolved. This is particularly important for an adduction contracture with abductor weakness. As strength and range increase then the apparent discrepancy will reduce. If this resolves to less than half an inch then no action should be taken, but wait at least 4 months before reassessment to ensure possible recovery.

The type of prosthesis and the incision site are the main dictators of the rehabilitation regime to be used. Both cemented and uncemented replacements follow a similar regime except for weight-bearing times. The patient with an uncemented prosthesis will remain partially or non-weight bearing for between 6 to 12 weeks postoperatively, or on some occasions up to 9 months (Engh & Bobyn 1985). Weight bearing with a cemented prosthesis usually begins on the first day postoperatively (Maihafer 1990).

Assessment

Problem-solving exercise 8.2

- What would you do for a preoperative assessment of a patient awaiting a total hip replacement?

If you have problems with this question look back at the case study for Mrs Jones in Chapter 5, and problem-solving exercise 5.11, for assistance.

Then, when you have tried to answer it yourself, check with the answer at the end of the chapter before reading on.

All these points (see Answer at end of chapter) are important but it is particularly important to gain knowledge of the preoperative range of motion, strength and functional ability. There are many studies which show that the successful outcome of a hip replacement is closely related to the preoperative motion available (Rowe et al 1989,

Stanic et al 1993). Stanic et al (1993) developed a successful and comprehensive evaluation of function for pre- and postoperative use with patients undergoing total hip replacement. The evaluation comprised passive hip movement, observational gait analysis, and kinemetric gait parameters (stride length, time, gait velocity, stance time, and joint kinematics). This team showed that all parameters changed significantly from pre- to postoperation, the most notable change being an increase in hip extension, reduction of a Trendelenburg gait and of adduction contracture.

Therefore it is particularly important to measure these aspects accurately. Advice on how to undertake a full clinical hip assessment can be revised in McRae (1990), Kendall et al (1993) and Norkin (1995). As mentioned previously, it is important to remember that a full clinical examination is not necessary for a preoperative assessment of a total hip replacement because the joint stability, range of motion, muscle power, proprioception will all change postoperatively. For the lower limb, obviously the weight-bearing functions are the most important to assess.

Problem-solving exercise 8.3

Go back to the chapter on assessment (Ch. 3) and that on fractures (Ch. 5) to review them before answering this question.

- How can the therapist measure the functions of: walking, stair climbing, sit to stand or forward flexion (e.g. to put on shoes or socks)?

After you have answered the question, review the answer at the end of the chapter.

Following surgery the postoperative assessment will be exactly the same as for a fracture around the hip joint. The greater risk of dislocation means that full range hip, knee, or lumbar spine motion should be avoided.

Self-assessment question

- **SAQ 8.2.** In what position does the hip joint

> dislocate after a total hip replacement? Try
> to answer this yourself and then check with
> the answer at the end of the chapter.

Postoperative treatment

Active postoperative therapy starts from day one. Remember that the abduction pillow or wedge should remain in situ whilst the patient is lying supine or on the non-operated side. Also keep in mind that the patient should be discouraged from performing a straight leg raise on the operated side until full quadriceps and iliopsoas control has returned.

The treatment goals at this time do not differ greatly from those of a patient following a fracture around the hip. These are:

- Restoration of:
  — Joint motion; hip extension, abduction and rotation are all lost preoperatively therefore these are the most important movements for which re-education should be begun.
  — Muscle strength; of hip abductors, extensors and rotators in particular, but hip flexors must be strengthened for climbing a stair or step or for putting on a shoe. Quadriceps and hamstrings activity should also be encouraged.
- Maintenance of:
  — Vascular function; foot and ankle pumps, quadriceps activity and deep breathing will all help.
  — Respiratory function.
- Education in:
  — Joint preservation techniques to prevent dislocation, loosening and fracture.
  — Bed mobility.
  — Weight bearing; gait and sitting to standing.

Bed mobility

The patient will need assistance to move up and down the bed and to go into the 'bridging position' for toilet purposes. If the patient has had a posterolateral incision then care must be taken to avoid too much hip extension in the early stages and it may be easier to get the patient out of bed for toileting. Getting the patient in and out of bed should have been taught in the preoperative stage, but if not, then this should be done on the first day of mobilising. Ideally the patient should be assisted out of bed on the operated side with the leg being held in abduction. If a posterior surgical approach has been used then the hip should also remain in extension as much as possible.

Muscle re-education

From day one postoperatively isometric exercises for the muscle groups highlighted above should be undertaken at least three to four times a day in the 'neutral' hip position in supine. The therapist will have to be present to assist the patient and to ensure that correct muscle activity is taking place. Because of misuse or complete lack of use of these muscles preoperatively then endurance will be limited and an appropriate low level programme should be initiated. Likewise active assisted or passive movements should be started at this time but only under the therapist's supervision.

Once grade II muscle activity has been achieved in the neutral hip supine position then isometric activity of the rotators, extensors and abductors can begin in hip flexion. Again the therapist must be present to control the hip position and check muscle function. In most cases 'good' muscle function returns quickly and most patients will have active grade III muscle power by 1 week postoperatively, but this will only be through the limited range of motion allowed during the early postoperative period.

Often the quadratus lumborum and the lateral trunk muscles will assist hip abduction activity by 'hitching' the pelvis on the side of abduction. This occurs as a compensatory activity to weak abductors and will appear in both supine and standing positions (Fig. 8.7). The therapist must encourage the patient to maintain a level pelvis whilst doing hip abduction. If 'hitching' occurs then more assistance should be given to reduce the weight of the limb and make abduction easier. Further explanation of this phenomenon may be found in *Muscles testing and function* (Kendall et al 1993).

It is very easy for the therapist to miss this compensatory action as the patient may have been doing this for many months preoperatively.

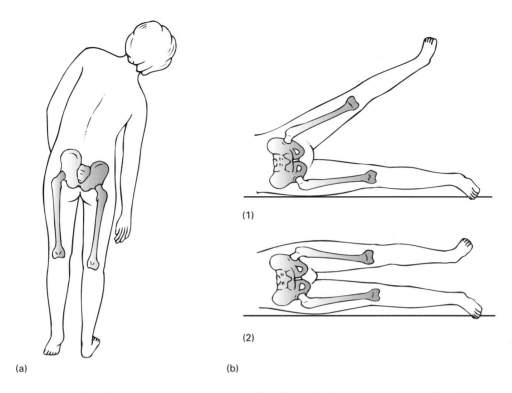

(a)   (b)

Figure 8.7 Hip abduction with weak gluteus medius. (a) Weak gluteus medius in standing. (b) Weak gluteus medius in side lying: (1) correct abduction; (2) use of quadratus lumborum to compensate. (Taken with permission from Kendall et al 1993.)

Another favourite compensatory action is the use of the abdominal muscles to help flex the hip in the supine and standing positions. Thus the pelvis is tilted in the posterior direction to gain more hip flexion.

Weight bearing
The start date for weight bearing depends on the incision used, any complications of surgery, and gaining a good postoperative check X-ray at approximately 24 hours. Patients with lateral or posterolateral incisions can start weight bearing from day one, but with patients who have antero-lateral incisions this may be delayed until 5 days postoperatively as extension is the dislocation position. Conversely, the start of sitting can be delayed for patients with a posterolateral inci-sion to prevent dislocation. Patients will be required to sit in a raised chair so that the hip is held at less than 90° of flexion.

Sitting and walking will become easier and more comfortable when the suction drain is removed and any intravenous drips are discon-nected (usually 24–48 hours postoperatively).

During the preoperative phase it is common for the patient to walk with limited hip extension range and weak hip extensors during the final stages of the stance phase of gait. This is compen-sated for by a rotation of the pelvis backwards, with forward flexion of the trunk and a shorter step length. This action allows the opposite side of the pelvis to rotate forward so that the oppos-ing leg can gain the correct position for weight bearing and achieve a reasonable step length (Perry 1992). This becomes a 'learned' response, but once the patient starts walking postopera-tively this compensation must be corrected as quickly as possible. Adequate strength in the hip extensors, flexors and abductors is required before this can be achieved.

When the patient is starting to weight bear a frame or crutches should be used to increase sta-bility, reduce the weight taken across the 'new' hip joint and reduce the load on the hip musculature. It is very common for the patient to flex forward at the hip and lumbar spine because of weak hip extensors and previous loss of hip extension range (Kendall et al 1993). This must be discouraged from the start, to help re-educate unused muscles and reinforce a 'correct' walking pattern (Perry 1992).

In cemented joints weight bearing is increased until minimal assistance is required from a walking aid. In the 1990 survey of 'normal' rehabilitation practice for a cemented hip arthroplasty most patients were discharged from hospital at 10–12 days postoperatively, walking with one or two sticks and able to climb a step or steps (Association of Orthopaedic Chartered Physiotherapists (AOCP) 1991).

Patients with an uncemented prosthesis will follow this pattern but will remain on crutches or a frame for much longer (from 6 to 12 weeks). It is even more important for these patients to be encouraged to walk with good hip extension during the stance phase of gait and to prevent forward flexion of the trunk, as walking aids will reinforce this posture.

Discharge

On discharge from hospital it is very unusual for patients with total hip replacements to be referred for outpatient physiotherapy. Therefore it is important that fact sheets on exercise, joint preservation and limitations should be given to the patient. The Arthritis and Rheumatism Council provide excellent leaflets on all of these subjects but most orthopaedic departments have developed their own advice sheets to accommodate their particular requirements.

Problem-solving exercise 8.4

■ What actions should the patient avoid until 6 weeks postoperatively?

Answer:
With an anterolateral and true lateral incision: excessive extension, external rotation and abduction, or a combination of all three.

With a posterolateral incision: excessive flexion, internal rotation and adduction, or a combination of all three.

Functions:
— *sitting in low chairs (under 21 inches (50 cm) in height)*
— *bending forward to put on shoes, socks, cut toenails*
— *crossing the legs in sitting or lying*
— *twisting the leg in sitting or lying*
— *driving*
— *jumping or running*
— *contact sport.*

These actions are self-explanatory but as the patient regains strength and motion and enjoys the loss of pain then they may carry out these actions without thinking. The surgeon will decide when the patient should return to driving and sport, but this very much depends on the activity and the person involved. In the past few years there has been an increase in patients wishing to participate in sport following joint replacement. In a survey of orthopaedic practitioners at the Mayo Clinic, McGrory et al (1995) highlighted that the sports recommended after joint replacement were: sailing, swimming, scuba diving, cycling, golfing, and bowling, after hip and knee replacement procedures, and also cross-country skiing after knee arthroplasty, that is low impact, non-contact sports. However, high impact or contact sports such as running, waterskiing, football, baseball, basketball, hockey, martial arts and soccer should be prohibited.

Mallon et al (1996) also suggested that golf could be resumed following hip or knee replacement surgery without increasing the risk of dislocation, loosening and hence revision.

Outcome

A patient with an uncomplicated cemented hip replacement should be able to achieve functional independence as defined by Zavadak et al (1995), that is:

● get in and out of bed with minimal assistance including raising from lying to sitting
● easily move from sitting to standing and vice versa

- walk approximately 100 yards (85 metres) with the assistance of one or two sticks, and
- be able to climb two or three steps with the use of a banister.

These may not be achieved by discharge as it takes a variable time to reach these goals (Zavadak et al 1995). It may be up to 6 months before the patient has the confidence to return to full function and by this time the musculature should be strong enough to support normal activity. The most problematic of activities is climbing stairs (Zavadak et al 1995).

Borstlap et al (1994) report that a single total hip replacement solves the problems of most people with a primary diagnosis of osteoarthrosis but only is partially helpful to those with rheumatoid arthritis because of their multiple joint problems. This fact is hardly surprising but does emphasise to whom rehabilitation efforts should be directed. There is no evidence, as yet, to show that the lack of a rehabilitation programme shortens the longevity of a total hip replacement, but only time and the number of revision arthroplasties being undertaken will illuminate this question.

Wykman & Olsson (1992) studied the outcome of single compared with bilateral hip replacements. The patients with bilateral surgery did not gain full functional independence until the second hip had been replaced. Even when good postoperative outcomes after the second replacement were attained, these were significantly different from the achievements of patients with a single joint replacement.

Treatment of surgical complications

External hip protectors
In some orthopaedic clinics hip protectors are being used to prevent falls and to offer stability to a 'new' hip replacement (Cameron & Quine 1994). For the patient with ongoing hip complications following a replacement or with a history of falling then these devices do offer assistance, but they are cumbersome and unsightly and it is not surprising that patients do not like to wear them (Cameron & Quine 1994).

Revision arthroplasty
If repeated complications arise, such as dis-

location, infection, or the natural end of the life of the prosthesis being reached with loosening, then a revision arthroplasty will have to be undertaken.

Mallory, in 1992, raised the concern that the hip replacement population was getting younger with an average age of 57 years, compared with an average age of 69 years in 1979. Therefore a greater number of hip replacements would need to be undertaken. More importantly, even with the advances in design and surgical technique, the number of hip replacements needing revision, through reaching the end of their natural life, will be immense (Mallory 1992).

Following a revision arthroplasty a period of bed rest may be needed. If this is the case then the role of the therapist is to maintain the motion and muscle strength of the lower limbs, maintain circulation and respiratory function and prevent complications of bed rest.

Specific treatment for the affected joint will depend on whether or not an excision arthroplasty has taken place. If this is the case then the therapist must maintain isometric muscle power around the joint and some active joint motion. The joints above and below the excised joints should be exercised as much as possible allowing for the fact that the patient has very little control of the excised joint in the early stages.

Once the revision joint has been inserted then the hip can be treated exactly as a primary replacement but greater care must be taken, particularly if the joint had been revised because of repeated dislocation. The muscles around the revised joint will take longer to regain their strength because of repeated surgical trauma. Therefore it will also take a longer time to gain functional independence.

Excision arthroplasty (Girdlestone's procedure) is now less common because of advances in revision surgery. Postoperative management of an excision arthroplasty requires the patient to have good muscle control around the hip. A knee–ankle–foot orthosis should be ordered to assist by taking some of the weight from the lower limb so that the hip can be loaded slowly over time. A considerable shoe raise (greater than 3 inches (7 cm)) will be necessary to accommodate for the leg length discrepancy which will increase as the end of the femur telescopes into the acetabulum on weight bearing. It is possible for the patient to mobilise with a frame or crutches but the outcome is not wonderful.

KNEE JOINT

The development of knee replacements was slower than for the hip, because of the complexity of the joint structure and biomechanics. The knee (tibiofemoral and patellofemoral joints) is the middle joint of the lower limb and therefore it acts as the link for all the forces on the lower limb. The knee joint relies heavily on its ligaments, joint surface congruity and muscle control for stability (Nordin & Frankel 1989). In knee pathology these three factors are altered; therefore the design of the knee replacement has to enhance the normal knee joint congruity to compensate for lost anteroposterior stability. This is particularly important as the anterior cruciate ligament is sacrificed in the operative procedure and in some cases the posterior cruciate will also be removed. The design of the prosthetic tibial replacement varies depending on the presence of the posterior cruciate ligament. The medial and lateral collateral ligaments are not removed during surgery, but may be stretched or damaged from previous pathology. If this is so, then operative repair may be necessary. There is controversy about the replacement or resurfacing of the patella, when the tibiofemoral joint is replaced. Surgeons hold differing beliefs depending on experience and the type of tibiofemoral replacement to be undertaken.

As a result of these issues the prosthetic knee will never totally replace the normal knee.

The aim of the orthopaedic surgeon therefore is to prolong the life of the natural knee joint before undertaking a knee arthroplasty, because of the known low longevity of the joint (Dandy 1993). A number of other surgical procedures can be undertaken prior to a total knee replacement. These are (Perrot & Menkes 1996):

- intra-articular lavage via an arthroscope
- debridement (trimming of soft tissue and wash out of joint)
- capsular and soft tissue repair
- meniscectomy or meniscal repair

- tibial osteotomy
- hemiarthroplasty or unicompartmental replacement.

Previously, if only one joint surface was affected then a MacIntosh surface replacement made from metal used to be inserted over the tibial plateau (Crawford Adams & Stossel 1992). It is now more common for a tibial osteotomy (realignment of the tibial joint surface) (Perrot & Menkes 1996) or unicompartmental arthroplasty to be performed (Figs 8.8 and 8.9). An unconstrained, unicompartmental arthroplasty is inserted when both joint surfaces of one compartment of the knee joint are affected by disease, usually osteoarthrosis. Goodfellow and O'Connor at Oxford designed and developed the unicompartmental joint using the concept of the Oxford meniscal knee replacement (Goodfellow et al 1988).

Non-surgical management is also encouraged including: patient education, psychological support, reassuring patients that the pain is a reversible state, use of splints, weight reduction, and non-conventional therapies such as homeopathy, acupuncture and transcutaneous electrical nerve stimulation (Perrot & Menkes 1996).

Types of knee joint

The first prosthetic knee designs were predominantly of the constrained type, utilising a metal hinge with a purely uniaxial motion, such as the Shiers or Wallidus type (Crawford Adams & Stossel 1992). Metal and plastic unconstrained total knee replacements such as the Polycentric, Freeman–Swanson, and Geomedic were first introduced in the late 1960s (Fig. 8.9) (Walker 1987). The evolution of the current designs of semiconstrained (see Fig. 8.10) and unconstrained prostheses mainly occurred because of advances in computer-aided technology. The precision and accuracy of these designs offer a greater chance of joint survival, but this is still dependent on surgical procedure where errors in alignment of as little as 3° can lead to failure (Dandy 1993).

Once again the fixation of the prosthesis to the bone can be with or without cement. Semi- and unconstrained prostheses have short stem or 'lug'

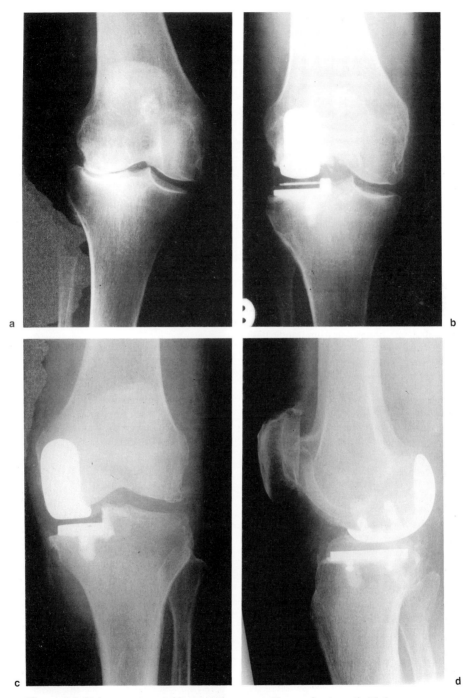

Figure 8.8 Unicompartmental knee replacement. X-rays of osteoarthritic knee (a) before, and (b) after knee replacement. (c) Anteroposterior and (d) lateral view of a different type of prosthesis. (Taken with permission from Dandy 1993.)

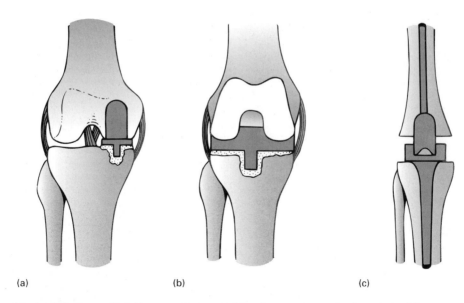

(a)   (b)   (c)

Figure 8.9 Types of total knee replacement: (a) unicompartmental arthroplasty; (b) unconstrained total knee replacement; (c) constrained hinge total knee replacement. (Adapted with permission from Dandy 1993.)

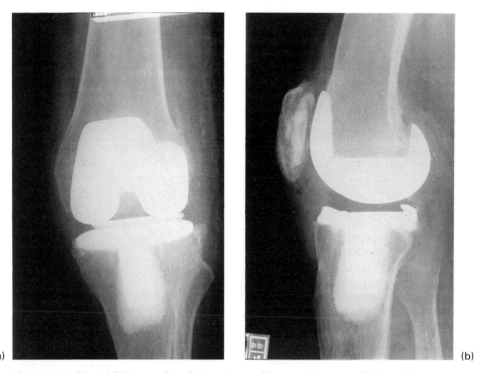

(a)   (b)

Figure 8.10 (a) and (b) X-ray of Insall–Burstein total knee replacement. (Taken with permission from Dandy 1993.) (c) Insall–Burstein knee replacement. (Taken with permission from Niwa et al 1987.)

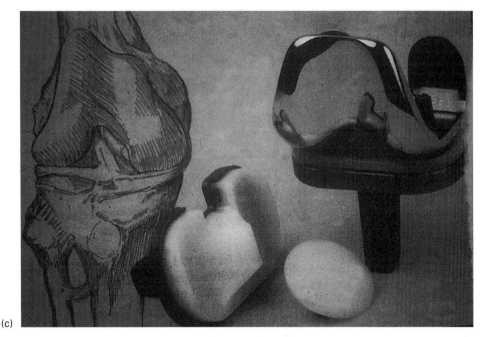

(c)

Fig. 8.10 (*cont'd*)

attachments to the underlying bone, whilst the constrained 'hinge' joints tend to have far longer stems into both the tibia and femur. Greater forces are taken across the knee joint surfaces than the hip; therefore the risk of loosening is far higher (Sahlstrom et al 1994). This is particularly so in the constrained joints where there is only one axis of motion, thus the rotatory and shear forces occur between the prosthesis–cement and cement–bone interfaces. In semi- and unconstrained joints the tibial component is often cemented in place but the femoral component is not, whilst both components of a hinge joint are usually held by cement (Fig. 8.10). Uncemented components are held by bone ingrowth around the roughened surface of the prosthesis.

Criteria for knee replacement

An un- or semiconstrained prosthetic joint is used if the patient complains of:

1. severe tibiofemoral pain, which may be accompanied by patellofemoral pain

2. loss of general function and / or knee joint mobility
3. severe deformity of the knee joint.

If severe loss of knee stability were present in combination with 1, 2 or 3 above, then a constrained joint would have to be utilised as it offers much greater internal control. A constrained or hinge joint would also be used as a revision arthroplasty following removal of a un- or semiconstrained joint. If a hemiarthroplasty were removed then a semiconstrained joint would act as the revision prosthesis.

Complications

Problem-solving exercise 8.5

■ What are the common complications specific to a joint replacement?

These are not dissimilar to the complications following a hip replacement, except that the risk of dislocation is far less in the tibiofemoral joint, although not uncommon at the patellofemoral joint. However because the knee has to endure far greater forces than the hip, the risk of loosening is much higher at the knee joint. The forces are much greater on the medial compartment compared with the lateral, and this can lead to specific loosening of the prosthesis (Sahlstrom et al 1994). Loosening of the tibial prosthesis can be noticed on X-ray or the patient may complain of continuing pain in the lower knee joint radiating down the tibia usually on the anterior aspect. This pain differs from deep infection pain, which is usually contained to the joint and is not as specific as the tibial pain.

Signs of 'wear' on the tibial plateau are also seen, particularly on the medial aspect. It is usual to have forces of up to four times body weight across the tibial plateau during normal walking (Nordin & Frankel 1989) and because of the normal adduction moment on weight bearing, the medial component has to endure more stresses (Sahlstrom et al 1994). Although the design of the prosthetic tibial component tries to limit the effects of wear by distributing the load more evenly, there will still be a greater stress on the medial side of the knee, particularly on weight bearing. If wear of the prosthetic surface does occur, then debris may be found within the knee joint and this may provoke an inflammatory reaction. Arthroscopy and joint wash-out can remove debris but this increases the risk of infection greatly, which is a far greater enemy to a knee joint replacement.

The risk of a deep vein thrombosis (DVT) or pulmonary embolus is also equally high for all total joint replacements. Swelling and pain in the centre of the calf, which increases with passive dorsiflexion in knee extension, must give concern that a DVT is present.

Lastly the risk of either a wound infection or a deep joint infection is as high as for the hip, but the consequences are far worse. If the joint becomes loosened or infected then removal and revision is the obvious choice, but it is far more difficult to undertake compared with the hip (Dandy 1993). Revision surgery requires that the prosthesis and all the cement be removed before

a new larger prosthesis is inserted (Goldie 1992). Thus bone stock is always sacrificed with a revision replacement, particularly in some cases when a custom-made constrained joint is inserted (Dandy 1993). Infection in a knee prosthesis is difficult to resolve and an excision arthroplasty does not share the same successful results as the hip operation. Once the knee joint has been excised then the gap is filled with antibiotic beads or antibiotic-impregnated cement for 6 weeks and then a new knee inserted.

Following excision arthroplasty of the hip the joint can gain some stability through good muscle control, but this is not so for the knee, where an external splint is always needed to give support to the knee. Following excision arthroplasty, either a compression or nail and graft arthrodesis can be undertaken to permit a stronger limb to bear weight. The vast loss of bone stock from the excision of the total knee replacement is not replaced when the arthrodesis takes place, therefore the leg ends up being considerably shorter than the other side (Crawford Adams & Stossel 1992). Cosmetically this is not pleasing particularly as a large shoe raise will have to be worn to provide compensation during weight bearing. Also the forces across the arthrodesed knee joint make success difficult to achieve and loosening of the internal metalwork or failure may occur. An external splint may have to be worn even after surgery.

The only option left if the infection is not treated successfully, or if an excision arthroplasty fails, is an above knee amputation. Even following amputation the patient does not necessarily return to a good level of function (Pring et al 1988).

Surgery and postoperative management

The knee is normally approached through a midline incision, curved slightly medially to avoid the patella (Crawford Adams & Stossel 1992). Suction drains will be inserted for at least 24 hours (Goldie 1992). During the operation, care is taken to align the joint correctly in all planes and that the soft tissue tension is balanced (Crawford Adams & Stossel 1992). Resurfacing of the patella may also take place. The posterior aspect of the patella is shaved until the entire roughened surface is removed and then a small high density polyethylene button is inserted. The button has to be of the correct dimensions, particularly width, so that it will run smoothly in the patellar groove of the femoral component.

Following surgery there are two main forms of management that can be chosen, namely the use, or not, of a continuous passive motion (CPM) machine. If a CPM machine is not used then the knee will be maintained in the extended position by a pressure bandage alone, or with either a splint or plaster of paris. The knee is kept straight for up to 7 days postoperatively limiting the start of an active exercise regime.

If a CPM machine is used then passive knee mobilising begins at some time from immediately following surgery, up to 4 days after the operation. The recommendation for an immediate postoperative start of CPM comes from many good researchers (Coutts 1983, Harms & Engstrom 1991, Johnson 1990, McInnes et al 1992, Wasilewski et al 1990). A few authors have advised delaying application until the second or third day postoperatively to allow the knee to 'settle' in extension prior to flexing (Gose 1987, Maloney et al 1990, Ritter et al 1989). The variation in length of time on the CPM machine during a 24-hour period ranges from 20 hours (Ritter et al 1989, Romness & Rand 1988) to 3 hours (Gose 1987). Basso & Knapp (1987) compared the results of treatment between two groups receiving either 20 hours or 5 hours of CPM immediately following knee replacement. No significant differences were found in range of motion, knee joint effusion, pain or length of stay in hospital; therefore they recommended the shorter application time. It is now common practice to limit CPM use to approximately 6 hours per day (Harms & Engstrom 1991).

Johnson (1990) indicates that if the range of flexion is controlled to a maximum of 40° over the first 72 hours then wound integrity will not be jeopardised. The flexion range should be increased by 10° per day until 80–90° of passive, and ideally active flexion is gained (Coutts 1983, Harms & Engstrom 1991, Johnson 1990).

The repeated motion on the CPM machine

will cause an increase in the volume of blood exuded via the suction drain and wound (Coutts 1983). The increased pumping action has a general effect on the vascular flow in the lower limb and this helps to reduce the tendency for postoperative DVT (Vince et al 1987) and will also reduce joint effusion (Harms & Engstrom 1991, McInnes et al 1992, O'Driscoll et al 1983).

There are many obvious differences between these two regimes, but the greatest is that the non-CPM regime promotes extension before flexion, and the CPM regime flexion before extension. The therapist must take this into account when preparing the rehabilitation programme and discuss the issues with the patient.

Rehabilitation

Preoperative

Prior to surgery the postoperative regime must be discussed with the patient and the range of knee motion, and quadriceps strength including lag, should be recorded. It is likely that a preoperative fixed flexion deformity of the knee will still be present after the operation. The patient should be shown any form of immobilisation, such as splint or POP back slab, prior to surgery and be advised on how, when and why it is to be worn.

If a CPM machine is to be used then the patient should try this before surgery and initial measurements can be made for ease following surgery. It is important that the CPM machine is set up correctly and that the patient understands how it works, and any problems that may occur, such as pressure under the ischial tuberosity, correct positioning of the knee and use of the emergency release switch, are explained (Coutts et al 1989).

If possible isometric quadriceps exercises should be encouraged preoperatively but these may be very difficult because of pain, effusion and deformity. If no walking aids have been used then the patient should be assessed for them and practise using them.

Early postoperative stage

Whether or not the CPM is used, isometric

quadriceps, glutei exercises and isotonic foot pumps should be started from day one postoperatively.

Treatment regime without CPM

If the knee is immobilised then no active exercise to the knee can begin until the immobilisation device is removed. During this period active motion of the ankle, toes and hip on the operated side should be encouraged, remembering that a straight leg raise will not be possible at this early stage. Indeed the straight leg raise should only be used as an isometric quadriceps exercise and not as a test of quadriceps function.

The immobilisation device may stay in situ for any time between 3 and 7 days (Harms & Engstrom 1991, Johnson 1990), but as soon as this is removed active assisted knee flexion should begin. A friction-free board, therapist assistance or pulley systems have all been used to promote assisted flexion, but the patient should try to undertake the action actively when possible.

Problem-solving exercise 8.6

■ **A.** Outline how you would expect the knee to be at the stage of release from immobilisation?

■ **B.** What should you be concerned about?

Answer:

A. *The knee will appear bruised, swollen and may be covered with antiseptic dye. A single or double suction drain will be protruding from the knee joint, and there will be an obvious surgical scar (as described earlier). The knee should lie in*

more extension than preoperatively but this may not be apparent because of swelling. The muscles around the knee will appear flaccid and the patient may feel the leg to be extremely heavy.

B. *Wound healing: are any parts of the wound open, infected or necrosed? This information can be gained from the nursing staff or doctors, but it is not uncommon for the therapist to be present when the immobilisation is removed. Also you will need to inspect the wound when flexion starts so that any leaking, bleeding or gaping can be observed and recorded. A pre-mobilisation look at the wound is essential.*

At this stage the patient may be very apprehensive about moving the limb and encouragement should be given as well as physical assistance. There is a great difference between the initial movements of hips and knees following replacement. Patients with hip replacements do not have the same anxieties about moving the joint or bursting the stitches and so on. This is partly because the patient cannot easily see the hip wound, but also because there is less inhibition to the surrounding musculature.

Once movement has started there will be an increase in pain and the patient may feel aching in the quadriceps/hamstrings muscles, or around the patella. Passive mobilisation of the patella and the scar may help to reduce pain in this area and enhance the ease of gaining flexion. Care must be taken if a patellar resurfacing has taken place and consultation with the surgeon may be necessary before doing mobilisation techniques to the patella.

A progressive exercise regime should be undertaken at least twice per day for at least 20 minutes but will vary depending on general strength, endurance and postoperative complications. By the seventh postoperative day the patient would normally have between 50–70° of active knee flexion and a fixed flexion deformity of 4–8° (Harms & Engstrom 1991, Johnson 1990).

Assisted weight bearing begins from day 3 postoperatively and is usually undertaken with an immobilisation device until good quadriceps control has been achieved (Harms & Engstrom 1991).

Treatment regime with CPM

As mentioned earlier the CPM may be applied in the surgical recovery room or ward during the first 24 hours after surgery (Fig. 8.11). If this is the case then the therapist may be responsible for the application and care of the machine. The patient should keep a record of the time spent on and off the machine and any problems experienced.

The CPM machine will only move the knee passively through the desired range; therefore from day one on the machine, there must be definite exercise times. The rehabilitation emphasis must be towards gaining static and controlled inner range quadriceps contraction. Therefore active knee flexion should not be encouraged

until quadriceps function is achieved (Coutts et al 1989). Passive mobilisation techniques to the patella may be necessary at this stage to ensure the return of flexion, but this is not as essential as for the non-CPM group. Active assisted knee flexion will always return much more quickly than with the non-CPM group (Coutts 1983, Harms & Engstrom 1991, Johnson 1990, McInnes et al 1992). By day 7 postoperatively then the patient should easily have 70–90° of flexion, but will have a degree of fixed flexion deformity similar to that of the non-CPM group (Gose 1987, Ritter et al 1989, Romness & Rand 1988). There is evidence that the longer the patient spends on the CPM the smaller the fixed flexion deformity (Basso & Knapp 1987). Maloney et al (1990) advocate the use of a bolster under the heel whilst the leg is on the CPM to ensure that the knee goes into full extension. Patients on CPM have a greater quadriceps lag (Ritter et al 1989) and should be advised to wear a splint at night, or

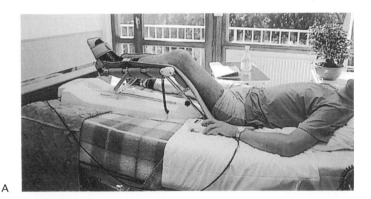

A

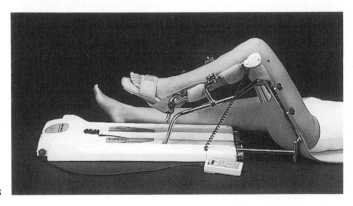

B

Figure 8.11 Continuous passive motion machine. (Kinetic CPM, courtesy of Smith & Nephew, Richards Ltd.)

when off the CPM, to reduce the possibility of holding the knee in flexion, encouraging the quadriceps lag (Harms & Engstrom 1991, Ritter et al 1989).

Once again weight bearing with a splint can start at day 3 postoperatively, and without the splint only when quadriceps control has been established. Unsupported weight bearing is often a day or two later than in the non-CPM group because of the presence of a greater quadriceps lag.

Harms & Engstrom (1991) indicate that following knee replacement, patients who achieve 60–70° of flexion by day 7, and 70–80° at day 14 postoperatively have 'the optimal rate of return of knee movement'. These guidelines should be used whether patients are on CPM or not.

Comparison of treatments with and without CPM

Comparison between regimes with and without CPM indicate that the CPM group will:

- always gain a greater degree of knee flexion (Coutts 1983), at an earlier stage (Vince et al 1987)
- have an easier return of knee flexion (Harms & Engstrom 1991)
- have less effusion (McInnes et al 1992)
- have smaller risk of manipulation (Coutts 1983, McInnes et al 1992)
- have a shorter stay in hospital (Coutts 1983, Johnson 1990), and
- have less risk of DVT (Vince et al 1987).

There will be a greater financial outlay, to purchase CPM machines, but this expense has been costed to be less than that incurred by the additional treatment (that is, manipulation) and length of hospital stay necessary when not using CPM (McInnes et al 1992).

By 1 year following the operation there is very little difference in the performance of the knee joint (Wasilewski et al 1990). An average of 101° of knee flexion is to be expected, with a minimal fixed flexion deformity of 4° and no extensor lag (Johnson 1990).

Disadvantages of CPM in the early stages relate to increased time in bed, loss of independence if on CPM for long periods, discomfort,

incidence of common peroneal nerve palsy, time taken to care and maintain the machine and non-compliance from the patient (McInnes et al 1992).

There have been no longitudinal studies of a CPM group to see if there are real disadvantages, either biomechanical or physical, at a later stage (i.e. longer than 1 year postoperatively).

Some possible problems following knee replacement

Problem-solving exercise 8.7

A patient with a 3-day-old new knee joint is complaining of a hot painful knee joint following inner range quadriceps exercise. On inspection the joint is slightly more swollen than prior to treatment.

- Why do you think this has occurred and what would you do about it?

After you have attempted this exercise, read the following section.

Hot painful knee joint after inner range quadriceps exercise
Possible causes of this are: infection, DVT or too much exercise too soon. The patient's body temperature needs to be checked to see if there are any systemic signs of infection.

Also check to see if there are any signs of a DVT in the calf (swelling, pain and discomfort). The knee also swells and becomes hot and painful if there is inflammation present. This could be part of the normal healing process but it is also possible that the patient was doing too much exercise too quickly.

All these signs should be reported to the nursing staff and recorded in appropriate medical/nursing or paramedical notes. Ice may be applied to the knee, if sensation is intact, and the leg elevated to help reduce the signs.

It is very difficult to know when and how hard to 'push' the patient, so start slowly and carefully progress from exercise session to exercise session; every patient is different.

The symptoms detailed above can occur at any stage of the rehabilitation process and the three possibilities 'infection, DVT, or too much too soon', should be kept in mind. At the later stages loosening or joint wear should be added to this list.

The knee can also become hot and painful if flexion is 'pushed' too much. This may happen in the non-CPM group because they are not moving into flexion as easily as the CPM group. If the knee joint flexion has not reached 60–70° by day 7 then it may be prudent to start the patient on CPM, taking knee flexion up to its maximum and keeping the machine on for a minimum of 6 hours a day to complement normal exercise sessions. The flexion range should be increased by at least 10° per day as for the CPM regime but this should be pushed as much as possible. On this 'added' passive flexion regime the knee should reach 80–90° by day 14. If a CPM machine is not available then a manipulation under anaesthetic (MUA) may be indicated. Under general anaesthetic the patient's knee is forced into flexion, stretching any intra-articular adhesions that have developed. Following an MUA, CPM should be used to augment therapy but if not then the therapist must work hard with the patient to maintain the passive flexion range before gaining active flexion and extension. Either following MUA or with the 'added' CPM regime some degree of active knee extension will be lost but this will return in time.

An extensor lag or fixed flexion deformity (FFD) does not resolve

This can be a particular problem for the CPM group and occurs if there is an imbalance between the gain of flexion to extension (Harms & Engstrom 1991). Progression of passive flexion on the CPM should be stopped until there is an increased range of active flexion and reduction of the extensor lag. To reduce the FFD the posterior aspect of the knee must be stretched and isometric quadriceps exercises encouraged in this new position.

Problem-solving exercise 8.8

■ How would you stretch the posterior aspect of a prosthetic knee replacement?

Whatever the technique used to gain extension the therapist should *not* force the knee into extension by applying a large posterior force down through the extended knee. Apart from causing excessive pain that will increase hamstrings spasm and therefore more flexion; the force may also affect the fixation of the joint. Gentle manual mobilisation techniques (Grade II Maitland mobilisations) can be used to help increase extension but only with caution.

An extensor lag will only decrease if the inner range quadriceps strength increases and any joint effusion is kept to a minimum. Therefore it is essential that the patient carry out specific inner range extension exercises on an hourly basis. The use of electromyographical (EMG) biofeedback may assist recovery of quadriceps activity. This becomes imperative when weight bearing is commenced, as often the patient is more anxious to get up walking than to undertake specific extension exercises.

Functional rehabilitation

In either group (CPM or non-CPM) functional retraining will take place once weight bearing without a splint commences. Wearing a splint will not encourage a normal walking pattern and therefore walking should be limited where possible until the splint is removed. Weight bearing without the splint will encourage quadriceps control as long as there is not a large extensor lag. Closed chain exercises in the parallel bars, such as foot placement, low level step-ups (2–3 inches (5–7 cm)) or small arc cycling in extension will all encourage extension without putting the joint under excessive strain. Practising sitting to standing from various heights and stair climbing will also promote muscle strengthening, joint mobility and proprioception.

All functional activities must be undertaken under supervision in the early stages and correction of compensatory patterns must be encouraged.

If there are ongoing difficulties with function gains, then loss of proprioception may be the main problem. The suggestion that the use of a CPM machine enhances the return of this sensation has not been supported by research evidence

(Coutts 1983). Barrett et al (1991) assessed the proprioception of patients following knee replacements and found that initially this was particularly poor but some degree of progression was made over time, although the preoperative level was not reached.

Problem-solving exercise 8.9

■ What compensatory patterns might occur when a patient with a knee replacement walks?

An overall leg length discrepancy may be present after surgery, but this is far less common than with hip joint surgery. The discrepancy is usually less than half an inch (1 cm) and can be accommodated, unless the patient has limited movement in the hip and lumbar spine. Only then should a temporary heel raise be applied.

Outcome

Dandy (1993) indicates that a knee replacement has been successful if:

- the knee straightens
- the knee gains flexion to 100°
- the leg takes the patient's weight, and
- the joint is stable.

These outcomes are far lower than those expected following a hip joint replacement and indicate the limited expectations of the joint. This must be made to clear to the patient, indicating that a good outcome would be that 80% of patients are still able to achieve these goals at 5 years following surgery (Dandy 1993). There are other beneficial outcomes from undertaking a knee joint replacement. Ries et al (1996) showed that in 13 patients there was 'a trend toward improvement in cardiovascular fitness one year after total knee arthroplasty and a significant improvement two years postoperatively for patients who had been able to resume routine functional activities because of the arthroplasty'. Even if full knee motion is not returned following surgery then the patient should gain an increase in general function and fitness after a period of time. A walking aid may be used by a number of patients but this is usually one stick; exceptions to this may be patients with rheumatoid arthritis whose general pathology may limit their full return to mobility (see Ch. 7). Often assistance is needed for stair climbing or descending and the patient may not feel confident doing this without using a banister.

Avoidance of twisting and turning, and high impact forces such as those sustained during jumping and running, and sudden jarring movements is essential for at least 3 months following the operation but some surgeons extend this to 6 months. Driving can be very difficult because of the repeated small arc motion needed to use the accelerator and clutch, not to mention the jarring movement of the brake pedal.

Loss of proprioception is normal with any joint replacement but removal of the anterior cruciate ligament and joint capsule, with joint effusion, exaggerates this loss following a knee replacement. Knee joint proprioception is definitely needed for driving and its return, along with inner range quadriceps strength and range of motion, may be used as a guide to when driving may be recommenced. As mentioned earlier, return to sporting activity may be possible following knee arthroplasty but consultation with the surgeon is essential before any sport is begun again or recommended to the patient.

Summary

Hip and knee replacement surgery have excellent outcomes for the majority of patients. Unfortunately when complications arise they can be major. Realistic expectations must be encouraged and the patient should be made aware of all possibilities – good and bad.

This must be particularly so for the younger patient (under 65 years) when the length of joint survival is especially important. The therapist must place emphasis on knowing the surgical regime to be used and the normal postoperative management. Understanding the complications, how they present, and informing the consultant or GP involved if you are anxious about the new joint or patient progression, are all important.

Return of full joint function will only be gained if the soft tissue length and strength are returned and this takes time, good physical therapy and compliance from the patient.

ANSWERS TO QUESTIONS AND EXERCISES

Self assessment-question 8.1 (page 205)

■ **SAQ 8.1.** How would you measure apparent and true leg length discrepancies?

Answer:

Apparent
The patient is in supine, lying with the head, shoulders, pelvis and lower limbs aligned. Place the end of the tape measure on the xiphisternum and extend it down to the medial malleolus and record the length on one side before measuring the other. If there is an adduction contracture then the 'good' leg should be adducted to the same degree as the contracture for comparison. Apparent shortening will demonstrate if there is a pelvic obliquity and may be accompanied by true shortening.

True
When the patient is in supine and the pelvis level the heels will not be level if a true discrepancy is present. To identify where the discrepancy is, three measures need to be taken:
● *From the anterior superior iliac spines on each side of the pelvis to the medial malleolus on the same side (complete limb length).*
● *From the greater trochanter to the lateral knee joint line (femoral length).*
● *From the medial knee joint line in flexion to the medial malleolus of that side (tibial length).*

Comparisons of measurements from each side and between apparent and true can then be made.

Leg length discrepancy may be present in the femoral neck, but this is very difficult to measure and may present as an apparent deformity. If the pelvis is mobile and can be levelled, and there is no true leg length discrepancy in the presence of an apparent difference, then there will be a shortening of the femoral neck (McRae 1990, Ch. 10, p 151–153).

Problem-solving exercise 8.1 (page 208)

■ To which of the common surgical complications mentioned in SAQ 5.7 do you think patients are most prone following total hip replacement?

Answer: *Infection, deep vein thrombus (DVT) or pulmonary embolus (PE), or respiratory problems.*

Problem-solving exercise 8.2 (page 211)

■ What would you do for a preoperative assessment of a patient awaiting a total hip replacement?

Answer:
Assess the following:

- *Joint movement and muscle tone around the joint: particularly the range of hip flexion and abduction, extension, rotation and abduction/adduction. Strength of hip glutei group (extension and abduction) and quadriceps group.*
- *General functional ability: walking, stairs, sitting to standing and bed mobility. Note the use of walking aids, handholds and how well the function is achieved.*
- *Respiratory function prior to surgery.*
- *Venous return in the lower limbs.*
- *What does the patient know about the surgery?*
- *Advise the patient about the postoperative regime.*

Problem-solving exercise 8.3 (page 211)

■ How can the therapist measure the functions of: walking, stair climbing, sit to stand or forward flexion (e.g. to put on shoes or socks)?

Answer:

Walking
Measure distance walked, time taken to achieve this (McNicol et al 1980). Observe and note any gait abnormalities (Perry 1992).

Stair climbing
Record the time taken, pattern used, and use of aids (e.g. banister or walking aid) to perform the function.

Sit to stand
Again the time taken and the pattern used should be noted. Here the position of the feet, use of the hands and the trunk motion are particularly important (Ada & Westwood 1992).

A video of the performance of any of these activities will be particularly useful and assist the patient to recognise improved performance of these activities.

Forward flexion
Remember that this can be measured preoperatively but not postoperatively until at least 3 months. *Measuring the distance from fingertip to floor represents both lumbar and hip movement, but if hip movement is to be recorded alone then a goniometer or electrogoniometer should be used. If this is not possible, then again a video of the activity will be helpful. Markers to the anterior superior iliac spine (ASIS), posterior superior iliac spine (PSIS), greater trochanter, lateral femoral condyle and lateral malleolus will assist observation of the video.*

Self-assessment question 8.2 (page 211)

■ **SAQ 8.2.** In what position does the hip joint dislocate after a total hip replacement?

Answer: *You would be correct if you answered: With an anterolateral and true lateral incision, the hip will dislocate if placed in excessive extension, external rotation and adduction, or a combination of all three. With a posterolateral incision, the hip will dislocate in excessive flexion, internal rotation and adduction, or a combination of all three.*

Problem-solving exercise 8.4 (page 214)

See answer following question in text.

Problem-solving exercise 8.5 (page 219)

■ What are the common complications specific to a joint replacement?

Answer: Dislocation, loosening, wound infection, deep joint infection, deep vein thrombus (DVT) or pulmonary embolus (PE), wear of the prosthetic surface.

Self-assessment question 8.3 (page 222)

■ **SAQ 8.3.** Why is it particularly important for a patient who has just had a total knee replacement to carry out isometric quadriceps exercises immediately postoperatively?

Answer:
— *To reduce joint effusion; contraction of the four components of the group compresses the suprapatellar pouch and so helps to remove excess fluid from the knee joint.*
— *Pain acts as an inhibitor to muscle activity, therefore early contraction of the quadriceps is important to overcome this.*
— *The patient is more than likely to have had a fixed flexion deformity preoperatively and the quadriceps function would be non-existent in the inner range. Encouragement of early activity will help to gain the return of inner range strength.*

Problem-solving exercise 8.6 (page 222)

See answer following question in text.

Problem-solving exercise 8.7 (page 224)

See the section immediately following the exercise.

Problem-solving exercise 8.8 (page 225)

■ How would you stretch the posterior aspect of a prosthetic knee replacement?

Answer: Immobilisation in plaster of paris, knee extension splint, serial casting or reversed dynamic traction, are each possible techniques.

— *Encourage passive knee extension stretch at all times, e.g. keep the feet elevated with knees straight when in bed or sitting.*
— *Encourage isometric quadriceps exercises in as much extension as is possible and inner range quadriceps exercises to maximum extension.*

Problem-solving exercise 8.9 (page 226)

■ What compensatory patterns might occur when a patient with a knee replacement walks?

Answer:
— *Dependent use of walking aids: because of limited balance and anxiety.*
— *Keeping the knee straight during stance: compensation for weak quadriceps.*
— *Reduced hip extension and push off during stance on the operated side: compensation for a generally stiff knee, and not wanting to move it.*
— *Excessive flexion of the hip and ankle on operated side during swing phase: compensation for limited knee flexion.*
— *Shortened step length: compensation for lack of extension.*

REFERENCES

Ada L, Westwood P 1992 A kinematic analysis of recovery of the ability to stand up following stroke. Australian Journal of Physiotherapy 38(2):135–142

Association of Orthopaedic Chartered Physiotherapists (AOCP) 1991 Survey of uncomplicated, cemented total hip replacements. AOCP, London

Barrett D S, Cobb A G, Bentley G 1991 Joint proprioception in normal, osteoarthritic and replaced knees. Journal of Bone and Joint Surgery 73B(1):53–56

Bartzokas C, Johnson R, Jane M et al 1994 Relation between mouth and hematogenous infection in total joint replacements. British Medical Journal 309:506–508

Basso D, Knapp L 1987 Comparison of two continuous passive motion protocols for patients with total knee implants. Physical Therapy 67(3):360–363

Borstlap M, Zant J, Vansoesbergen M, Vanderkorst J 1994 Effects of total hip-replacement on quality-of-life in patients with osteoarthritis and in patients with rheumatoid arthritis. Clinical Rheumatology 13(1):45–50

Brinker M, Reuben J, Mull J et al 1997 Comparison of general and epidural anaesthesia in patients undergoing primary unilateral THR. Orthopedics 20(2):109–115

Cameron I, Quine S 1994 External hip protectors – likely noncompliance among high-risk elderly people living in the community. Archives of Gerontology and Geriatrics 19(3):273–281

Coutts F, Hewetson D, Matthew J 1989 Continuous passive motion of the knee joint: use at the Royal National Orthopaedic Hospital, Stanmore. Physiotherapy 75(7):427–430

Coutts R 1983 The effect of continuous passive motion on total knee rehabilitation. Orthopaedic Transactions 7(3):355–356

Crawford Adams J, Stossel C 1992 Standard orthopaedic operations, 4th edn. Churchill Livingstone, Edinburgh

Dandy D 1993 Essential orthopaedics and trauma, 2nd edn. Churchill Livingstone, Edinburgh

Echternach J 1990 Clinics in physical therapy: physical therapy of the hip. Churchill Livingstone, New York

Engh C, Bobyn J 1985 Biological fixation in total hip arthroplasty. Slack, Thorofare, New Jersey

Engh C, Bobyn J, Glassman A 1987 Porous-coated hip replacement; the factors governing bone in-growth, stress shielding and clinical results. Journal of Bone and Joint Surgery 69:145

Fernandez-Galinski D, Puig M, Rue M et al 1996 Pain evaluation in elderly patients after orthopaedic surgery under regional anaesthesia. Pain Clinics 9(3):303–309

Goldie B 1992 Orthopaedic diagnosis and management. Blackwell Scientific Publications, London

Goodfellow J, Kershaw C, Benson M, O'Connor J 1988 The Oxford Knee for unicompartmental osteoarthritis. Journal of Bone and Joint Surgery 70B(5):692–701

Gose J 1987 Continuous passive motion in the postoperative treatment of patients with total knee replacements. Physical Therapy 67(1):39–42

Harms M, Engstrom B 1991 Continuous passive motion as an adjunct to treatment of the total knee arthroplasty patient. Physiotherapy 77(4):301–307

Hasheminejad A, Birch N, Goddard N 1994 Current attitudes to cementing techniques in British hip surgery. Annals of the Royal College of Surgeons of England 76(6):396–400

Hull R, Raskob G, Pineo G et al 1997 Subcutaneous low-molecular-weight heparin vs warfarin for prophylaxis of deep vein thrombosis after hip or knee implantation – an economic perspective. Archives of Internal Medicine 157(3):298–303

Johnson D 1990 The effect of continuous passive motion on wound healing and joint mobility after knee arthroplasty. Journal of Bone and Joint Surgery 72A(3):421–426

Kendall F, McCready E, Provance P 1993 Muscles testing and function. Williams and Wilkins, Baltimore

Kessel L, Bayley I 1986 Clinical disorders of the shoulder. Churchill Livingstone. Edinburgh

McGrath D, Dennyson W, Rolland M 1996 Death rate from pulmonary embolism following joint replacement surgery. Journal of the Royal College of Surgeons of Edinburgh 41(4):265–266

McGrory B, Stuart M, Sim F 1995 Participation in sports after hip and knee arthroplasty – review of literature and survey of surgeon preferences. Mayo Clinic Proceedings 70(4):342–348

McInnes J, Larson M, Daltroy L et al 1992 A controlled evaluation of continuous passive motion in patients undergoing total knee arthroplasty. Journal of the American Medical Association 268(11):1423–1428

McNicol M F, McHardy R, Chalmers J 1980 Exercise testing before and after hip arthroplasty. Journal of Bone and Joint Surgery 62B(3):326–331

McRae R 1990 Clinical orthopaedic examination, 3rd edn. Churchill Livingstone, Edinburgh

McRae R 1994 Practical fracture treatment, 3rd edn. Churchill Livingstone, Edinburgh

Maihafer G 1990 Rehabilitation of total hip replacements and fracture management considerations. In: Echternach J (ed) Clinics in physical therapy: physical therapy of the hip. Churchill Livingstone, New York, ch 6

Mallon W, Liebelt R, Mason J 1996 Total joint replacement and golf. Clinics in Sports Medicine 15(1):179

Mallory T 1992 Total hip replacement in the 1990s: the procedure, the patient, the surgeon. Orthopedics 15(4):427–430

Maloney W, Schurman D, Hangen D et al 1990 The influence of continuous passive motion on outcome in total knee arthroplasty. Clinical Orthopaedics and Related Research 256:162–168

Niwa S, Paul J P, Yamamoto S 1987 Total knee replacement. Springer-Verlag, Tokyo

Nordin M, Frankel V 1989 Biomechanics of the musculoskeletal system. Lea and Febiger, Philadelphia

Norkin C 1995 Measurement of joint motion: a guideline for goniometry, 2nd edn. F A Davis, Philadelphia

O'Driscoll S, Kumar A, Salter B 1983 The effect of the volume of effusion, joint position and continuous passive motion on intra-articular pressure in the rabbit knee. Journal of Rheumatology 10(3):360–363

Perrot S, Menkes C 1996 Nonpharmacological approaches to pain in osteoarthritis – available options. Drugs 52(S3):21–26

Perry J 1992 Gait analysis: normal and pathological function. Slack, Thorofare, New Jersey

Pettine K, Aamlid B, Cabanela M 1991 Elective total hip arthroplasty in patients older than 80 years of age. Clinical Orthopaedics and Related Research 266:127–132

Pring D, Marks L, Angel J 1988 Mobility after amputation for failed total knee replacements. Journal of Bone and Joint Surgery 70B(5):770–771

Ries M, Philbin E, Groff G et al 1996 Improvement in cardiovascular fitness after total knee arthroplasty. Journal of Bone and Joint Surgery 78A(11):1696–1701

Ritter M, Gandolf V, Holston K 1989 Continuous passive motion versus physical therapy in total knee arthroplasty. Clinical Orthopaedics and Related Research 244:239–243

Romness D, Rand J 1988 The role of continuous passive motion following total knee arthroplasty. Clinical Orthopaedics and Related Research 226:34–37

Rothman R, Hozack W 1988 Complications of total hip replacements. W B Saunders, Philadelphia

Rowe P, Nicol A, Kelly I 1989 Flexible goniometer computer system for the assessment of hip function. Clinical Biomechanics 4(2):68–72

Sahlstrom A, Lanshammer H, Wigren A 1994 Ground

reaction force and its moment with respect to the knee joint centre in a total condylar arthroplasty series. Clinical Biomechanics 9:125–129

Stanic U, Herman S, Merhar J 1993 Evaluation of rehabilitation of patients with total hip replacements. IEEE Transactions on Rehabilitation Engineering 1(2):86–93

Vince K, Kelly M, Beck J, Insall J 1987 Continuous passive motion after total knee arthroplasty. Journal of Arthroplasty 2(4):281–284

Walker P S 1987 Computer graphics design of total knee replacements (keynote lecture). In: Niwa S, Paul J P (eds) Total knee replacement. Springer-Verlag, Tokyo 3–22

Wasilewski S, Woods L, Torgerson W, Healy W 1990 Value of continuous passive motion in total knee arthroplasty. Orthopedics 13(3):291–295

Woolson S, Watt J 1991 Intermittent pneumatic compression to prevent proximal deep vein thrombosis during and after total hip replacement. Journal of Bone and Joint Surgery 73A(4):507–511

Wykman A, Olsson E 1992 Walking ability after total knee replacement. Journal of Bone and Joint Surgery 74B(1):53–56

Zavadak K, Gibson K, Whitley D, Britz P, Kwoh C 1995 Variability in the attainment of functional milestones during the acute-care admission after total joint replacement. Journal of Rheumatology 22(3):482–487

9

Orthopaedics in paediatrics

■ Paediatrics ■ Orthopaedics ■ Child development ■ Assessment
■ Traumatic injury ■ Congenital conditions ■ Juvenile chronic arthritis
■ Physiotherapy intervention ■ Areas of conflict ■ Management strategies

Objectives

By the end of this chapter you should:

1. Have an overview of the types of orthopaedic condition that affect children.
2. Start to appreciate the different perspective that needs to be adopted when working with children as opposed to other groups of clients.
3. Recognise how you can use your problem-solving and clinical reasoning skills in this different, but related, area of orthopaedics.

INTRODUCTION

The speciality of paediatrics covers a large range of conditions and philosophies of management that are beyond the scope of this book. This chapter aims to give an overview of the areas where physiotherapists may come into contact with children whose management involves some orthopaedic intervention. It also aims to give some guidance regarding the use of problem-solving and clinical decision-making skills in these situations.

Physiotherapists come into contact with children in many areas of practice which can include primary care settings, health centres, outpatient departments and hospital wards as well as nurseries and schools. These children range in age from babies born prematurely through to adolescents, with all of the concomitant developmental and psychosocial changes that occur as they grow up. This is in addition to any physical, mental, developmental, learning or emotional problems they may have.

The most important point to remember whenever treating children is that they are not just small adults, they are developing human beings (Association of Paediatric Chartered Physiotherapists (APCP) 1995). There are issues that need to be addressed at all stages. It is essential to see the child first, and the child with problems second (Eckersley 1993).

> *To become a fully integrated and mature person a child must develop a vast array of skills, both personal and social, to which many factors are contributory. Children's physical and mental potential, their family, and their environment are of primary importance (APCP 1995).*

One of the issues, as alluded to in the above quotation, is that members of the health care team are not just dealing with the child, but also with parents, and possibly, the rest of the family, as well as other carers such as teachers. As mentioned earlier in this book, these carers must, in fact, be part of the health care team. If any intervention is to be successful, the child must be seen in the context of the family who have a key role in this team. It is essential that everyone works together with agreed management plans. If this consistent approach is not taken, the child and the parents may become confused and find it difficult to comply with any intervention.

There must also be a balance between the needs of the child and the family.

It is important to remember that whatever problems a child has, he or she has 'special needs for fun, play and love' and parents and other professionals are partners with the physiotherapist in this enterprise (APCP 1995).

WHAT DOES THE PHYSIOTHERAPIST NEED TO WORK SUCCESSFULLY WITH CHILDREN?

It is important for the physiotherapist to consider the needs of both the parents and the child, and to be able to communicate effectively. Table 9.1 gives an indication of the skills and knowledge necessary.

Many of the skills and much of the knowledge used when treating children is the same as for physiotherapists in other settings. This relates very much to the overall philosophy of this book: where the actual 'condition' can be almost secondary, the important aspect is to focus on the patients and their needs and expectations. The physiotherapist must assess the child and then use the same problem-solving and decision-making skills as used with any other category of patient (based on an existing knowledge and skills base) in order to plan the intervention. Techniques must be appropriate for use with infants and children and may need to be modified. However, one major difference here is that the therapy is often carried out via another person, such as a parent.

Table 9.1 Skills and knowledge needed by the physiotherapist to work successfully with children and their carers (adapted from Grimley 1993)

1. A sound base of core physiotherapeutic skills.
2. Specialist skills which can be built onto this core.
3. Regular updating of knowledge and skills.
4. A knowledge of normal child development to facilitate recognition of any deviations from this.
5. Knowledge of the specific pathologies of childhood disorders and their common signs and symptoms.
6. Knowledge of the theories and philosophies of different approaches to the treatment of children.
7. Knowledge of, and skills in, the use of treatment modalities.
8. A variety of handling skills specifically for use in the management of children must be acquired and refined.
9. Knowledge of any specialist equipment.
10. An understanding of any statutory obligations.
11. Counselling skills.
12. Good interpersonal skills.
13. An awareness of social, environmental and cultural variables which influence family structure, dynamics and motivation.

Table 9.2 Development of motor skills in the first 12 months (Bedford 1993)

Age	Skill
2 months	Lifts head in prone
4 months	Lifts head in prone, weight on forearms Brings hands to midline Head kept in line with trunk when pulled to sitting
5 months	Lifts head in supine Lifts bottom in supine Rolls to side Pushes up on straight arms in prone Reaches with one arm in prone
6 months	Sits with hands in front for support Rolls supine to prone Takes both feet to mouth Helps pull self to sitting
7 months	Pivots and pushes self backwards in prone
8 months	Creeps forwards on forearms Sits unsupported with straight back Can reach in sitting Can get into lying
8–10 months	Crawls on all fours Pulls to standing
10–12 months	Gets down from standing Walks with both or one hand held
12 months	Some children walk independently

DEVELOPMENT

Development goes on from the moment the embryo is formed until the time that growth is complete. The term 'growth' indicates an increase in size, but 'development' relates to much more than this and involves an increase in complexity. It includes change and adaptation due to predetermined genetic factors and the experience of the child in interacting with the environment. Growth and development are closely related, but whereas growth can be quite reliably measured in such terms as height and weight, development manifests itself in many different ways; it is very individual, and so more difficult to quantify.

It is important to remember that children develop at different rates, albeit in a predictable sequence. Although certain developmental 'milestones' are available, these often give wide time ranges to allow for these different rates of change in each child. For example, one child may

be walking at the age of 9 months, whereas another may not walk until the age of 18 months. There are also some children who miss out certain stages, for example, the child who stands and walks without going through a crawling stage, and then there are those who perform different actions such as bottom shuffling (which is usually familial) (Bedford 1993).

A summary of the development of motor skills in the first 12 months is given in Table 9.2. From the orthopaedic point of view the most important milestones are the following:

1. Head held unsupported at around 3 months.
2. Sits unaided at around 6 months, with hands in front.
3. Stands up unaided between 9 and 12 months.
4. Walks between 12 and 18 months.

If the child is unable to sit by the age of 9 months, pull him/herself upright by 12 months or walk by 20 months, this should alert carers that something could be amiss and that a paediatric opinion may be required (Dandy 1993).

Although this book concentrates on musculoskeletal issues, it is important not to forget about other areas of development which can have profound effects on that of the musculoskeletal system. Neither the nervous, nor the respiratory systems, are fully developed at birth. Acquisition of motor control and skill follows progressive change in the nervous system: the growth of nerve fibres, formation of new synapses and activation of neurotransmitters (Shepherd 1995). During the first year of life the weight of the brain increases threefold, mainly due to an increase in size of the neurons and myelination of the axons. As the myelination occurs, antigravity control develops in a particular sequence, that is, the baby will develop control over antigravity neck movements before similar trunk movements. Similarly control over the shoulder girdle occurs before hand function and so on. The more distal development is dependent upon the maturation of the more proximal/central muscles. Related to this, there is a predictable sequence in the development of erect positions from the lower, more stable ones such as prone and supine, to higher, less stable positions such as four-point kneeling, sitting and eventually standing (Hinderer & Hinderer 1993).

One of the explanations put forward as a main reason for this process of functional connections forming in the central nervous system, is that it occurs as a response to stimulation and use. Sensory and motor development are interdependent and so it is essential for the child to be interacting with the environment in order for normal neuromuscular development to occur.

Normal development of bone and soft tissue depends partly on the stresses applied to them. If the stresses are abnormal for any reason, then development may also be abnormal. For example, if a child has poor posture, this could lead to muscle imbalance which could, in turn, lead to abnormal stresses on bone and so problems in development. These muscle imbalances will have more serious implications at this early stage in life, possibly causing more severe deformity than the same imbalance would cause in an adult. It is also important to remember that the consequences of these problems will persist into adult life, and this may have implications for further physiotherapy intervention.

Normal musculoskeletal development may also be affected if there are problems with the respiratory system. If a disease causes delayed development or irreversible damage in the respiratory system, this will have implications for the amount of activity the child is able to perform. Reduced exercise tolerance could well delay or alter musculoskeletal development. Again, the disease occurring at this stage in life will have more wide-ranging effects than the same disease in an adult where growth and development are complete, as well as the possibility of the problems extending into adulthood.

Although a knowledge of motor development is essential for the orthopaedic paediatric physiotherapist, many other changes occur as a child grows up. It is useful to have some knowledge of these in order to understand the child as a whole. The psychological and emotional environment in which the child grows up will have far-reaching effects on general development. Other important areas to be aware of are mentioned below.

Hearing

Normal babies babble, beginning at about 1 month. The quality of this starts to change at around 6 months when they start to imitate sounds that they hear. They also start to use intonation, which shows that they hear and take note of adult intonation. The child's listening and verbal skills can give an indication of hearing ability. There are also hearing tests which are usually carried out at intervals during the child's development.

Communication

This involves verbal and non-verbal aspects. Non-verbal communication is the most important before a child is able to speak, and mothers are often able to discern what their child wants or needs from cries, movements and facial expressions.

Later on, the child starts to realise that his/her behaviour has an effect on other people's reactions and this is the beginning of meaningful communication. But as communication is a two-way process, the child also has to learn to attend to what is being done or said by others. This takes some time to develop as babies are very easily distracted by other stimuli.

Verbal communication starts to develop as mentioned in the previous section on hearing. Babies understand many more words than they are able to say at first (receptive language). By 15 months a child can use two to six words meaningfully and this is the start of the development of expressive language. By 18 months the number of words has increased to up to 20. Speech is usually fluent by the age of 5 years (Bedford 1993).

Vision

Development of vision will inevitably have an effect on the child's general functional abilities, as well as affecting the development of the psyche (Morse 1983). At birth, the lens has a fixed focus (about 20 cm). The development of binocular vision, accommodation and acuity occur over the first 6 months as long as there is no abnormality in the eye. Visual stimulus is necessary in order for the visual pathways to form normally in the brain.

If the level of vision is limited for some reason, this may affect the early bond usually formed between mother and child, 'necessary for feelings of security, the transmission of empathy, and the establishment of trust' (Morse 1983). An adequate body image may not be established if there is a lack of visual input regarding the functioning of the child's body or the feedback from significant adults. This may have an effect on the child's level of mobility and so, in turn, on musculoskeletal development.

Perception

This involves development of figure–background discrimination, appreciation of depth and distance, a recognition of the constancy of size and shape, and closure. In order for these areas to develop, the child will use more than one sensory modality, for example vision and touch at the same time.

Cognitive skills

This involves the development of thinking, perceiving and reasoning skills. There are many theories of cognitive development, which are beyond the scope of this book. This area of child development will inevitably have an effect on the other types of development already mentioned. But it is important to remember that each child will progress through the stages at different rates, and some will ultimately achieve higher levels than others. The type of cognitive skills developed may also vary depending on the background and culture in which the child is immersed.

Play

Play is a social activity, the objective of which is that the participants should enjoy themselves. However, it has a major influence on the development of motor, perceptual, communication and social skills (Bedford 1993).

It is particularly important for the physiotherapist to be aware of how children play at different ages, as this may be the main way in which therapy is delivered. Interventions need to be interesting, stimulating and fun, otherwise the child may become bored and there will be a lack of compliance with treatment.

COMMON AREAS OF ORTHOPAEDICS WITH REGARD TO PAEDIATRIC PATIENTS

As mentioned earlier, physiotherapists in all areas of practice may come into contact with children who have orthopaedic problems. However, the role of the physiotherapist has changed in recent years. Much time used to be spent dealing with problems such as knock knees, bow legs and flat feet but the majority of these conditions have now been recognised as transitory, and so unlikely to be treated with physiotherapy. If something does turn out to be more serious, such as a developmental abnormality or dislocated hip, then the physiotherapist may be involved in rehabilitation. But, generally, the main input is likely to be in reassuring and educating the parents. The management of conditions such as tuberculosis of the hip and spine and Perthes' disease used to involve long periods of immobilisation where physiotherapy intervention would have been important. However, tuberculosis is now much rarer and Perthes' disease is treated much more actively with early mobilisation being encouraged. The physiotherapist may be involved with the latter.

Poor posture is seen quite often, particularly in adolescents, but again this is usually transitory. Physiotherapists may be involved in general educational programmes in schools relating to back care and manual handling, depending on the local situation. This may help to avoid some of these problems. If a child does present with poor posture, the most effective way to deal with this is probably to encourage general exercise such as swimming, gym work or other sports-related activities, rather than trying to instigate a home exercise programme for which there would be little enthusiasm or adherence (Dandy 1993, Shepherd 1995).

Orthopaedic problems may be primary, for example, where a child has a soft tissue injury, a fracture, a rheumatic disease or a deformity due to a congenital condition. A congenital condition is a disease that develops during fetal life which can be due to a genetic factor or can be acquired. Conversely the orthopaedic elements of the child's condition may be secondary; for example, many children with cerebral palsy do have orthopaedic problems but these may not be the primary concern of the physiotherapist.

Traumatic injury

Young children, due to their intensely curious natures, are prone to accidents. They are constantly exploring and do not always realise the danger of the situations they encounter. This is compounded by their lack of coordination and judgement, which in an older child or adult, would probably enable avoidance of injury. With a certain amount of luck and much parental vigilance, accidents may only result in fairly minor cuts and bruises which require little, if any, treat-

ment, but unfortunately this is not always the case.

The most common injury in young children which involves a physiotherapist's intervention, is fracture. Some mention of childhood fractures was made in Chapter 5. A little more detail will be given later, but unless there are complications, many children recover fully with only minimal physiotherapy input. As the child gets older, into the teens, the treatment for fractures will become more like that of adults, and so the physiotherapist may be more involved.

Self-assessment question

■ **SAQ 9.1.** a. How do the union and consolidation times of fractures in children relate to those in adults? b. Approximately how long does it take for callus to form in a child following a fracture?
(Hint: see Chapter 5 if you can't remember.)

Fractures may occur as a result of other pathology. This could be localised, such as a bone cyst, or more general, for example, in the familial disease, osteogenesis imperfecta, or if a child has osteoporosis due to rheumatoid arthritis.

Soft tissue injuries are rare in young children. The type of trauma which, in an adult, would cause damage to soft tissue, is more likely to cause separation of an epiphysis (Shepherd 1995). An example of this is slipped femoral epiphysis which is more common in boys than girls. This can occur as a result of trauma, but there are other elements involved such as hormonal disturbances (McRae 1990).

Some older children are very keen on particular sports. There is the possibility of soft tissue injury occurring here; for example, low back pain, ankle and knee injuries in young, female gymnasts (Homer & Mackintosh 1992).

If a physiotherapist is working with children on a regular basis, it is important to be aware of the possibility of non-accidental trauma. Child abuse is usually carried out by an adult who is in charge of the child and the injuries can be physical, emotional or sexual.

In child abuse cases where injuries are sus-

Table 9.3 Physical factors which may indicate child abuse (adapted from McRae 1994)

- Fracture with no history of injury, or vague history not in keeping with the nature or extent of injuries
- Presence of multiple fractures or other injuries especially at different stages of healing indicating that they have occurred as separate incidents
- Presence of multiple soft tissue injuries including swelling, bruises, burns, welts, lacerations and scars. Again they may be at different stages of healing
- If there is head injury, X-rays may show a fracture or widening of the sutures. The latter may be due to raised intracranial pressure because of cerebral oedema or subdural haematoma
- Evidence of failure to thrive, growth retardation, fever, anaemia, or seizures

tained, 80% are found in children under the age of 3 years (McRae 1994). Some of the factors which might alert a medical professional to the symptoms of child abuse are listed in Table 9.3.

Physiotherapists may be involved in treating the effects of abuse, but may also play an important role in the detection of signs that abuse is taking place (Griffiths 1993). A paediatric physiotherapist should only breach confidentiality in exceptional circumstances and it is important that local child abuse policies are adhered to. These are normally agreed with a number of agencies such as social services, the local health authority, local education authority and the police. Paediatric physiotherapists have a duty to be aware of what information is relevant to pass to other team members or to the other agencies as appropriate, in order to prevent further damage occurring (APCP 1995). This may be done by being in close contact with other professionals, such as paediatricians, who are experienced in this area.

Rheumatic conditions

One child in a thousand will have some form of arthritis during the childhood years. These are chronic conditions with variable aetiologies, most of which are uncertain or unknown. Generally the child will complain of pain and swelling in the joints with reduction in range of motion. There may also be systemic features such as a rash, a raised temperature and/or fatigue. The outcome of these conditions depends very much on how the child is managed by the health care team. The physiotherapist has an important role in working with the child and his/her carers, to provide education about the optimal ways in which to live successfully within the limits of the disease.

There are usually some periods of active physiotherapy treatment which may involve hydrotherapy and land-based exercises and/or splinting, but much of the management will be carried out by the parents. With appropriate intervention and cooperation from the children and their families, many reach adulthood with little, if any, disability.

Juvenile chronic arthritis is one of the most common rheumatic disorders, making up approximately 30–50% of new cases referred to specialist paediatric rheumatology clinics (Leak 1991).

Congenital conditions

As mentioned earlier, the term 'congenital' relates to diseases appearing at birth, having developed during fetal life (Anderson 1985, Sheldon 1992). An example, and one of the most common congenital abnormalities, is spina bifida which occurs when the neural tube fails to close (Shepherd 1995).

Congenital conditions can be genetic disorders which may be due to heredity (that is, inherited from one or both parents), or mutation (which can occur spontaneously or as a result of contact with radiation, chemicals or infective agents). These disorders can be chromosomal, that is, where there is an extra chromosome, parts of chromosomes missing or duplicated, translocation (material rearranged) or mosaics where only some cells have abnormal chromosome patterns. Genetic disorders can also be due to single gene alterations (mutations). Over 4000 disorders of this type have been identified.

There are many disorders which have multifactorial causes and genetic factors often play a part here. But other elements are important, such as the environment. This group of disorders is less well understood and the link to genetic aspects less clear.

The known causes of congenital disorders are called teratogenic factors which can be hereditary, environmental or a mixture of the two. There are critical time periods which dictate the type and severity of the effect the teratogenic factor may have on the fetus. Most defects arise during the second and third months of development when the major organ systems are forming.

It is important to remember that although congenital problems may be due to genetic conditions, not all genetic conditions manifest themselves at birth. The diseases produced can vary enormously, from life-threatening defects to mild disorders which may only manifest in adulthood. Lastly, not all of these conditions will have orthopaedic elements (Anderson 1985, Donnai et al 1993, Govan et al 1996, Sheldon 1992).

Self-assessment questions

- **SAQ 9.2.** What skills and knowledge are needed by the physiotherapist in order to work successfully with children and their carers?

- **SAQ 9.3.** What are the important orthopaedic milestones in child development?

ASSESSMENT

Many of the general features covered in the earlier assessment chapter will be of relevance when dealing with children; however, there are some areas that need to be modified, and there may be specific tests or techniques that need to be carried out.

Self-assessment question

- **SAQ 9.4.** Review the role of assessment within the overall physiotherapy management of a patient. (That is, why is assessment essential?)

Review points

Before reading this section, using your previous knowledge and experience, try to think through any similarities and differences in your approach to assessing patients in the following categories: (a) a 70-year-old adult; (b) a 20-year-old adult; (c) a 14-year old adolescent; (d) a 5-year-old child, and (e) a newborn baby.

It is essential that assessment of children at any age is an holistic and ongoing process, and not a procedure that is 'got out of the way' when the patient is first seen. This is particularly important in younger children where many developmental changes are occurring at the same time as any intervention. This approach to assessment is necessary in order to ensure that any treatment outcomes are successful. (It should be noted that this principle applies to different degrees in the assessment of all patients.) Many children referred to the physiotherapist have continuing problems, which require ongoing intervention over a long period (APCP 1995). A knowledge of the changes in performance which occur due to growth and development becomes even more important here.

Accurate and appropriate assessment is necessary to enable the following processes to take place (adapted from Bastow et al 1993):

1. development of initial plan of intervention
2. prioritisation with regard to future therapy
3. monitoring of any changes and progress
4. evaluation of effectiveness of treatment
5. evaluation of outcomes.

Screening

Physiotherapists tend to be involved mainly with rehabilitation situations providing treatment and management for acute and chronic disorders, although some may work in a preventative and educational role with children. On the whole, this means that much of the screening has been performed outside of the physiotherapy environment. But it is still important that the physiotherapist is aware of the available screening procedures that are available to detect and identify paediatric problems both pre- and postnatally.

Before the birth, this involves routine surveillance of mothers during pregnancy (health education and clinical examination), and if necessary more complex investigations to test the baby in utero. These include: ultrasound for growth, development and the detection of certain congenital abnormalities; amniocentesis to detect neural tube defects, and chorionic villus sampling to detect some sex-linked conditions.

Just after birth, the baby is given a physical examination where height, weight and head circumference are checked. Ortolani's test (McRae 1990) is used to check for congenital dislocation of the hip and a simple neurological test is carried out. This is repeated at 6 weeks and any abnormalities found can be followed up. There are also a number of biochemical tests, performed routinely, for conditions such as phenylketonuria. Developmental screening then continues regularly throughout the pre-school years (Griffiths 1993). Probably the most reliable developmental warning sign is a mother's suspicion that her child is not seeing, hearing, moving or taking notice like other children of a similar age (Sheridan 1975).

Self-assessment question

■ **SAQ 9.5.** What are the broad areas of child development that the physiotherapist should be aware of?

Physiotherapy assessment

Environment

The environment in which the assessment takes place is an important factor, as it can affect how well the child performs. If possible, the surroundings should be familiar and comfortable to help the child to feel as secure as possible, but should also be appropriate for the assessment process. If the room and contents are familiar to the child before the assessment, it will mean that there is less distraction. If these points are considered, any behaviour, responses to different stimuli and ability to perform activities observed by the physiotherapist will more closely mirror the 'normal situation'. With the increasing move towards primary care, the physiotherapist's first contact with the child and family may be in the home, unless specific equipment is necessary or there is a need to attend a specialist clinic. This is

the most familiar situation in which the assessment can take place – but the physiotherapist must be aware of any distractions. There may also be other situations where assessment could take place such as nursery or school.

It is not absolutely necessary to see previous medical records before the initial contact. This avoids preconceptions and may mean that observations are more objective. The main issue is for the physiotherapist to regard the child as a whole.

Developmental assessment

Child development was discussed briefly earlier in this chapter. Depending on the situation and the age of the child, the physiotherapist may have to carry out some form of developmental check along with the more specific orthopaedic examination. Many schedules are available to guide these checks and an example is shown in Table 9.4.

A more comprehensive test battery often used by health professionals is the Sheridan Stycar (Sheridan 1975) which includes the following elements:

- posture and large movements
- vision and fine movements
- hearing and speech
- social behaviour and play.

Schedules of this type usually give the age of the child and a range of activities/abilities expected at that stage. The child attending for assessment can then be observed, compared and monitored against this body of knowledge considered to be the 'norm'. The available schedules give a guide for this, but the physiotherapist will also benefit from possessing a good background knowledge of child development in order to be able to quickly and effectively identify any problems.

Subjective assessment

Discussion with parents or carers is essential in the subjective assessment. This should also continue throughout any intervention the physiotherapist suggests. It is important to find out how much the parents know and understand about the child's condition. During any discussion it should also be possible to obtain some indication

Table 9.4 Developmental screening: the Birmingham Chart. (Reproduced with permission from Eckersley 1993)

Date	Month	Motor	Social	Hearing and speech	Eye and Hand	Month
	1	Head erect for few seconds	Quieted when picked up	Startled by sounds	Notices bright objects close to	1
	2	Head up when prone (chin clear)	Smiles	Listens to ball or rattle	Follows ring up, down and sideways	2
	3	Kicks well	Alert. Follows person with eyes	Searches for sound with eyes	Glances from one object to another	3
	4	Lifts head and chest in prone	Returns examiner's smile	Laughs	Clasps and retains cube	4
	5	Holds head erect with no lag	Frolics when played with	Turns head to sound	Pulls paper away from face	5
	6	Rises on to wrists	Turns head to person talking	Babbles or coos to music	Takes cube from table	6
	7	Rolls from front to back	Friendly with strangers	Makes four different sounds	Looks for fallen object	7
	8	Tries to crawl vigorously	Shows toy	Shouts for attention	Passes toy from hand to hand	8
	9	Turns around on floor	Helps to hold spoon	Says 'Mama' or 'Dada'	Manipulates two objects at once	9
	10	Stands when held up	Rings bell in imitation	Listens to watch, responds to talking	Clicks two bricks together	10
	11	Pulls up to stand	Finger feeds	Understands 'No'	Pincer grip	11
	12	Walks or side-steps round furniture	Plays 'Pat-a-cake'	Three words with meaning	Points with index finger	12
	13	Stands alone	Waves 'Bye Bye'	Looks at picture	Picks up small object	13
	14	Walks alone	Uses spoon	Knows own name	Makes mark with pencil	14
	15	Climbs upstairs	Shows shoes	Four to five clear words. Points to familiar toy	Places one object upon another	15
	16	Pushes pram, toy horse etc.	Curious	Knows 'give', 'show', 'get'	Scribbles freely	16
	17	Climbs onto chair	Manages cup well	Babbled conversation	Watches from window	17
	18	Picks up toys without falling	Takes off socks and shoes	Enjoys pictures in books	Constructive play with toys	18
	19	Climbs stairs up and down	Knows one part of body	6–20 words	Tower of three bricks	19
	20	Jumps	Imitates activities	Echoes words	Removes wrapper from sweet	20

Table 9.4 (*cont'd*)

21	Runs	Puts on garment	Two-word sentences	Circular scribble	21
22	Walks up stairs	Tries to tell experiences	Listens to stories	Tower of five or more bricks	22
23	Seats himself at table	Knows two parts of body	Demands by pointing	Copies perpendicular stroke	23
24	Walks up and down stairs	Knows and names four parts of body	Names four toys	Copies horizontal stroke	24

Notes
1. Test items in each parameter, placing √s or Xs in adjacent right-hand columns, and starting at child's chronological age
2. Carry on until three Xs consecutively are marked. If necessary, go back and check earlier items.
3. Add √s in each column.
4. Compare number of √s with chronological age in months. Marked divergence in column suggests a specific problem in an area of delay which should be checked.
5. A tape-slide set 'Developmental Screening' 81/24, explaining the use of the chart, is obtainable from Graves Medical Audiovisual Library, Chelmsford.

about how well they are coping and whether or not they have any support from relatives, friends and other professionals. Depending on the gravity of the situation and the personalities involved, this may take time and sensitivity on the part of the physiotherapist, who should try to create a supportive atmosphere. It is essential to build up as good a relationship as possible with the parents, particularly if they will be carrying out any part of the physiotherapy intervention. If they understand the underlying reasons for any techniques or exercises, they will be able to help in a more informed way. Overall compliance may also be improved.

In babies and younger children, any background information will have to be obtained from the parents or carers. This will include basics such as name, address, age, date of birth, gender, ethnic group, number of children and whether they are born to the family, adopted or fostered. It may also be useful to investigate family history and any past medical history of note. Some of the data may be obtained from medical notes, but it is useful to check them with the child's parents/carers for accuracy. As with the assessment of any patient, this information needs to be obtained at some point during the investigation of the present condition. An older child or teenager may be able to give some or all of the

information to the physiotherapist, or it may be a joint procedure.

After the background has been established, the present condition can be addressed. The type of questions asked may be very similar to those used in any orthopaedic assessment, but again, in babies and younger children, much of the information will come from the parents.

Objective assessment
Depending on the age of the child, the collection of objective data will be undertaken in various different ways. In an older child or teenager, the physical assessment may be very similar to that of an adult patient. However, in younger children the objective assessment may involve a mixture of observation of free play, physical examination and the use of a series of specific tasks or activities, plus questioning of the parent or carer (APCP 1995).

Any test techniques used must be modified especially when assessing children younger than 6 years old. For infants and toddlers much information has to be obtained by observation and palpation whilst they are involved in age-appropriate developmental/functional activities. When looking at neonates and infants, their state of alertness is important because if they are sleepy, it is not possible to elicit optimal performance. Most activity, particularly in the muscles, is observed when the child is alert, hungry and/or crying. Due to these differences in behaviour it may be necessary to repeat observations at various times of the day. The child's level of alertness should be recorded. It may be possible to look at the more passive elements early in the assessment, followed by observation of spontaneous movements before any handling occurs. Then tactile and/or auditory stimuli can be used to arouse more active responses. Some resistance can be given to normal activities such as crawling to give an idea of muscle strength. For accurate assessment, it is very important that a physiotherapist can distinguish between active and reflex movements (Hinderer & Hinderer 1993).

For older children, between the ages of 2 and 5 years, more functional tests can be carried out. This is suggested as they probably will not cooperate with usual assessment procedures. Examples of the sort of activities that can be used particularly to look at muscle strength are shown in Table 9.5.

Children of school age and older are usually more able to participate in standard testing procedures. It is important that the physiotherapist explains each test carefully and, if possible, ascertains that the child understands what each one is for. This helps to ensure that effort is maximal, although it is essential to remember how easily young children can be distracted. It may also be necessary to demonstrate certain movements or

Table 9.5 Activities which can be used in the assessment of muscle strength in children (Hinderer & Hinderer; taken from Harms-Ringdahl 1993, Muscle strength, with permission)

Position	Observations
Standing	
1. Posture (posterior and lateral views)	Symmetry and alignment, postural curves, scapular position
2. Walking	Gait deviations indicative of muscle weakness
3. Heel walking	Bilateral dorsiflexor strength
4. Toe walking	Bilateral plantarflexor strength
5. Stepping up and down a step	Leg lifted onto step via hip flexors and hamstrings (concentric contraction). Body elevated via quadriceps and hip extensors (concentric contraction). Leg and body lowered down onto step via eccentric contraction of the same muscle groups
6. One-legged stand	Strength of hip abductors (gluteus medius and minimus). Pelvis should remain level. If the pelvis drops on the non-weight-bearing side, or if the trunk leans toward the weight-bearing side, hip abductor weakness may exist
7. One-legged stand on tiptoes	Unilateral plantarflexor strength
8. Toe touching, rising and lowering	Eccentric and concentric contractions of back extensors and gluteus maximus
9. Squat to stand, rising and lowering	Eccentric and concentric contraction of gluteus maximus and quadriceps femoris (watch for Gower's sign, where child pushes on thighs to assist)
10. Scapular stability, arms extended against wall	Ability of serratus anterior to stabilise scapula against thoracic wall
Prone	
1. Wheelbarrow position	Triceps, latissimus dorsi, serratus anterior and neck extensors
2. Flying position (head, trunk, arms and legs extended)	Back and neck extensors, middle trapezius and posterior deltoid
3. Prone kicking (hips alternately extending)	Gluteus maximus and hamstrings
Supine	
1. Sit-up	Neck flexors and abdominals
2. Pull to sit	Neck flexors, finger flexors, biceps
3. Bridging	Gluteus maximus, hamstrings
4. Bicycle in supine	Hip and knee flexors and extensors
Sitting	
1. Sitting push-up	Upper and lower trapezius, lattissimus dorsi, triceps, hip flexors

positions. Any commands given should be short, clear and above all, consistent, to avoid confusion. As with any assessment, issues such as comfort, posture and correct positioning need to be addressed. If any equipment is used, further simple explanation is necessary to reassure the child and to allay any fear or anxiety which could affect performance (Hinderer & Hinderer 1993).

Gait

In children with orthopaedic problems, it is important to be particularly aware of their method of locomotion, that is, how they get around, if at all. Children become increasingly skilled in locomotion as they develop, and move through a recognised progression from rolling through crawling to walking (although some children have interim stages such as bottom shuffling or 'walking like a bear' on hands and feet). Sensation for movement comes from the eyes, vestibular system, joints, muscles and skin. In order for normal gait to occur the following are necessary:

- an intact neuromuscular system for balance and coordination
- efficient levers to transmit muscle force into movement
- a desire to move and an awareness of quality of the desired movement
- energy to fulfil the aim (adapted from Jones 1993).

If a child has an orthopaedic problem then some of the above prerequisites for gait may be affected. In the simplest terms a fracture will affect the lever system (that is the skeleton) and so forces produced by the muscles will not be transmitted correctly and movement will be abnormal. In another situation, a child may have a long-standing condition affecting the skeleton, including the joints which may have reduced general mobility. This may mean a reduction in muscle strength and general debilitation, which would again have a major effect on locomotion.

In a normal child, gait begins with the feet wide apart, flat feet, knees stiff, arms slightly flexed and held above the head or at shoulder height for balance. This gradually develops into an adult gait pattern at approximately 7 to 9 years (Jones 1993, Sheridan 1975).

The physiotherapist assessing a child's gait should be familiar with the normal gait cycle and any differences there may be due to each stage of development. It will probably be necessary to look at the child's walking on a number of occasions, and for fairly long periods to obtain a full picture of any problems. It is important for the child to be undressed sufficiently for the physiotherapist to be able see what is going on. The most useful observations usually occur when the child is unaware that an assessment is taking place. As well as looking at the quality of the gait, a note should be made of the distance the child is able to walk and any pain or discomfort complained of. A useful strategy may be to use video to record walking and other activities, to allow repeat viewing, which may reduce stress on the child and parents. Other tests could be carried out if the physiotherapist has access to a gait laboratory, but this will depend upon facilities and the compliance of the child.

If the child has a walking aid, gait should be assessed both with and without it if possible. In a child with gait problems who has not had a walking aid before assessment, it may be necessary for the physiotherapist to provide one. In this case, it is important to remember that this could be difficult for the child and/or parents to accept and so needs to be handled sensitively (Jones 1993).

General assessment point

In their Standards of Practice, the Association of Paediatric Chartered Physiotherapists recommend that the following points are recorded in writing as evidence of a full assessment (APCP 1995):

- Child's history and relevant developmental milestones
- History of presenting problem
- Family history
- Child's abilities and inabilities, physical and functional, appropriate to age
- Child's own perception of any difficulties
- Parental anxieties
- Family interaction
- Social conditions.

PHYSIOTHERAPY INTERVENTION

Once the assessment has been completed, the next step is to identify areas suitable for intervention by the physiotherapist, and to plan an appropriate treatment programme keeping in mind the needs and expectations of the family and the child. They need to be kept informed at all times regarding the proposed intervention, and encouraged to be involved and to make active choices. The treatment should be offered rather than imposed. It is important to ensure that any information is modified in order that the child as well as the parents/carers can understand it. For the child, possible ways of modification may be:

- by simple understandable explanation
- by demonstration
- through story telling using visual and/or verbal methods
- by the use of toys
- through games
- by the use of appropriate signing systems such as Makaton or Bliss.

The Children's Act 1989 requires the child to give informed consent before any intervention can occur. This means that once an explanation has been given the child should be encouraged to respond. This may be verbal or non-verbal. In order for this process to be successful the physiotherapist needs to modify and adapt communication to an appropriate level of comprehension and pace. Where the child is unable to give consent, the parents or guardians may take on this role (APCP 1995).

> ### Self-assessment question
>
> ■ **SAQ 9.6.** Review the main points that should be recorded as evidence of a full paediatric assessment.

FAMILY ISSUES

Unless there is an overriding need for a stay in hospital, much the preferred option is to manage the child at home. 'The trend of managing childhood illness at home, in preference to hospital admission, is now firmly established' (Whyte et al 1995). The extent of the responsibility that parents take for this management will depend, to a certain extent, on the actual problems the child has. The chronicity of the condition is also a factor; for example, the management of a child after a fracture will only last for a few weeks, which will be very different from involvement of the parents in managing a child with a long-term disease such as juvenile chronic arthritis. Another determinant of how well parents may cope with a child at home is the level of professional support available in the community. This tends to be less consistent, and the nature of the support necessary not clearly understood (Whyte et al 1995). Even if support is available, it may not be easy to find out how it can be accessed or for the precise help required to be obtained (Marks 1985). This point is reinforced by Cameron (1987) who notes that parents of children with special needs are often critical of the services they receive. This seems to be due to lack of practical support and advice, difficulties in getting information and assistance from service agencies and a lack of sympathy and sensitivity from professionals involved in management.

Much of the work on the care of children in the home (rather than in a hospital base) has been carried out in relation to those with chronic problems such as cerebral palsy, cystic fibrosis and learning difficulties. However, many of the important points are also relevant to children with orthopaedic conditions.

Parents do encounter a wide range of problems in obtaining a child's cooperation with home physiotherapy programmes. Management of children with special needs of any sort, be they temporary or long-term, can be complex and so support from health professionals is vital. According to Woods (1987) 'the definition of a home based service for the families of children who have special needs is one where the family is visited at regular fixed intervals by a professional providing support, a planned programme of treatment and appropriate materials or equipment'.

Much work has been undertaken to study the impact on the family, of caring for a chronically ill or disabled child. It can place considerable demands upon particular family members and/or on the family as a unit, and the therapy itself can cause much disruption to family life (Ross & Thomson 1993, Whyte et al 1995). There is a fine balance to be struck between the demands on the parents of any therapy programme and the demands of siblings, partners, work, social commitments and so on. It is also important to remember that no two family situations are exactly alike and so there is no convenient 'blueprint' of management (Marks 1985). This is where problem-solving and clinical decision-making skills are so important for the physiotherapist.

The ability and willingness of the parents to take on responsibility for home supervision of any therapy must be carefully assessed. It is vital that they believe the advice given to them by physiotherapists regarding their child's care will be of benefit, otherwise compliance will be low. Realistic and developmentally appropriate goals should be planned jointly with the child, or the child and the family. These should be based on the child's lifestyle, and should be relevant and achievable, but flexible enough to be modified on monitoring and review. It is important to be aware of family circumstances when organising visits and treatment sessions. For example, appointment times should be flexible and arranged to suit parents/carers wherever possible, and alternative venues could be considered where access is difficult (APCP 1995).

Alongside the goals, the management programme designed for the child, in negotiation with those involved, must also be relevant, achievable and flexible. The physiotherapist has a role in helping the parents to develop any skills which may be necessary, for example, hands-on techniques or use the of certain equipment, and these need to be monitored and evaluated throughout the management period. Here the physiotherapist is acting as an educator, and so must be able to modify his/her communication in order to ensure that any instructions are easily understood. This could involve the use of written information, diagrams, audiovisual methods or simply verbal description and demonstration.

With regard to interaction with the child during any contact, the APCP (1995) highlights the importance of encouraging confidence and self-worth by using the following strategies:

- Highlight the child's assets rather than difficulties.
- Handle the child's behaviour consistently.
- Reward the child for effort made rather than final result. (This recognises that children are not encouraged by excessive praise of something they have not done well.)
- Show appreciation of achievements, however small.
- Make every effort to boost the child's confidence.
- Allow the child responsibility during the therapy sessions.

Self-assessment question

■ **SAQ 9.7.** In what ways can the physiotherapist modify information about proposed management to make it understandable for the child?

Areas of conflict and management strategies

It is inevitable that in many cases there will be some conflict between parents and child, or sometimes between the parents themselves. In a long-term condition such as juvenile chronic arthritis for example, the child must usually perform daily exercises and wear splints. It is not always easy to convince the child that these things are necessary, particularly if some parts of the process are painful or difficult. Children often do not understand the reason behind exercises and this means they will be reluctant to perform them (Puddefoot et al 1997). This can cause distress if the parent has to battle with the child each time treatment time arrives, and resentment of the 'therapist' role can build up if it causes alienation between them. Distress can also be increased if parents are very anxious to follow a professional's instructions, and resort to threat or punishment in order to gain the child's cooperation.

There might be an issue if partners do not support each other in relation to the child's therapy. Occasionally one parent might insist on taking the whole responsibility for the child's treatment programme which could cause problems with the other partner feeling isolated. Conversely one parent might consciously or unconsciously opt out of the therapy sessions which would shift the responsibility onto the other person. This could again result in alienation between child and the 'therapist' parent as well as giving mixed messages to the child about the importance of the treatment. Either of these scenarios would cause dissonance between the parents and add extra stress to what may be an already difficult situation. The child could well sense this and become more anxious.

The issues may be different for older children who are able to understand the importance and relevance of their therapy. Even though they are able to appreciate these points, it may still be difficult to motivate them to do their exercises as extra pressures come to bear, such as homework and social life. There are other factors involved as these children move into adolescence. They are finding their own identities and becoming more independent, while at the same time trying to come to terms with implications of having a chronic orthopaedic condition. This can lead to feelings of anxiety, guilt, anger or depression, as well as to a realisation of being different from their peers.

In the young child, external enforcers may be useful as incentives to encourage cooperation with the treatment programme. These could include star charts, prizes or certificates of bravery as appropriate (Hartley 1993). This should be done in conjunction with explanations suitable to the child's level of understanding, and support for the parents.

Adolescents tend to become less compliant if parents try to use reasoning, threats or persuasion to gain cooperation with the therapy programme. As restrictions on social activity increase, so compliance decreases. Teenagers are thought to respond best to negotiation, and written contracts can sometimes be helpful. It has been found that compliant adolescents have a greater sense of autonomy and self-esteem than those who are non-compliant (Litt et al 1982).

The physiotherapist should give support to the parents in these situations whenever it is possible or appropriate.

SPECIFIC ORTHOPAEDIC PROBLEMS

Fractures

As with adults, fractures in children can be due to a wide range of causes. Think back to the chapter on fractures and answer the following SAQ:

> **Self-assessment question**
>
> ■ **SAQ 9.8.** Review the causes of fracture.

A common type of fracture in children is known as greenstick (although not all fractures in children are of this type). Due to the bones being less brittle than those of an adult, they tend to buckle rather than break. The buckling occurs on the side of the bone opposite to the force and the periosteum can tear on the same side (Fig. 9.1).

Other soft tissue damage is usually minimal, and reduction of the fracture is helped by the absence of displacement and the tissue which remains intact. The periosteum on the buckled side is undamaged and very springy. Because of this, a recurrence in the angulation could occur if fixation is not applied carefully. As long as immobilisation is satisfactory, healing is very rapid (Dandy 1993, McRae 1994).

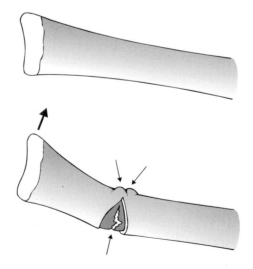

Figure 9.1 A greenstick fracture. (Reproduced with permission from McRae 1994.)

More severe violence can cause a total break in the bone, and this can have more serious consequences if it occurs through an epiphysis.

Self-assessment question

■ **SAQ 9.9.** What could the implications of an epiphyseal fracture be?

Epiphyseal separation can occur due to trauma in childhood, as a result of birth injury, secondary to a joint infection or diseases such as rickets. Endocrine disturbance is thought to be an important factor in the slipping of the upper femoral epiphysis, and here avascular necrosis is quite common if forced reduction is attempted after a delayed diagnosis. Other types of trauma may result in part of an epiphysis being damaged. If diagnosis and reduction are rapid, prognosis is usually good. Failure of reduction or a delay in diagnosis could cause growth disturbance in part or all of the epiphysis, which could result in either an overall reduction in the length of a bone and/or an angulation deformity. The magnitude of these problems depends on the age of the child and on which epiphysis is damaged (McRae 1994).

If the shaft of a long bone is fractured, the rate of healing is much faster than in an adult. For example, if a 3-year-old child sustains a fractured femur, union will occur in approximately 4 weeks. The same injury in an 8-year-old will unite at around 9 weeks and so on. Remodelling of bone in children is excellent and can correct moderate shortening and angulation. In fact, bone growth in the affected limb is greater than on the other side which helps in this process. Internal fixation is used occasionally but only when it is difficult to control angulation and/or rotation at the fracture site (Dandy 1993, McRae 1994).

Self-assessment question

■ **SAQ 9.10.** Review the complications that might adversely affect the rate at which a fracture heals.

Given the speed with which fractures heal in children, the physiotherapist will probably have limited input. This may involve discussions with the parents and child regarding exercise, and the safe use of walking aids as appropriate. Hydrotherapy may be indicated particularly if the child is non-weight-bearing for some time.

Congenital dislocation of the hip (CDH)

The term CDH is very well established, but would in fact be more correct if the condition were known as infantile dislocation or displacement, as very few babies actually have dislocated hips at birth (Robb 1993, Stoker 1985). However, the hips can be subluxed or dislocated manually. Some are extremely unstable, and can dislocate in the first few weeks after birth (McRae 1990). This is a serious condition particularly if it is not diagnosed and treated within the first week of life (Dandy 1993). The routine screening after birth should pick the laxity up, but if it is missed, it can lead to abnormal development of the hip and possibly early osteoarthrosis (Mollan 1985, Stoker 1985). It is important that the tests used (Ortolani, described in detail by Mollan 1985, and the Barlow tests) are repeated, as not all babies with lax hips at birth have CDH; this may be a transient phase from which they recover spontaneously.

Even though routine screening is carried out, some cases of CDH are missed, or occasionally the head of the femur can slip out of the acetabulum slowly over the first year of life. The problems may only become apparent when the child starts to walk and an abnormal gait is noted. There may also be asymmetrical abduction, with range of motion being reduced on the affected side due to shortening in the adductors and iliopsoas. It has remained undiagnosed up to the age of 3 years in some children (Dandy 1993, Mollan 1985, Robb 1993).

CDH occurs in approximately 1.5 per 1000 live births, the incidence varying in different races, and it is more common in girls. There does seem to be some genetic predisposition as the incidence is higher if a relative is affected (Dandy 1993, McRae 1990, Mollan 1985).

In CDH, laxity is found in the structures surrounding the hip joint. In some cases there may be primary maldevelopment of the acetabulum which allows the head of the femur to slip out. This is an inherited defect and can be associated with conditions such as spina bifida or cerebral palsy. Conversely, there may be a normal acetabulum and head of femur with anteversion of the neck of femur. In an undiagnosed CDH, the abnormal relationship of the head of the femur to the acetabulum can cause secondary dysplasia. Soft tissue such as the capsule and labrum will also be affected (Robb 1993).

Although it is hoped that CDH would be noted at an early age by the screening processes, it is useful if the physiotherapist is aware of the signs that may indicate the condition at a later stage. These are as follows (Dandy 1993):

- shortening of the affected limb
- foot laterally rotated
- asymmetrical skin creases
- positive Trendelenburg sign
- unequal hip abduction.

Management

Treatment is easiest and most effective when started early. This consists of a harness or splint which holds the hips in abduction and flexion. An example of this can be seen in Figure 9.2

which illustrates the Cambridge splint. The Pavlik harness is another type of splintage.

These should not be too rigid to allow movement but should limit extension and adduction. They should not put the hips into more than 60° of abduction as this could cause avascular necrosis of the femoral head. The splintage normally remains on for approximately 12 weeks. Once reduction is satisfactory, the child is free of splintage but observed until walking begins. (Blaney 1985, Dandy 1993, McRae 1990, Robb 1993).

If diagnosis is later (2–12 months), the treatment is more radical and may include manipulation of the femoral head into the acetabulum, a period of traction and immobilisation in plaster. Once in the plaster, the child would probably be managed at home. It is possible that reduction is still not satisfactory, in which case surgery may be necessary.

Case study 9.1

Sophie
Sophie is a 2-year-old girl who had been diagnosed with left CDH at 6 months. After initial conservative treatment of 6 weeks of immobilisation in plaster (managed at home), followed by a Cambridge splint, reduction had

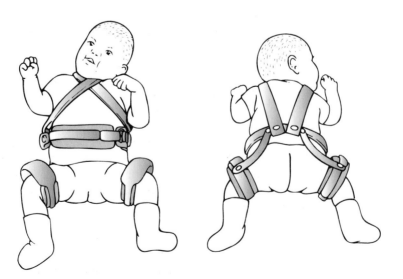

Figure 9.2 The Cambridge splint. (Reproduced with permission from Dandy 1993.)

been felt to be satisfactory. But when she was 2 years old the orthopaedic surgeon decided that development of the left hip was not sufficient and that an upper femoral osteotomy was necessary. Sophie returned from theatre in a hip spica which slightly flexed and abducted her hips, and laterally rotated the left hip. There was a V-shaped hole cut in the spica to allow for toiletting. Once stable she was to be sent home in the spica for 6 weeks.

Problem-solving exercise 9.1

- ■ After you have done this exercise, compare your ideas with those in the following section.

- ■ Think through the issues that Sophie's parents may have to deal with when they take her home, and come up with any advice you feel the health care team could give to help them manage.

Approach to problem-solving exercise 9.1

The following discussion is based on Blaney (1985).

Sophie is 2 years old and is in a hip spica for 6 weeks due to unresolved CDH. There are a number of issues that her parents will have to deal with at home which the physiotherapist may be able to help with.

Care of the plaster

If Sophie is not yet toilet-trained, it is essential to change her nappies frequently and to place them carefully to minimise soiling of the plaster. It may be necessary to use other products such as nappy rolls or incontinence pads. Pieces of plastic sheeting could be tucked around the edges of the plaster in an attempt to keep it as dry as possible. She would probably sleep in prone and so pads and towels would need to be placed on the cot/bed to soak up any leakage.

Skin condition

This needs to be considered carefully, and a watch kept for any rubbing or sore areas. It is important to keep the edges of the plaster smooth, and to keep the skin under the plaster as dry as possible. Any accessible skin should be washed, preferably a number of times during the day. A cool hair dryer could be used to dry the skin rather than towels or tissue paper, thus avoiding friction. Sophie would need to be moved frequently to avoid pressure areas.

Sitting

This may be quite difficult. She may be able to sit on someone's lap for a short time but this would probably not be comfortable. A large bean bag might be very useful for Sophie to recline on. She would be able to play with her toys or watch television. If a table with a sloping top and non-slip surface can be obtained or made, it can be placed over her whilst she is on the bean bag so allowing independence in eating and drinking.

Lying

This is possible in supine as long as her head is supported. In prone a foam wedge can be used to support her. It is important to ensure that her toes do not rub on the ground or the wedge. The foam must be of an appropriate height to allow her to carry out activities.

Moving around

She may be able to move around independently on a 'tummy trolley'. This is a shaped, padded board, on castors. She would push herself using hands and arms.

Carrying Sophie will be awkward and her parents may need to be inventive in order to be able to transport her in a car.

In order to take her out, there are some trolleys available which are similar to large pushchairs. It may be possible to borrow one of these from a local organisation. It would be very useful for Sophie's parents if the physiotherapist had this kind of information available.

Sleeping

Prone is probably most comfortable particularly if this is Sophie's habitual sleeping position. Support from pillows will be needed to fit the shape of the plaster and to keep her in position overnight.

Perthes' disease

This is a condition where the child will present with an 'irritable hip' which may be difficult to distinguish from transient synovitis in the early stages (or tuberculosis, but this is very rare in Britain). It may be classified as an osteochondritis or osteonecrosis. Initially the main symptoms are a limp, decreased range of movement (particularly abduction and medial rotation) and sometimes pain in the joint. There may also be pain in the thighs or knees. The cause is unknown, it is more common in boys than girls and occurs in children between the ages of 4 and 10 years.

There is a disturbance of the blood supply to the epiphysis of the femoral head, causing avascular necrosis. If a large portion of the epiphysis is affected, it can cause flattening of the femoral head. There may also be changes in the acetabulum. Radiographic changes may be well established before the child complains of any pain. It is a self-limiting condition in which the femoral head will heal, but there is usually residual deformity (Evans & Draycott 1984).

Management

Management is variable, but if there is pain it usually involves bed rest with skin traction. The aim is to contain the femoral head within the acetabulum whilst it re-forms. For those cases where more than half of the femoral head is affected, an osteotomy may be carried out or some sort of immobilisation may be considered (for example a brace or plaster cast) (Dandy 1993, McRae 1990, Robb 1993).

Problem-solving exercise 9.2

■ How might the physiotherapist be involved (remembering that treatment could be long-term) if a child is: a. on bedrest, or b. put into a plaster cast to hold the hip in position?

Slipped femoral epiphysis

This is yet another condition affecting the hip joint, but in this case, occurring in adolescence.

As with Perthes', it is more common in boys and due to their delayed growth spurt, it occurs about 2 years later than in girls. It presents most commonly around the age of 11 or 12, but can be found in individuals up to the age of 17.

The specific cause is unknown, but there is sometimes preceding trauma, there seems to be a hormonal factor involved in a high proportion of cases, and also a familial link (Evans & Draycott 1984, McRae 1990).

A separation occurs at the bone–cartilage interface in the upper femoral epiphysis which is thought to be structurally weaker during the adolescent growth spurt. There is also some atrophy of the periosteum which is an important stabiliser in this area. As the head of the femur is held into the acetabulum, the neck of the femur rotates externally and slides upwards, so that on X-ray the appearance is of the femoral head apparently sliding downwards.

Presentation varies from acute (after an injury), where pain is severe and weight bearing impossible, to chronic where there may be a limp, loss of range of abduction/medial rotation and some aching in the hip coming on over a number of weeks. There may also be shortening of the leg. Once identified, the other hip should also be examined and kept under regular surveillance.

Management

Weight bearing is not allowed and the child may be admitted to hospital for a period of bed rest and skin traction. This would only be used temporarily to relieve spasm and pain. If the slip is acute, a manipulation may be attempted but this could cause avascular necrosis and so is not always considered to be an option. The main aim is to stabilise the head of the femur in whatever position it is in, and to maintain range of motion. The stabilisation is achieved surgically by internal fixation, using pins which pass across the epiphysis. Figure 9.3 shows the displaced femoral epiphysis and the appearance of the surgical fixation of the epiphysis.

The main role of the physiotherapist here is to encourage movement postoperatively, starting with active assisted exercise, and progressing as appropriate. The child will be non-weight-bearing for a period of weeks and so help will be

A

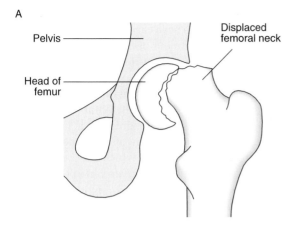

Pelvis

Head of femur

Displaced femoral neck

B

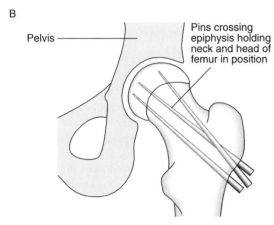

Pelvis

Pins crossing epiphysis holding neck and head of femur in position

Figure 9.3 A Displaced femoral epiphysis; **B** surgical fixation of a slipped femoral epiphysis.

required with gait and walking aids. Hydrotherapy is also useful at this stage as many exercises can easily be carried out in a non-weight-bearing position. The most important aspect will inevitably be in the education of the patient and his or her parents regarding exercise, functional activities and gait. Whilst the child is in hospital, the physiotherapist is also in a good position to observe the opposite hip for any sign of symptoms, particularly as more stress may be put on the 'unaffected' joint during the non-weight-bearing phase.

Congenital talipes equinovarus

This is the commonest of the major congenital abnormalities to affect the foot in children. All newborn babies should be examined to exclude it. The deformity is quite complex with a varus position of the heel and adduction, inversion and plantar flexion of the forefoot. Accompanying this, there is shortening of soft tissue structures on the posterior and medial aspects of the ankle, and muscle wasting.

Management

It is not possible to return the foot and ankle to normal with treatment. Corrective passive stretching and splinting, however, should be begun as soon as possible, in order to prevent bony deformity and to keep the foot plantigrade. The physiotherapist may be responsible for this part of management. The foot is progressively stretched and then strapped in an overcorrected position using adhesive tape and felt (Fig. 9.4).

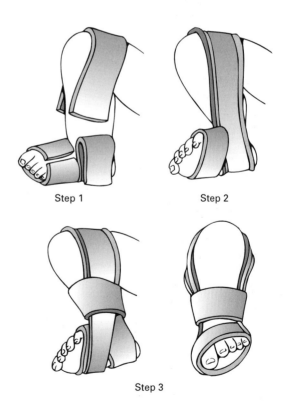

Step 1   Step 2

Step 3

Figure 9.4 Strapping for congenital talipes equinovarus. (Reproduced with permission from Eckersley 1993.)

The strapping remains in place for approximately 6 weeks with periodic removal for more stretching. If it is not successful, surgery may be considered which would involve release of tight soft tissue. If the results of this are not satisfactory, then bony operations such as osteotomy or arthrodesis (usually a triple arthrodesis if the position is still unsatisfactory after growth is complete) may be necessary.

Self-assessment question

- **SAQ 9.11.** List the signs that you would look for if a child was suspected to have late-diagnosed CDH.

Arthrogryposis multiplex congenita

This is another condition that may be seen in children who are in contact with the physiotherapist. It is fairly rare (1 in 3000 live births). Another, clearer term which can be used to describe it is multiple congenital contractures. It is characterised by the replacement of skeletal muscle with fibrous tissue. The soft tissues are contracted, with the joint capsule and periarticular structures being thickened (Dandy 1993, Robb 1993).

The clinical features include rigid joints (for example the elbows fixed in extension and the wrists in flexion), and deformities which tend to be symmetrical, such as talipes, medial rotation in the shoulders and fixed flexion at the knees. Some joints are dislocated, particularly the hips. Muscle groups may be totally absent, and many of those that are present, are atrophied. There is a general reduction in subcutaneous tissue. If there is atrophy in the respiratory muscles, there may be some respiratory insufficiency which can be life-threatening. This condition has no effect on intelligence or cutaneous sensation.

Management

The most immediate management for these children is surgery involving soft tissue release and osteotomy, performed in an attempt to bring the limbs into their most functional positions. The soft tissue release needs to be followed up with firm support using orthoses, otherwise there

may be recurrence of the contractures. Stretching and splinting has been carried out by physiotherapists in the treatment of these children, but the effect seems to be transitory and contractures return. The physiotherapist will be most involved postoperatively as a member of the health care team in the rehabilitation phase. A very useful type of treatment here is hydrotherapy as it allows freedom of movement and a measure of independence which may be impossible on dry land. This could also enable the child to be water-confident and to swim as a recreational activity which is something that the rest of the family can be involved in.

Osteogenesis imperfecta (the brittle bone syndrome)

This is a rare disease found in approximately 1 in 20 000 live births (Robb 1993). The cause is unknown and the incidence sporadic, but it is an inherited disorder of varying severity (Catto 1985). The most obvious feature is osteoporosis which means that the bones are more fragile and liable to fracture. The defect lies in the synthesis of Type I collagen, and this means that connective tissue throughout the body may be affected, not just the bones. Examples of this are blue sclerae, laxity of ligaments, abnormal teeth, thin skin, thin aortic valves and early onset deafness (Catto 1985, Dandy 1993).

Four types are identified as follows.

Type I (autosomal dominant). This makes up the majority of cases (approximately 80%). These patients have mild bone disease and so stature is normal. Although there is still an increased incidence of fracture, they do not develop severe deformities or become dwarfed. They may show more of the extraskeletal abnormalities such as deafness and the blue sclerae.

Type II (probably autosomal recessive). In general this is a lethal form of the syndrome. Multiple fractures occur in utero. At birth there are gross deformities in the limbs. The most severely affected children die due to intracranial haemorrhage resulting from the poor protection offered by the largely unossified skull, and/or from respiratory failure due to many rib fractures.

Type III (due to sporadic mutation or autosomal recessive). This is less severe than type II. Fractures may be present at birth and progressive deformity occurs. Stature is small and a kyphoscoliosis can often develop. These patients are usually unable to walk.

Type IV (rare, autosomal dominant). This has a similar presentation to type III. The children are severely affected with small stature and fragile bones (Catto 1985, Dandy 1993, Robb 1993).

Although this classification is not ideal, it can be helpful in genetic counselling.

The shafts of the long bones are shorter than normal and very slender. The cortex is thin and the epiphyses appear broad. The bones are more plastic than normal and this, plus the multiple fractures, tends to cause bowing. Compression fractures can occur in the vertebrae giving them a wedged or biconcave appearance (Catto 1985, Dandy 1993).

Management

Fractures heal well, although sometimes more callus is formed than usual. In mild cases, repeated fractures can cause deformity for which stabilisation with intramedullary rods may be necessary. This is more usual in the lower limbs. Management needs to be careful as immobilisation can increase the amount of osteoporosis and so the liability to further fractures. Severely affected children often use wheelchairs for mobility (Robb 1993).

The physiotherapist may be involved with the health care team dealing with these children postoperatively. If any passive or active assisted movements are performed, it is essential to remember that joints will be hypermobile due to the laxity of soft tissues. Again, hydrotherapy is an ideal medium for these children as long as they are happy in water. Gentle, finely graded exercises can be performed. The effect of gravity is counterbalanced by the buoyancy and so weight bearing is not an issue. The environment is relaxed and treatment is fun.

The physiotherapist may also be involved in provision of seating and wheelchairs for these children. This should involve a multidisciplinary approach. Careful assessment will be necessary, taking into consideration the wide range of areas of the patient's life where the seating will be used. Correct positioning is essential, but especially so if the child has any trunk involvement. This relates to the optimal posture (or postures) for the child, and the support required from different elements of the seating to provide this (Bardsley & Jones 1993). Once the assessment has been carried out, the most suitable seating can be devised. It is advisable to have a 'fitting' stage which allows for adjustments to be made. It is imperative that regular review of the seating takes place as alterations will need to be made for growth and / or any progressive deformity.

Achondroplasia

This condition is due to a failure of endochondral ossification. All bones ossified from cartilage are small, whilst intramembranous ossification occurs normally. The condition is present when the child is born and can actually be diagnosed in utero, by the use of X-rays.

The person with achondroplasia has the following typical features (Catto 1985, Trivella et al 1991):

- prominent forehead
- reduced nasal bridge, root of the nose drawn in
- short limbs in proportion to the trunk
- often a varus deformity present at the knees, giving a curved appearance to the lower limbs
- increased lumbar lordosis
- skin folds due to the soft tissues growing more than the bones
- broad hands with fingers of equal length
- height rarely exceeding 140 centimetres.

Apart from the shortened limbs, the pedicles of the vertebrae are shorter than in the normal vertebral column. This can lead to stenosis and some neurological problems (Dandy 1993).

Management

Many children with this condition do not have any medical intervention. However, the physiotherapist is most likely to encounter them when they have surgery for leg lengthening.

Leg lengthening

This procedure is available to two categories of patient:

1. Those with 'disproportionate small stature' resulting from conditions such as achondroplasia. This would be bilateral surgery carried out for both function and cosmesis.
2. Children with a discrepancy in the length of the legs resulting from a variety of conditions. The procedure here is to produce or regain symmetry (Burton 1991).

The surgical techniques used to perform the lengthening are either 'chondrodiatasis' which involves distraction of the epiphyseal plate, or 'callotasis' which is lengthening through the healing callus of an osteotomy (Trivella et al 1991). During the operation an external fixator or lengthener is applied to the appropriate bone via screws proximal and distal to the segment to be lengthened. If callotasis is the method, distraction does not begin until the seventh postoperative day as the callus forms (in older patients this time may be longer). The rate of lengthening is approximately 1 mm per day carried out in four increments of 0.25 mm (Burton 1991).

In bilateral lengthening, fixators may be placed in the following ways:

- on both femora at the same time
- the femur and the tibia of the same leg
- the tibia of one leg and the femur of the other
- on both tibiae at the same time.

Leg lengthening takes a long time and is complicated. This is even more so if the process is bilateral. Postoperatively, much of the lengthening procedure takes place at home and the parents take a large amount of responsibility. This can cause problems as discussed earlier in the chapter, and members of the health care team need to be aware, and available for support if necessary. Self-help groups may be set up if enough parents are interested and have the time and opportunity to take it forward: it may be something that could be suggested.

Problem-solving exercise 9.3

- Read the following section and try to formulate a list of physiotherapy aims/objectives for each stage of treatment following a leg-lengthening procedure.

Leg-lengthening procedure

This section is based on a paper by Burton (1991); for more detail please refer to the original paper.

The physiotherapist will be involved during the preoperative assessment period, and then postoperatively, there are a number of interventions for which he or she will be responsible.

For the first few days, the limb(s) may be placed on a continuous passive movement machine to maintain range in the knee(s). Active or active assisted exercises should be taught for circulation and to maintain muscle length.

Those undergoing bilateral or femoral lengthening often use a wheelchair, whilst those with a unilateral fixator are allowed to get up, partially weight bearing.

Stage 1
Lengthening begins after a number of days. This will put tension on the soft tissues and so range of movement in the joints may reduce during the lengthening period.

Stage 2
After the desired length has been achieved (remember much of this process has taken place at home with some outpatient attendance), the fixator is locked for a period of 'neutralisation'. Soft tissue is at maximum stretch at this point but the tension does reduce once lengthening is stopped. Callus begins to form.

Stage 3
The third stage is known as 'dynamisation'. Here the fixator is unlocked to allow compression forces along the length of the bone(s). This helps to strengthen the structure of the bone. Partial weight bearing is gradually increased to full as the child's confidence increases.

Stage 4

Once the fixator is removed, some extra support may be necessary such as a cast brace or a hip spica. In this case the patient is treated similarly to those with fractures. Once the support is removed, intensive rehabilitation begins.

After you have formulated your own list of physiotherapy aims, read the following section.

Physiotherapy objectives during a leg-lengthening procedure

This answer to problem-solving exercise 9.3 is based on Burton (1991).

Answer:

Physiotherapy aims during leg lengthening:
- maintain joint ranges
- maintain muscle power
- encourage independence in locomotion, either weight-bearing or in a wheelchair
- monitor posture.

Physiotherapy aims during neutralisation:
- increase joint range
- increase muscle power
- either increase weight bearing or introduce it in those who have been in a wheelchair
- correct/maintain posture as necessary.

The physiotherapist's aims during dynamisation are the same as for the neutralisation phase.

Aims of physiotherapy in the rehabilitation phase:
- restore joint range to preoperative levels
- regain maximal muscle power in affected muscles
- to assess and restore proprioception in the lower limb as necessary
- to re-establish balance reactions as necessary
- re-education of gait
- maintain/regain good posture.

Scoliosis

Scoliosis is an excessive lateral spinal deformity. It has a higher incidence in adolescence and often has no known origin, and so is known as adolescent idiopathic scoliosis (AIS) (Coutts 1992). But it can also occur idiopathically in infants (infantile) and in children after the age of 3 years and before puberty (juvenile) (Robb 1993). Scoliosis of the structural type may also occur for more specific reasons, listed below (Coutts 1992):

- neuromuscular, as a result of neuromuscular diseases such as cerebral palsy or poliomyelitis
- congenital, secondary to malformation of the vertebral elements of the spine
- trauma, such as fracture
- disease processes, infection or rickets for example
- tumours, causing direct damage to the spinal structure.

Scoliosis is also classified by the direction, magnitude and location of the abnormal curves. These curves can present as single or double, either being two major curves or a single major curve with a smaller compensatory curve. They can occur in different regions of the spine. In AIS, the abnormal curves tend to be in the thoracic, lumbar or thoracolumbar regions.

Idiopathic scoliosis is the most common diagnosis (approximately 70%). AIS presents around the time of puberty and before maturity. It is commoner in girls, and the female to male ratio increases with the size of the curve (Coutts 1992, Dandy 1993). Approximately 2–3% of the population have a scoliosis of 10° or more, but this drops to 0.2–0.3% for curves of 30° or more. Progression of the curves can continue after skeletal maturity (Coutts 1992).

As well as the bones and joints of the spine, the curves will also affect the thorax, the pelvis, associated muscles, other soft tissues and internal organs. Posture is affected with a decrease in the volume of the thorax and a reduced respiratory capacity. The first indications are changes in the contour of the trunk such as a rib hump posteriorly and asymmetry in the levels of shoulders and/or pelvis (Robb 1993). Figure 9.5 shows the appearance of scoliosis.

Management

The management of scoliosis is aimed at decreas-

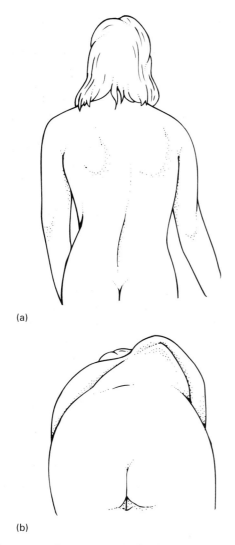

(a)

(b)

Figure 9.5 The appearance of scoliosis: (a) in standing, and (b) in forward bending where the rib hump becomes more prominent. (Reproduced with permission from Dandy 1993.)

ing or stabilising progression of the curvature, and may involve conservative or surgical methods. At early ages and at less than a 25–30° curve, the general consensus seems to be a 'watch and wait' policy, but review needs to be regular in order to check on progression. Exercise, postural correction and electrical stimulation are all used as treatment methods. There seem, however, to be differences in opinion as to whether or not

these have any effect on progression of the curvature.

Corrective casts are said to stop progression in infantile scoliosis if applied early enough (Dandy 1993). Bracing can be used and the aim is to halt the curvature rather than to correct it. These orthoses are either active or passive. An active brace has pressure areas applied to specific anatomical points, with relief areas opposite so the patient can pull the spine into the corrected position. Examples of these are the Boston and Milwaukee braces. Passive braces have total body contact and allow no movement, for example, the Wilmington brace. The amount of time a brace needs to be worn is also a point of contention, with some authorities claiming that it should be worn for 23 hours, whilst others claim similar results with the brace being worn for 16 hours. There is an issue of compliance here, and it may be that the brace is not worn for 23 hours especially if the child is at school, and it is a particularly visible orthosis. This type of factor could explain the similarity in results. There is agreement, however, that the braces should be worn until skeletal maturity is reached. Braces are the most common conservative treatment, even though some evidence suggests that they have no effect and are only apparently successful in those patients whose scoliosis would not have progressed anyway (Coutts 1992, Dandy 1993, Robb 1993).

Surgical treatment is used when the curve presents at, or progresses to, 45°. This consists of posterior or anterior fusion using internal fixation of different kinds but usually involving rods, screws and wires. If Harrington rods are used, the patient has to wear a cast or orthosis postoperatively for 3–6 months. If Luque rods or Cotrel-Debousset instrumentation is used, no immobilisation is necessary postoperatively (Coutts 1992). Anterior and posterior methods are sometimes combined (O'Brien & Draycott 1984, Robb 1993).

If the surgery is uneventful, results are usually good. Complications can occur such as broken rods, neurological damage or infections.

Physiotherapy intervention is important in assessment as part of the monitoring process in those curves where a 'watch and wait' policy is being used. There will also be a role with these patients where exercise and active postural correction are undertaken. Pre- and postoperative care and rehabilitation are important when the patient undergoes a surgical procedure.

Problem-solving exercise 9.4

■ What factors would you need to take into account in achieving your aims of treatment with a child undergoing leg lengthening, given that much of the therapy might be performed by the parents?

Juvenile chronic arthritis (JCA)

JCA is defined as an inflammatory arthritis beginning before the 16th birthday. It is fairly uncommon, affecting approximately 1 in 1000 children, but as mentioned earlier in the chapter, makes up 30–50% of all new cases referred to specialist paediatric rheumatology clinics (Leak 1991, Robb 1993).

There is no known cause, but there seems to be some relationship to viral infections such as rubella or mumps. There may also be some genetic predisposition; in fact, this is a similar mechanism to the aetiology of arthritis in adults. In order for a rheumatic condition in a child to be classified as JCA, there has to be the presence of at least two of pain, swelling or limitation of movement, in at least one joint, for at least 3 months, in a child under 16 years. However these criteria are extremely general and not of particular use in diagnosis.

There are three possible types of onset:

- systemic
- polyarticular
- pauciarticular.

The ages and patterns of onset are summarised in Table 9.6 (Leak 1991). Most children do fit in to one of these categories at onset, and the patterns are well recognised. However, later on the distinction may become less clear.

Systemic
This accounts for approximately 10–20% of affected children (Robb 1993).

Table 9.6 Typical clinical features of subgroups of juvenile chronic arthritis. (Adapted with permission from Leak 1991.)

	Age of onset, years		
	0–5	6–10	11–16
Pauciarticular	F >> M Knees, ankles, wrists especially Often ANA positive* Chronic uveitis	←——— F = M Overlap ———→ either way	M >> F Lower limb arthritis. Enthesitis Acute uveitis, ± later sacroiliitis
Polyarticular	F > M Small and large joints Flexor tenosynovitis (spares metacarpophalangeal joints)	F > M Similar to under 5 years	F >> M Symmetrical Often RhF positive† with erosive arthritis
Systemic onset		All age groups	
	Fever, rash Variable arthritis Acute phase response ++		M = F Auto AB negative

M, male; F, female
* ANA positive: antinuclear antibodies found on immunological assay
† RhF: rheumatoid factor found in the blood, detected by latex haemagglutination

As well as the fever and rash mentioned in Table 9.6 those children with systemic onset may also present with lymphadenopathy, hepatomegaly, splenomegaly, pericarditis and other general symptoms of inflammation, with little or no joint manifestation. But in order for a definite diagnosis to be made, they do have to exhibit the required signs of arthritis eventually. The systemic features are often in evidence for some time before joints are affected (Barnes 1988, Leak 1991).

While 50% recover almost completely, the rest will go on to develop polyarticular symptoms with the resulting disability. These children are in most danger of life-threatening complications and general growth problems (Barnes 1988).

Polyarticular

Here, five or more joints are affected in the first 3 months. About 50% of all children with chronic arthritis have this presentation. There may be some systemic symptoms, but not as severe as in the previous case. The most commonly affected joints are the knees, wrists and ankles (Barnes 1988, Robb 1993). There may also be involvement of the small joints of hands and feet, plus shoulder, hip and temporomandibular joints (Leak 1991).

Morning stiffness is common. There may be problems with bone growth due to the epiphyses maturing early (Barnes 1988).

Pauciarticular

This accounts for approximately 30–40% of cases. Here, four or fewer joints are affected in the first 3 months. Of these children, 25% will go on to develop polyarticular JCA. It most commonly affects the knee, wrist, hip, elbow or ankles. If only one joint is affected, it is likely to be the knee (75% of cases). Systemic symptoms are rare and the disease seems almost to be ignored by some children.

Uveitis is uncommon and completely asymptomatic in the early stages. A child with pauciarticular onset is most likely to develop this eye problem and so should be screened regularly, as it can lead to visual loss if undiscovered, and total blindness in the worst case scenario (Barnes 1988, Leak 1991, Robb 1993).

Prognosis

The majority of children go into permanent remission and have no serious disability. Probably 70% are in remission 10 years after onset. Mild disability persists in approximately 45% of those assessed after the age of 18 years. The overall prognosis, therefore, is considered to be good, but 10–30%, however, do have severe residual problems, the worst functional outcome being in those with major involvement of the hip.

With this fairly optimistic outlook for children with JCA, prevention of joint deformity during active disease phases becomes a high priority (Barnes 1988, Leak 1991).

Case study 9.2

Rosie

Rosie is 2 years old. Her mum and dad became concerned when she was reluctant to use her hands when playing, she had also started to limp and was rather reluctant to walk. In the previous few weeks they had noticed a rash appearing on her back, tummy, thighs and upper arms which seemed to come and go with no particular pattern. She had also had a spiking fever in the late afternoon for a few days, which then returned to normal. At these times she seemed rather poorly but then was fine for the rest of the day, and during the night.

Sometimes she was unusually tired later in the day, and her movements appeared to be stiff when she first got up in the morning.

On examination by her GP, Rosie was found to have some swelling in the metacarpophalangeal joints of both hands, both wrists and both knees. Although there was no apparent tenderness or pain, the range of movement was decreased.

A tentative diagnosis of polyarticular JCA was made. This was confirmed on a visit to the rheumatology clinic. The decision was made to admit Rosie to the rheumatology ward for a short period for thorough assessment, and to begin drug treatment. She was prescribed a non-steroidal anti-inflammatory drug (NSAID).

Problem-solving exercise 9.5

■ **A.** Which members of the health care team would be involved in Rosie's management?

■ **B.** You are Rosie's physiotherapist and are going to see her for the first time. After obtaining subjective information from the notes and from talking to her parents, what areas would you include in your objective assessment?

■ **C.** What useful information do you think any professional member of the health care team should be able to ascertain from observing Rosie with her parents?

After you have tried to answer this exercise for yourself read the following section for the approach to parts **B** and **C**.

Assessment and observation of Rosie and her parents

Objective assessment
The points made earlier in this chapter in the section on assessment should be carefully considered here, particularly as Rosie is so young.

Observation. Rosie should be undressed sufficiently to allow you to clearly observe the affected and unaffected areas. Swelling may be quite obvious in the hands, wrists and knees. You should also look at her movements and general activities, as they may give you more information about limitations due to pain and stiffness than some specific tests.

Palpation. You may use gentle palpation to test for any tenderness around the joints. Pain is rarely complained of, but this may be due to the natural tendency of young children to complain less of pain than adults. They also seem to find it difficult to localise pain to a specific area. Some of her joints may feel warmer than normal.

Movements. You may be able to perform passive range of movement if Rosie is willing, but active movements may need to be observed when she is playing or moving around. It may be very difficult to use a goniometer to measure range of movement unless Rosie is particularly tractable. With knee involvement, it is important for you to consider leg length, as there may be flexion deformities. Her hands may show reduction in flexion and radial deviation at the metacarpophalangeal joints. You might also find some ulnar deviation at the wrists. As Rosie is only a short time from onset, there may not have been time for these deformities to occur. It would still be important for you to note the range and position of these joints to give you a baseline against which to monitor progress.

Muscle testing. It will probably be impossible for you to do specific muscle tests with a child as young as Rosie. So again, functional activities can be used to estimate these (look back to Table 9.5). It is an important area to look at as muscle atrophy occurs quickly in children with JCA.

Functional activities. These may involve going up and down stairs, getting up from the floor and walking on tip toe, as well as dressing and play activities.

Observation of Rosie and her parents
Observation is an important skill for any health professional. It is important to watch Rosie and her parents as they come into the room. From facial expression and movement, it may be possible to get an idea of how Rosie is feeling. Is she being allowed to walk in or is one of her parents carrying her? Do they allow her to take her own clothes off or insist on doing it for her?

If Rosie's parents are being extremely protective, it may make it more difficult for you to carry out an assessment. This may change, however, when you have had the opportunity to explain what the assessment is all about. Watching Rosie with her parents may also give you some idea as to how they might manage the home programme.

If both parents are present, you may also get some feeling about who is going to take on the responsibility for Rosie's treatment. Will it be an equal partnership or is one parent much more dominant?

These and other similar issues are extremely important for the physiotherapist to consider. They may enable you to modify your approach in order to facilitate a successful implementation of the treatment programme.

Self-assessment question

■ **SAQ 9.12.** Using the information already given in this and earlier chapters, plus your own experience, list the aims of physiotherapy for Rosie.

Management

The main aim of management in JCA is to control the inflammatory process; this is essential if deformity and loss of function are to be avoided. It is generally accepted that the care of children with this condition should have a multidisciplinary approach, and the team must be experienced in the field. Ideally a rheumatologist and a paediatrician should be involved plus a physiotherapist, occupational therapist, ophthalmologist, social worker, nurse, orthotist and orthopaedic surgeon as necessary or appropriate. It is also essential to remember that the child and the parents must be part of this team approach, and should be consulted and included in discussions when decisions are made.

As discussed earlier in the chapter, the team must have a background knowledge of child development in order to be able to produce an appropriate, age-related plan of management.

Drug therapy

The majority of children with JCA benefit from the use of NSAIDs. It is now more common for non-aspirin NSAIDs to be used as they are easier to administer and some are approved specifically for use with children. Unfortunately they can take a long time to have their maximal effect: 2 weeks to 3 months. They are well tolerated, but all of the usual side-effects have been observed (Leak 1991).

The use of disease-modifying antirheumatic drugs is rather more contentious. They all tend to have serious side-effects, and so with the fairly frequent incidence of natural remission in JCA, they may be avoided if possible. If they are prescribed they need to be carefully monitored by the rheumatology clinic.

Corticosteroids may be used as intra-articular injections in the case of persistent active arthritis. In small children this is usually performed under a light general anaesthetic and the joint may need to be rested in a splint for 24–48 hours afterwards (Leak 1991).

Systemic steroids are used sometimes, but tend to be avoided because of the side-effects such as osteoporosis, water retention and growth retardation. If their use is deemed to be unavoidable (that is usually in extremely severe or life-threatening JCA), then the dose should be tapered down at the earliest opportunity (Barnes 1988).

Physiotherapy

The central aims of physiotherapy are to prevent deformity and to maximise function. (These should be the aims of the whole health care team once the inflammation is being reduced by the drug therapy.) The overall philosophy should be to encourage the parents to assume and maintain responsibility for the child's physiotherapy programme as soon as possible. Care can then be transferred home, with monitoring and updates of advice occurring at regular clinic visits (Hartley 1993).

The overall programme of physiotherapy usually involves providing information to the parents about JCA and its management. Then specific exercises for the affected joints are taught, plus a daily general exercise regime for all joints which needs to be introduced as early as possible. It will involve active exercises and stretching. This has a number of uses, as it:

- maintains/improves mobility
- maintains/improves exercise tolerance
- maintains/improves muscle strength
- monitors joint range and allows early detection of any problems with other joints, or regression in those joints already affected.

A certain amount of activity regulation may be necessary in older children. Younger children often regulate their own activity depending on the state of their disease. However, teenagers may perceive that they need to 'keep up' with their peers and be tempted to do too much, which would exacerbate the condition. Therefore, some external structure may relieve this situation, helping the child to avoid getting overtired and putting too much stress on the joints. Increased levels of rest may be necessary at times, but bedrest is not appropriate. Certain positions and activities may be discouraged in the interest of joint protection such as:

- high-impact activities such as jumping/road running
- use of pillows holding the neck into flexion
- supporting total body weight on non-weight-bearing joints, for example in press ups, cartwheels, chin ups and so on
- activities/positions putting stress across the joints such as skiing, sitting cross-legged.

Hydrotherapy is an ideal form of therapy for children with JCA, as long as they are happy and confident in water. This can lead on to swimming which is a good all-round exercise and is suitable as it does not involve weight bearing or over-stress the joints.

Part of the management of JCA involves wearing splints in many cases. These are provided in order to support and maintain joints in a good position. The most commonly used are either resting splints, usually worn at night, or functional splints which support a joint during activity.

Self-assessment question

■ **SAQ 9.13.** Rosie's physiotherapy management will be supervised at home by mum and dad, and this may involve exercises, splinting and the application of temporary pain-relieving modalities (heat or cold) as necessary. Thinking back over the information given in the chapter, review the areas you might need to discuss with her parents in order to facilitate this process. (Remember: she is only 2 years old.)

An approach to this question is outlined in the following section, but as ever, it is important that you should first try to answer it yourself.

Areas to discuss with Rosie's parents

There are many issues which the physiotherapist should discuss with parents who are about to take on responsibility for the home programme of their child with JCA. The content and direction of the discussion will vary greatly, depending

upon the situation, the resources available, the existing support networks and the personalities involved.

It is vital for the parents to have adequate information. The physiotherapist must ensure that they understand the purpose of any exercises, activities, hands-on techniques and/or splinting they have to carry out. They must also be prepared to perform the treatment daily, on a regular basis.

The main aims of physiotherapy intervention are to prevent muscle weakness and loss in range of movement, so preventing deformity, particularly during the active disease phases.

The programme designed by the physiotherapist must cause the minimum possible disruption to family life and routine. This is where discussion with the parents is essential. It is also important to be aware of any home programmes designed by other members of the health care team. This will avoid unnecessary duplication. In fact, a more preferable team approach would be to formulate a combined programme.

It is well known that compliance with therapeutic home programmes is fairly poor for a number of very valid reasons (see text). If the health professionals involved in the design of the programme try to incorporate the following characteristics, it may help to improve compliance levels. The programme should be:

- as simple as possible
- the most efficient in time and effort
- the least painful
- the least expensive
- designed to achieve individual goals which are relevant, achievable, realistic and developmentally and age-appropriate
- regularly monitored and modified as necessary in discussion with parents and child.

Compliance may also be enhanced if the parents can be shown a simple method of checking range of motion at home.

The physiotherapist could suggest to Rosie's parents that they try to make the programme part of her daily routine. It is extremely important to explain that a number of the exercises (particularly the stretches) will cause some discomfort.

But this does not mean that they are damaging her joints or muscles. It is quite likely that a 2-year-old child like Rosie, will cry during some of the exercises. Her parents should be reassured that this is not a contraindication to treatment. This situation can be very difficult for the parents to accept as they may already feel guilt associated with having a child with a chronic illness. Reassurance by the physiotherapist and any other professionals involved, is therefore of paramount importance (Barnes 1988).

Rosie should be involved in the treatment as much as possible. Strategies such as counting up to 10 for the stretches may help her to feel more in control. As mentioned in the earlier text, sometimes external reinforcers are useful, such as star charts and certificates of bravery.

This section has given you some suggestions with regard to discussion with parents prior to starting a therapeutic home programme. As you gain more experience and discuss options with other physiotherapists who are experts in the field, you will gradually develop a larger background database to use in these situations.

Surgery
This is generally only used in very severe cases of JCA, but would be considered if joint deformity has occurred despite drug and physical therapy. Procedures that may be undertaken include soft tissue release (most commonly of hip or knee), or joint replacement. These are performed more to regain function than to relieve pain.

Summary

This chapter has given you an overview of the issues involved in the treatment of children, including background information on a number of common orthopaedic conditions. It has also briefly highlighted key areas which physiotherapists need to consider when involved in the management of children, such as a knowledge of child development, assessment and the approach that needs to be adopted to intervention, given that parents are closely concerned with treatment.

There are a great many situations where you may come into contact with children. The information you have gained from this chapter should have given you a basis to build on. Inevitably the condition that each child has will be different, and you will need to be aware of any local philosophies and programmes of management that are in place with regard to particular pathology, surgical intervention and so on. It is, however, important for you to remember that you should focus on each patient as an individual. Assess carefully, and discover what the particular problems and issues are (almost irrespective of the 'condition') for that child and his or her family, within the developmental framework discussed earlier.

On reading this summary, do you feel you have grasped the above points? If not, perhaps you should go back and reread any appropriate parts of the chapter before moving on.

ANSWERS TO QUESTIONS AND EXERCISES

Self-assessment questions 9.1–9.3

See information in text.

Self-assessment question 9.4 (page 240)

The information to answer this can be found throughout the book, but particularly in Chapter 3 on assessment.

Self-assessment questions 9.5–9.7

See information in text.

Self-assessment question 9.8 (page 248)

The information can be found in Chapter 5 on fractures.

Self-assessment question 9.9 (page 249)

See information in text.

Self-assessment question 9.10 (page 249)

The information can be found in Chapter 5 on fractures.

Problem-solving exercise 9.1 (page 251)

See the following section in the text.

Problem-solving exercise 9.2 (page 252)

■ How might the physiotherapist be involved (remembering that treatment could be long-term) if a child is: a. on bed rest, or b. put into a plaster cast to hold the hip in position?

Answer:
a. If bedrest is chosen as the non-weight-bearing method of treatment, the child with Perthes' must be taught static and active resisted exercises as appropriate, to avoid muscle wasting. It is important to try to make these as much fun as possible otherwise compliance may be poor.

b. The role of the physiotherapist will be different if the child is put into a plaster cast
or some other form of immobilisation such as a brace. Weight bearing is allowed, and the physiotherapist will be instrumental in helping the child to become independent in walking. The child will go home in the cast and so communication with the parents is essential. Depending on the type of immobilisation used, a child may return periodically to hospital to have it removed to allow joint mobilisation (non-weight-bearing). If this is the chosen regime, then hydrotherapy is an extremely useful treatment modality. After mobilisation, the cast or brace will be reapplied and the child discharged home again. This would be continued until healing is shown to be complete on X-ray.

Self-assessment question 9.11 (page 254)

See information in text.

Problem-solving exercise 9.3 (page 256)

See the section 'Physiotherapy objectives during a leg-lengthening procedure' (p. 257).

Problem-solving exercise 9.4 (page 259)

■ What factors would you need to take into account in achieving your aims of treatment with a child undergoing leg lengthening, given that much of the therapy might be performed by the parents?

Answer: *Many of the issues to be considered by the physiotherapist when treating a child undergoing leg lengthening are similar to those already mentioned elsewhere in the chapter. It is a very protracted procedure and, therefore, it is important that both parents and the child understand this. In some centres a 'cooling off' period is allowed and assessment is carried out over a year to allow all involved to carefully consider the decision being made. This is especially pertinent in the case of lengthening for short stature, which is considered to be non-essential surgery.*
As for children with chronic conditions,

the wearing of one or two external fixators will cause disruption to home life, school and social activities. The actual lengthening process is carried out by the parents, so it is essential that the family unit is secure enough to cope with the daily care and any problems that may occur.

Information is important for the family in order that they understand what the procedure entails. Initial assessment of the patient and the family is carried out by a number of health professionals (such as the surgeon, physiotherapist, social worker and psychologist). If they are found to be suitable then further, more detailed, assessment occurs. They may also be introduced to other families who are undertaking the procedure, to allow time for discussion.

If the child has particular weaknesses in relevant muscle groups before the operation, the physiotherapist may be involved in designing a home programme to rectify this as much as possible.

Before the operation, it is important that expectations for the postoperative period are considered, and any practical arrangements put into place. For example, if the child will be in a wheelchair postoperatively, then factors such as ramps, showers, furniture location and door widths should be considered in the home. Access to school and leisure facilities also needs to be addressed.

Many of the points made in the answer to SAQ 9.13 (p. 263), regarding the characteristics of a successful therapeutic home programme, will apply here when considering the physiotherapy input during the lengthening, neutralisation, dynamisation and rehabilitation periods.

Problem-solving exercise 9.5 (page 261)

For the answer to part **A**, see information in text. For the answers to parts **B** and **C**, see the following section in the text.

Self-assessment question 9.12 (page 262)

See information in text.

Self-assessment question 9.13 (page 263)

See the following section in the text.

REFERENCES

Anderson J R (ed) 1985 Muir's textbook of pathology, 12th edn. Edward Arnold, London

Association of Paediatric Chartered Physiotherapists (APCP) 1995 Standards of practice: paediatric physiotherapy. Chartered Society of Physiotherapy, London

Bardsley D G I, Jones M 1993 Aids and appliances. In: Eckersley P M (ed) Elements of paediatric physiotherapy. Churchill Livingstone, Edinburgh, ch 21

Barnes L W 1988 Physical therapy management of juvenile arthritis. In: Bamwell B F, Gall V (eds) Physical therapy management of arthritis. Churchill Livingstone, Edinburgh, ch 9

Bastow V, Clegg M, Jones M, King L 1993 Common assessment procedures. In: Eckersley P M (ed) Elements of paediatric physiotherapy. Churchill Livingstone, Edinburgh, ch 17

Bedford S 1993 The developing child. In: Eckersley P M (ed) Elements of paediatric physiotherapy. Churchill Livingstone, Edinburgh, ch 4

Blaney A R 1985 Practical problems of managing a child at home in splints and plasters. Physiotherapy 71(9):395–398

Burton M 1991 Regimes of leg lengthening at Sheffield Children's Hospital. Physiotherapy 77(11):727–732

Cameron R 1987 Helping parents to help children. Physiotherapy 73(4):172–175

Catto M E 1985 Locomotor system. In: Anderson J R (ed) Muir's textbook of pathology, 12th edn. Edward Arnold, London, ch 23

Coutts F 1992 Scoliosis and thoracolumbar motion. Unpublished dissertation, University of East London, London

Dandy D J 1993 Essential orthopaedics and trauma, 2nd edn. Churchill Livingstone, Edinburgh

Donnai D, Kerzin-Storrar L, Wigmore P 1993 Genetics and embryology. In: Eckersley P M (ed) Elements of paediatric physiotherapy. Churchill Livingstone, Edinburgh, ch 3

Eckersley P M (ed) 1993 Elements of paediatric physiotherapy. Churchill Livingstone, Edinburgh

Evans G A, Draycott V 1984 Disorders of the hip and inequality of leg length. In: Downie P A (ed) Cash's textbook of orthopaedics and rheumatology for physiotherapists. Faber and Faber, London, ch 8

Govan A D T, Macfarlane P S, Callander R 1996 Pathology illustrated, 3rd edn. Churchill Livingstone, Edinburgh

Griffiths M I 1993 Accidents and child abuse. In: Eckersley P M (ed) Elements of paediatric physiotherapy. Churchill Livingstone, Edinburgh, ch 13

Grimley A M D 1993 A historical perspective. In: Eckersley P M (ed) Elements of paediatric physiotherapy. Churchill Livingstone, Edinburgh, ch 1

Hartley J 1993 A survey to identify problems with home exercises and splint wear in children with juvenile chronic arthritis. Unpublished project, University of East London, London

Hinderer K A, Hinderer S R 1993 Muscle strength development and assessment in children and adolescents. In: Harms-Ringdahl K (ed) Muscle strength. Churchill Livingstone, Edinburgh, ch 7

Homer S, Mackintosh S 1992 Injuries in young female elite gymnasts. Physiotherapy 78(11):804–808

Jones M 1993 Assessment of gait. In: Eckersley P M (ed) Elements of paediatric physiotherapy. Churchill Livingstone, Edinburgh, ch 17

Leak A M 1991 Juvenile chronic arthritis. Topical reviews no. 19 – Reports on Rheumatic Diseases (Series 2). The Arthritis and Rheumatism Council, London

Litt I F, Cuskey W R, Rosenberg B A 1982 Role of self-esteem and autonomy in determining medication compliance among adolescents with juvenile chronic arthritis. Pediatrics 69(1):15–17

Marks L 1985 Parents: how much help? Physiotherapy 71(4):170–172

McRae R 1990 Clinical orthopaedic examination, 3rd edn. Churchill Livingstone, Edinburgh

McRae R 1994 Practical fracture treatment, 3rd edn. Churchill Livingstone, Edinburgh

Mollan R A B 1985 Screening for congenital dislocation of the hip. Physiotherapy 71(12):511–513

Morse J L 1983 Psychosocial aspects of low vision. In: Jose R T (ed) Understanding low vision. American Foundation for the Blind, New York, ch 2

O'Brien J P, Draycott V 1984 Spinal deformities. In:

Downie P A (ed) Cash's textbook of orthopaedics and rheumatology for physiotherapists. Faber and Faber, London, ch 15

Puddefoot T, Hilliard H, Burl M 1997 Effect of verbal feedback on the physical performance of children. Physiotherapy 83(2):76–81

Robb J 1993 Orthopaedic aspects of childhood disorders. In: Eckersley P M (ed) Elements of paediatric physiotherapy. Churchill Livingstone, Edinburgh, ch 12

Ross K, Thomson D 1993 An evaluation of parents' involvement in the management of their cerebral palsy children. Physiotherapy 79(8):561–565

Sheldon H 1992 Boyd's introduction to the study of disease, 11th edn. Lea and Febiger, Philadelphia

Shepherd R B 1995 Physiotherapy in paediatrics, 3rd edn. Butterworth Heinemann, Oxford

Sheridan M D 1975 From birth to five years – children's developmental progress. Routledge, London

Stoker D J 1985 The radiologist's approach to hip disorders in children. Physiotherapy 71(9):391–394

Trivella G, Zambito A, Aldegheri R, Leso P, Burton M 1991 Functional and aesthetic results of leg lengthening in achondroplastic patients. Physiotherapy 77(11):724–726

Whyte D A, Baggaley S, Rutter C 1995 Chronic illness in childhood: a comparative study of family support across four diagnostic groups. Physiotherapy 81(9):515–520

Woods M 1987 Impressions of home based portage services. Physiotherapy 73(4):175–176

10

Bone diseases

■ Orthopaedics ■ Bone disease ■ Tumours ■ Infections ■ Nutrition
■ Metabolic disorders ■ Degenerative conditions
■ Physiotherapy management ■ Assessment

CONTENTS

Objectives

By the end of this chapter you should:

1. Have gained insight into the various classifications of bone diseases.
2. Have gained an understanding of the different ways in which the physiotherapist can contribute to this area of orthopaedics.
3. Have gained some confidence in how you can draw on your previously acquired knowledge and experiences by using problem-solving approaches.

Prerequisites

In order to get the most out of this chapter you need to refresh your knowledge of the problem-solving approach (you may want to refer to earlier chapters). Browsing through available orthopaedic journals will help you to develop an insight into the current debates in this area with regard to medical and surgical management. This will help you to appreciate the differing roles of the physiotherapist in the varying arenas of rehabilitation.

INTRODUCTION

Bone diseases cover an enormous area in the field of orthopaedics as will become clear when you look at their classification. While many of our patients have a frank diagnosis of a specific bone condition (such as Paget's disease) others will often present with less obvious signs of the problem which need careful eliciting in a skilful assessment (such as osteoporosis). This aspect of our practice – yet again – is the most important one when dealing with patients who have bone problems. If in doubt, go back to Chapter 3 on assessment to refresh your own ideas and convictions in this area. Without good assessment skills it would be very difficult to plan a reasonable and cohesive management strategy for and with patients who are in need of problem solving that not only addresses their immediate musculoskeletal problem but also their future outlook on life and its management. As this latter point recognises, in this area we are dealing with long-term difficulties rather than 'one-off' episodes.

In contrast to people with soft tissue injuries who often refer themselves to a physiotherapist or are referred by their general practitioner, this group of patients will most probably be referred by a specialist (orthopaedic surgeon, paediatrician or physician). Communication with the referrer about assessment findings, treatment goals and outcomes and long-term management is absolutely vital. In this case the physiotherapist is not an isolated practitioner but a member of a multidisciplinary team which should of course include the patient and/or their carers. Physiotherapy management therefore has to take team issues into account. Worthington (1994) explored the different aspects of the multidisciplinary team (MDT).

Self-assessment question

■ **SAQ 10.1.** What is your own experience of working in an MDT? Try to be specific about who was part of it and in which area of practice it occurred.

What do you think was special about this setting which led to the involvement of an MDT?

Who was perceived to be the leader of the MDT and did that reflect his or her contribution to the overall management of the patient, or was a more established hierarchical set-up followed?

How were decisions arrived at?

It is important to remember that people with a diagnosis of one of the many bone diseases can belong to any age group. We see babies and young children who might be diagnosed as having, for example, neurofibromatosis (von Recklinghausen's disease); we might see adults with metabolic problems (such as osteoporosis) or tumours and we often see older patients with, for instance, Paget's disease.

Bearing in mind these different client groups, you will recognise that we, as physiotherapists, could meet them in all sorts of different settings. We might see them in our own hospital departments or wards, in the GP's practice, in their own homes as we work in a domiciliary capacity or in private practice settings. All of these contexts naturally require quite different approaches from the physiotherapist. Good communication skills, therefore, are absolutely vital. It is good to remember at this point that these skills, like any others, need practice and supervision if they are to be of a high order (Thomson et al 1997).

Self-assessment question

■ **SAQ 10.2.** How will you be able to detect whether your communication skills are effective and appropriate?

It was mentioned earlier that people with bone diseases might have to live with a long-term, at times irreversible problem, in contrast to patients, for instance, with soft tissue injuries or other short-term problems. The physiotherapist will have to change his or her approach in order to allow for this. Many of the necessary skills are of course exactly the same as in other physiotherapy encounters, but obviously the goal setting and treatment planning carried out with the patient must be different given the lifelong nature of the condition. Lifestyle questions must therefore be addressed, work positions must be explored and the changing nature of the problem with regard to the future, for instance with ageing, has to be attended to.

This lifelong aspect makes it particularly important to view the patient as a participator in goal setting and assessment of outcome, and Ramsden (1975) advocated this collaborative approach a long time ago. Does it really happen and what are the patients' experiences of this? Payton & Nelson (1996) interviewed a group of patients about their views on whether they believed that they had an important input in goal setting and treatment planning. Most of their sample felt that their participation was not great, but they believed that they gave important and influential feedback on the outcome of the actual therapy. When asked whether they valued the physical therapy input, they were very positive and felt that they had confidence and trust in their physiotherapists. Payton & Nelson's interesting study seems to indicate that goal setting and treatment planning with patients are the weakest aspects of our interaction with them, while the patient's participation in treatment evaluation is the strongest.

This is an important area for us to consider as there seems to be strong evidence that patient compliance is directly related to the non-authoritarian and cooperative approach of the therapist (Lloyd & Maas 1992).

THE ANATOMY AND PHYSIOLOGY OF BONE

Before discussing the classification of bone diseases, a short review of the anatomy and physiology of bone will be useful.

Long bones consist mainly of articular cartilage at the top covering the bone of the epiphysis, below which the epiphyseal plate is located (in growing bone). The bone of the diaphysis protects the marrow cavity of the bone which of course is the site of blood cell production.

Sherwood (1995) gives a good and concise overview of the physiology of bone as follows.

The structure of bone
Bones are made up of a kind of connective tissue which consists of cells on the one hand and an extracellular matrix on the other that is produced by these cells which are known as osteoblasts. The matrix is made up of collagen and hence is responsible for the tensile strength of bone. Clearly though, bone is not really rubbery as this description might imply. Bone is made hard by the calcium phosphate crystals within this matrix. However if bones were composed mainly of these crystals they would be hard, brittle and easily breakable. In fact, they are incredibly strong, are light and not brittle, due to the structural interweaving of an organic scaffolding hardened by inorganic crystals.

The important elements of bone therefore are calcium carbonate, calcium phosphate, collagen and water. The relative proportions of these vary with age and health. Calcium carbonate and calcium phosphate make up nearly 60–79% of bone weight. Water makes up about 25–30% of the total bone weight (Hall 1991) and is directly related to its strength.

Not all bones are made up in the same way. The smaller the proportion of calcium phosphate and calcium carbonate and the greater the proportion of non-mineralised bone tissue the more porous the bone is going to be. If 5–30% of bone tissue is occupied by non-mineralised tissue (thus the bone is less porous) it is termed cortical bone. If 30–90% of bone volume is occupied by non-mineralised tissue the bone is cancellous bone which is rubbery and spongy. Most bones have an outer layer of cortical bone and internal layer of cancellous bone. Cortical bone is stronger and hence more able to sustain stress, while cancellous bone is more flexible and hence more able to deal with deformation (Hall 1991).

How does bone grow in thickness?
Sherwood (1995) explains how new bone is added to the outer surface of the bone as a result of osteoblast activity inside the sheath of connective tissue which covers the outer part of the bone. While this is happening on the outside, osteoclasts situated inside the bone are engaged in breaking down bone tissue nearest the marrow cavity. In other words, as the shaft circumference is enlarged the marrow cavity is also enlarged to keep pace with these changes.

How does bone grow in length?

This happens via a different mechanism compared with that responsible for the increase in thickness. Sherwood (1995) describes how this process is located mainly in the epiphyseal plate where a proliferation of cartilage cells can be observed. Cell division on the outer edge of the plate immediately next to the epiphysis causes thickening of the cartilaginous plate and hence a pushing away of the epiphysis from the diaphysis. As this process happens near the epiphyseal border the old cartilage cells close to the diaphyseal border die off and are replaced by osteoblasts which move upwards towards the epiphysis. These osteoblasts then model new bone around the persistent survivors of the disintegrating cartilage, until the inner aspect of the diaphysis where it meets the epiphyseal plate is entirely replaced by bone. Once this process is completed, the diaphysis has increased in length and the epiphyseal plate has resumed its original thickness.

Once the osteoblasts have carried out their bone-creating role, they becomes buried inside the extracellular matrix as this calcifies. They do not really die off, however, but turn into osteocytes and lay down an extensive tunnel system to receive their nutrients and to get rid of waste. In the new bone one therefore sees a multitude of little canals which the osteoblasts themselves have formed.

What is the role of growth and other hormones?

The processes discussed above are made possible by growth hormone, which is responsible for the increase in thickness as well as length in bone. It works directly on the proliferation of epiphyseal cartilage. As we have seen, this allows for more bone formation and osteoblast activity. Growth hormone works on the epiphyseal plate, hence allowing an increase in bone length. For this to happen though, the epiphyseal plate must remain open, that is cartilaginous. This plate closes or ossifies under the influence of the sex hormone once adolescence is completed, and so people do not grow in height after this period.

Bone formation and removal normally happen all the time. This is important for:

1. keeping the skeleton in a state of maximum efficiency for its mechanical functions and the demands on it
2. maintaining the free plasma calcium level.

This leads to the conclusion that mechanical factors are the most important factors for adjusting the strength of bone, as the greater the mechanical or physical stress on it the greater the rate of bone formation. Athletes' bones are more massive than those of sedentary people (Sherwood 1995). The other side to this is that loss of mechanical stress, as in prolonged bed rest, for example, results in loss of bone mass.

However, the actual rate of bone formation and removal is again controlled by hormones. The actions of the growth and sex hormones have already been discussed. The other important hormone with regard to bone is the parathyroid hormone. It takes calcium out of the bone fluid which is found in the multitude of little canals in between the buried osteoblasts (now called osteocytes). (In contrast to plasma, bone has calcium in abundance.) In this way the actual integrity of the bone is not interfered with at all and all the necessary plasma calcium comes from this bone fluid.

If by any chance there is an acute lack of calcium, for instance in diet problems, the parathyroid hormone stimulates the local dissolution of bone and promotes the transfer of calcium, as well as other ingredients, from the bone itself into the plasma. On the whole this process does not leave any discernible effects on the bones. This is clearly a potentially life-saving mechanism for the body. Once the plasma calcium levels have become higher again, the superfluous calcium is redeposited in the bone. However, if this process were to be maintained over many months there would be a widening of the fluid-filled canals, and they would eventually cluster together as cavities.

CLASSIFICATION OF BONE DISEASES

Many different classifications appear in the literature but the one that is still most frequently referred to was established by Wynne-Davies & Fairbank (1976):

1. Bone dysplasias and malformations
   — achondroplasia
   — osteogenesis imperfecta
   — diaphyseal aclasis
   — Ollier's disease
   — Paget's disease
   — polyostotic fibrous dysplasia
   — neurofibromatosis
   — fibrodysplasia ossificans progressiva
2. Inborn errors of metabolism
   — Gaucher's disease
   — histiocytosis X
3. Metabolic bone disease
   — hyperparathyroidism
   — nutritional rickets
   — other forms of rickets
   — nutritional osteomalacia
   — other forms of osteomalacia
   — vitamin C deficiency
4. Endocrine disorders
   — senile osteoporosis
   — hypopituitarism
   — gigantism
   — acromegaly
   — hypothyroidism
   — glucocorticoid excess.

Another way of classifying these abnormalities may be found in Dandy (1993). He suggests an ordering based on the probable cause of the abnormality.

1. *Abnormalities of bone structure*
These may be influenced by the following hormones and vitamins:

- growth hormones
- sex hormones
- thyroid hormones
- parathyroid hormones
- vitamin C
- vitamin D plus calcium
- calcitonin.

Collagen forms part of bone and abnormalities here can lead to:

- scurvy
- osteogenesis imperfecta.

The bone structure can further be influenced by abnormalities of mineralisation which in turn leads to bone loss by:

- osteomalacia – decreased mineralisation
- osteolysis – increased removal by osteoclasts
- osteopenia – decrease in osteoid tissue.

Often these three occur together and are referred to as osteoporosis.

Abnormalities of the osteon structure are involved in:

- Paget's disease
- fibrous dysplasia
- other dysplasias.

Abnormalities of cartilage include:

- mucopolysaccharidoses
- achondroplasia
- diaphyseal aclasis.

2. *Osteochondritis*
This may be caused by vascular abnormalities, as in:

- Perthes' disease
- Kienboeck's disease
- Koehler's disease.

It may be caused by damage to the apophyses as in:

- Osgood–Schlatter's disease
- Sever's disease
- Sinding Larsen's disease
- Scheuermann's disease.

Others causes are:

- osteochondritis dissecans
- Calvé's disease.

3. *Bone infections*
These include:

- osteomyelitis
- septic arthritis.

As you can see the field of bone diseases is enormous and not easily classified.

Self-assessment question

■ **SAQ 10.3.** Which of the above have you

come across? Try to remember as much as possible about these with regard to the following:

1. The age and sex of the patient.
2. The part of the body affected or was the entire body involved?
3. The general physical condition of that patient.
4. Where you met this patient? In hospital? As an outpatient? In the community?

Table 10.1 Bone diseases which the physiotherapist may encounter

1. Dysplasia	Paget's disease
2. Degenerative	Osteoarthritis
	Osteochondritis
3. Nutritional/metabolic	Rickets
	Osteoporosis
	Osteomalacia
	Vitamin C deficiency
4. Infections	Tuberculosis
	Osteomyelitis
	Periostitis
5. Tumours	
Benign	Osteoma
	Chondroma
	Osteochondroma
	Giant cell tumour
Malignant	Osteosarcoma
	Chondrosarcoma of bone
	Fibrosarcoma of bone
	Ewing's tumour
	Multiple myeloma
	Secondary (metastatic)

Reading through the lists given above you will immediately recognise some conditions and not others. While any of these might come the physiotherapist's way, some will do so more frequently than others, and now that you have reflected on your encounters with patients with bone diseases, you might have already formed an opinion as to the frequency of some of these conditions as well as concerning their preferred sites and behaviours.

This chapter will concentrate on the manifestations of bone disease in adults which we as physiotherapists come across. Paediatrics, and the particular occurrences and demands of that age group have been covered in Chapter 9.

A shorter list of the principal bone diseases which physiotherapists come across more frequently than others is given in Table 10.1. You will immediately recognise that this is not a complete list, compared with the classifications given previously.

PHYSIOTHERAPY REFERRALS OF PATIENTS WITH BONE DISEASES

The diagnosis of bone disease in itself is not usually a reason for referral. In fact as stated previously, the actual diagnosis is often secondary with regard to rehabilitation. What is important are the actual findings in terms of loss of function or pain and what these mean to the patient.

We may meet patients with bone disease after surgery, which might have been aimed at correcting a deformity, for instance, or replacing a 'worn out' joint, salvaging a limb (on account of a tumour) or following a fracture. All of these are encountered more often in a ward situation within a hospital.

On the other hand we might come across patients from this group when they complain of pain or an inability to live life in the same way as they have been used to. These patients might be met in our outpatient departments as well as GP practices or community settings.

As medication and surgical approaches change, so does the role of the physiotherapist. Where there might once have been regimes involving lengthy stays in hospital, where the physiotherapist might have been needed to combat the effects of prolonged bed rest, our role now is mostly much more proactive, taking advantage of a more active general management.

Strong bones are needed to provide a lever for muscles and ligaments. When these are weakened for whatever reason, postural problems will automatically follow. This will result in functional losses due to muscle weakness and perhaps gait abnormalities. The analysis of gait patterns and their rehabilitation is an area physiotherapists are involved in all the time. We therefore need to see these patients in our gyms and departments for general strengthening, muscle imbalance work or gait re-education, for instance.

Prevention of future problems is of course a major aspect of our work in habilitation – a more holistic approach than straightforward rehabilitation. Prevention is usually much easier than the treatment needed once a problem has occurred. It therefore makes a lot of sense to spend time and expertise homing in on this. Clearly in someone with a lifelong locomotor problem this is vital, and no management approach is acceptable that does not focus on this point.

General conditions of the skeleton

Most of these are very rare and hence not often seen by physiotherapists. Many are congenital, such as achondroplasia or osteogenesis imperfecta, and hence are usually first seen in paediatric settings (see Ch. 9). It seems that most of these are caused by a dominant mutant gene (Crawford Adams & Hamblen 1990) in the fetal stage of development. As mentioned in Chapter 9, it is important to remember that not all of these conditions manifest themselves at birth but might only become apparent later on.

Self-assessment question

- **SAQ 10.4.** By remembering the child's developmental milestones and from your observation, how would you as a physiotherapist know that a bony abnormality has manifested itself?

Apart from these genetically caused bone diseases, metabolic changes can have a general effect on the skeleton. A good example of this might be rickets, which is caused by a deficiency of vitamin D leading to defective calcification of growing bone (Crawford Adams & Hamblen 1990). The sight of thin children with weak and very bendy bones is now very rare in western societies as diets and exposure to sunlight have improved.

Osteomalacia, another vitamin D-deficiency problem, is a condition frequently encountered by physiotherapists. This is often seen as a side-effect of Crohn's disease which involves a resorption problem leading to bone mineral loss. Vogelsang et al (1995) tried to determine whether long-term dietary supplementation with low doses of vitamin D helps to prevent bone loss and the development of osteomalacia in patients with Crohn's disease. They concluded from their positive results that long-term oral vitamin D supplementation seems to be an efficient means of preventing bone loss in these patients and hence of preventing osteomalacia.

Finally, a large group of patients who show general bone changes are those whose problems have an endocrine cause. Patients with osteoporosis are the biggest subgroup. It is caused amongst other factors by a general decrease in calcium in bone.

Self-assessment questions

- **SAQ 10.5.** What are the mechanisms involved in bone growth? If in doubt reread the physiology review at the beginning of this chapter.

- **SAQ 10.6.** How would you expect the presence of bone disease to influence the healing time of a hip fracture in an elderly woman?

Local diseases of bone

These might not all be caused by genetic problems. The most important ones are infections, tumours, osteochondritis and cystic changes.

These can manifest themselves in childhood, for example in osteomyelitis when organisms reach the bloodstream, or on the other hand at any stage in life as a consequence of an open fracture or surgical intervention.

Tuberculosis which used to account for a large number of local bone infections is much rarer in the western patient population now, though still a major problem in some countries. This infection is chronic, develops slowly and is much more subtle than many conditions which develop more quickly, such as osteomyelitis. It is often confined to a particular joint, such as the hip, but can spread to other parts of the body where all sorts of complications can arise, for example compression of the spinal cord by an abscess of the spinal column. In contrast to many other patients with bone diseases this group of patients will have general malaise with high temperatures, raised ESR levels and a positive Mantoux test (Crawford Adams & Hamblen 1990).

Tumours are either benign or malignant. As physiotherapists we come across them as either a primary cause or as a metastatic occurrence. Both of these situations are regularly found in any orthopaedic practice.

Osteochondritis usually occurs in young people or children and seems to be caused by the development of bony nuclei inside the bone which leads to a softening of the bone structure.

ASSESSMENT

Specialised tests

X-rays are of course the primary specialised tool for the doctor. Of particular interest are the length and width of bones, the state of the epiphyses, the size of the spinal canal, the symmetry of the vertebrae, any outgrowths of bone and translucency of bones. Magnetic resonance imaging (MRI) is the routinely used, modern, non-invasive, reliable screening which has the advantage of giving a good view of the soft tissues. When a tumour is suspected, a biopsy might be necessary. Blood tests show whether the plasma calcium levels are normal or low, whether alkaline phosphatase is increased (for instance in osteomalacia) and whether the calcium balance is normal or negative. Bone (radioisotope) scans are invaluable in the detection of Paget's disease, for example.

It is important that the physiotherapist is able to interpret these results as possible clues to the background diagnosis. However, our forte is physical assessment rather than specialised tests.

It is important that you have a good idea about your assessment priorities as a physiotherapist before you begin to evaluate someone with a bone disease problem. You might want to quickly reflect on some of the issues raised in the chapter on assessment. This area is often dominated by highly specialised technological tests and screening which focus on a particular area of the skeleton. In the presence of all this technological information it can be easy to forget, though, that some of the patient's problems will be entirely hidden, and it is only through a skilful assessment that suspicion of a problem connected to bone disease will be aroused.

Subjective assessment

The aim of the subjective assessment is to gain an insight into the patient's problem. One needs to ascertain the mechanical, social and psychological elements which might contribute to the whole picture. The patient's lifestyle and the way he or she uses the body has to be established by careful interviewing. Patients must have the opportunity to express their own thoughts and feelings about the problem and what they are hoping to gain from physiotherapy. It is all too easy to jump to particular conclusions after having read the diagnosis of the referrer. As physiotherapists we should attempt to build up a relationship with patients enabling them to focus on particular aspects of the wide variety of possibilities. We do not really treat a condition. The patient is likely to experience problems which will have to be tackled in the light of the rest of his or her lifespan rather than involving a few weeks of treatment. It may be necessary for a patient's partner to be involved in this aspect of the assessment.

Remember to introduce questions focusing on possible mineralisation loss, for instance, as a result of hysterectomy, gastrectomy or long-term use of steroids or any blood thinning agent. The resulting deficit of bone mineralisation might become visible on X-ray only when more than 30% has been lost. Thus the clinical interview might raise suspicions before radiographic findings can confirm the problem.

Usually our assessments try to identify a mechanical pattern and hence a mechanical cause for the patient's problems. With this patient group, however, where we are concerned with permanent changes rather than an injury, you need to make absolutely sure that you understand hints the patient might give you which have little to do with the mechanical aspects of their problem. Considering the lifelong nature of these conditions, it is important that a measure of disability which uses subjective as well as objective markers can be introduced. Disability is experienced in very different ways by different patients and depending to their diagnosis. Clearly someone with osteoporosis will feel themselves to be differently affected from someone with cancer. There are, therefore, very different disability measures which should be employed for each of these client groups.

Objective assessment

The aims of this are not really very different from any other aspect of orthopaedic assessment inasmuch as it is an attempt to elicit and isolate the patient's main problem through focused tests and examinations. Special physical tests are dictated by the physical findings rather than the diagnosis. They are altered to suit the different client groups, for instance children, adults or the elderly, and to take account of possible contraindications.

Bone structure and alignment are a very important area on which to concentrate with these patients.

Posture

As mentioned earlier in this chapter, a change in bone strength, length or shape is bound to have an effect on muscles and ligaments and hence on posture. Posture is probably one of the most difficult areas of any physical assessment. In order to assess abnormalities of posture you must refamiliarise yourself with the hallmarks of normal posture.

Roaf (1978) defined posture as the position the body assumes in preparation for the next movement. Mere uprightness, he continued, is not a valid definition of posture since the latter involves balance, muscular control, coordination and adaptation. With this definition in mind it becomes clear that postural defects are very common. Barlow (1952) assumed that about 70–80% of adolescents presented with postural problems and he considered this number to rise with increasing age.

Grieve (1981) comments on the monumental task of classifying and meaningfully assessing the rich variety of emotional, hormonal, mechanical, neurophysiological and social factors that might all influence posture.

On the whole, one assumes that postural problems can be abolished. If, however, permanent soft tissue shortening, bone and joint changes have manifested themselves, postural problems may have clearly led to a deformity. Congenital and acquired deformities tend to produce asymmetry and thus predispose to degenerative changes. On the other hand, however, degenerative changes can produce changes of body contour and attitude. These can manifest themselves at every level, and therefore need careful attention in an assessment.

Grieve (1981) reminds us that the interpretation of our objective findings is very important. Things are not always what they seem and a deformity might not result in pathology.

SPECIFIC BONE DISEASES

Osteoporosis

Osteoporosis is a metabolic disease of bone which is characterised by reduced bone mass resulting in an increased risk of fractures. It is by far the commonest bone disease (Ritson & Scott 1996). Dinan & Rutherford (1994) reported that in the UK 1 in 12 men over the age of 70 years and one in four women over 60 years have osteoporosis. Pettifor (1981) reported that one in four of all white women in the USA and South Africa have sustained one or several osteoporotic fractures after the age of 65.

Bone mass increases throughout childhood and early adult life reaching a peak in the third decade. As discussed earlier it is dependent on hormones, exercise, diet, genes, lifestyle and illness (Adami 1994). In the assessment of the level of bone turnover in women with vertebral osteoporosis, serum osteocalcin and urinary pyridinoline appear, so far, to be the most sensitive markers (Delmas 1993). On the other hand, at present there appears to be no specific and reliable test for the measurement of general bone resorption and formation, and hence patients are usually asked to undergo a whole battery of tests to determine these two general indicators. Osteoporosis is characterised in the spine by a thinning of the cortices of the vertebrae and a thinning of the individual trabeculae with a resultant widening of the vertebral canal.

Turner (1991) reminds us that fractures of the proximal femur and distal radius are regarded as typical osteoporotic fractures. These mostly seem to occur in elderly women. On the other hand Spector (1990) reports vertebral fractures as occurring three times as often as hip fractures but remaining undetected more frequently. These can occur almost spontaneously after a cough or sneeze and can lead to chronic pain, a crushing down of vertebrae on top of each other and hence an increased thoracic kyphosis and loss of height. A wedge-shaped vertebra is a classical radiological finding in osteoporosis (Fig. 10.1).

Turner (1991) lists the following groups who may be at risk of accelerating bone loss:

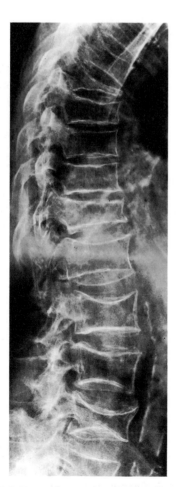

Figure 10.1 X-ray of osteoporotic spine. (Reproduced with permission from Crawford Adams & Hamblen 1990.)

- post-gastrectomy patients who have poor calcium absorption
- people who diet excessively or who have diets deficient in calcium or vitamin D
- post-hysterectomy patients
- people who suffer from anorexia nervosa and related diseases
- females who exercise excessively, affecting normal menstruation
- people with a history of osteoporosis
- people receiving long-term steroids
- people with metabolic or glandular disorders, such as hyperparathyroidism
- people who have to submit to immobilisation, such as patients with spinal cord injuries
- post-menopausal women.

Problems start when bone resorption exceeds bone formation. It seems that oestrogen can prevent accelerated bone loss (Pettifor 1981). On the whole obese women seem to be less susceptible to osteoporosis. Schnitzler (1987) explains that adipose tissue can convert the precursors of gonadal hormones, which are secreted by the adrenal glands after menopause, into oestrogen and oestradiol.

Management
Turner (1991) discusses this in three stages: primary prevention, secondary prevention and tertiary management.

Primary prevention
This is aimed at young women and usually takes the form of specifically targeted advertising. It covers the known factors of diet and exercise.

Secondary prevention
This is aimed at the high-risk group, that is women in their forties. In this pre- or perimenopausal period it is important that women are informed about hormone replacement therapy and correct diets especially concentrating on vitamin D and calcium. Weight-bearing exercise or activities are essential but the high impact jarring of some sports might be counterproductive. Postural exercises and general fitness to promote good posture should be encouraged.

Tertiary management

Here symptoms have occurred and actual treatment is necessary. This could happen at any stage in life and is mainly concerned with the relief of pain and the possible loss of mobility and deformity. The initial spinal deformity can make it difficult to treat patients in the usual treatment positions of supine or prone lying. Clearly, other positions need to be explored. Any change in spinal shape will obviously cause a change in respiration which needs to be checked and if necessary addressed in a treatment plan. Walking is a good self-treatment method, as is any kind of fitness and strength training.

Sinaki & Mikkelson (1984) looked at the effect of flexion versus extension exercises on postmenopausal osteoporotic women and demonstrated that the extension group had a significantly lower number of osteoporotic fractures compared with the flexion group. The aim of exercise is to maximise the bone mass by loading the skeleton and contracting muscles. Revel et al (1993) demonstrated that a 1-year programme of psoas training can reduce bone loss.

Ritson & Scott (1996) investigated the treatment techniques commonly used amongst Scottish and Swedish physiotherapists. These also included electrotherapy (especially transcutaneous nerve stimulation) for pain relief and hydrotherapy for general mobility. These authors drew up a list of 10 exercises obtained from the literature, ranked in order of benefit to those at risk of osteoporosis:

1. runing/jumping
2. walking
3. strength training
4. extension
5. postural exercise
6. flexibility
7. swimming
8. cycling
9. flexion
10. bed rest.

None of these approaches, however, really addresses the disability experienced by women with osteoporotic spinal fractures.

Helmes et al (1995) reported their initial results in trying to validate the Osteoporotic Functional Disability Questionnaire (OFDQ). The domains of the OFDQ include: quantitative indices of pain, a standard two-dimensional-item scale, 26 items relating to functional disability, a scale of social activities, and an indicator of confidence in the efficacy of prescribed osteoporosis treatment in reversing disability. The authors reported the test–retest reliability to vary between 0.76 to 0.93 with internal consistencies from 0.57 to 0.96. They also reported that the OFDQ correlated significantly with relevant spinal pathology, and it detected significant improvements in activities of daily living and socialisation indices when active exercisers were compared with inactive patients with osteoporosis. Helmes et al (1995) therefore concluded that the OFDQ is a reliable instrument which correlates well with objective measures of osteoporotic spinal damage. It is also sensitive to changes in disability brought about by participation in an aerobic exercise programme. As physiotherapists we are in need of a more biopsychosocial measuring tool and might investigate this further.

Self-assessment question

■ **SAQ 10.7.** What sort of pointers might you come across in your assessment that would alert the physiotherapist to the fact that disability is a bigger problem than the measured impairment?

Often a drug regimen including fluoride, calcium and vitamin D needs to be included. Research with tiludronate has shown that it is capable of preventing disuse osteoporosis, for instance in spinal cord patients (Chappard et al 1995), without impairing the mineralisation process.

Case study 10.1

Daisy Bell

Mrs Daisy Bell is a 58-year-old mother of three grown-up children. She has started to notice pain in her lumbar spine over the past year or so. She particularly finds any static posture or position extremely uncomfortable. On the whole short rests help her, but she now feels severely curtailed in her activities.

Problem-solving exercise 10.1

■ **A.** After reading carefully through this chapter so far, what do you think are the main concerns the physiotherapist must address in his or her assessment?

■ **B.** Are there any special questions/tests that the physiotherapist should include?

■ **C.** What is the problem list likely to be?

■ **D.** What might be the main aims of treatment?

■ **E.** What treatment management might the physiotherapist discuss with Mrs Bell?

■ **F.** What advice would the physiotherapist need to include to look to the future?

Paget's disease

Case study 10.2

William Jones
This patient is a 60-year-old man who has been referred to you by his physician who diagnosed him as having Paget's disease. Mr Jones complains of a painful (R) thigh. While this has been going on for quite a few years, lately it has interfered with his job as a carpenter.

During the subjective assessment you find out that while it had been the leg pain that made Mr Jones seek medical help, he suffers from all sort of distressing symptoms: in particular headaches, some deafness and generalised stiffness. He is also concerned that his appearance seems to have changed a lot. From being a man of medium height and upright posture he appears to have lost height and to be quite bent forwards.

Self-assessment question

■ **SAQ 10.8.** Listening to Mr Jones' story, what characteristic features of Paget's disease have you identified so far?

Paget's disease is a common condition which is also referred to as osteitis deformans. About 3% of the population over 40 years of age (Apley 1977) can show signs of it. In spite of much research its cause is unknown, although it is interesting to note that it is virtually never found in some areas, such as Norway and Japan. It is a slowly progressive problem, affecting one or several bones but never crossing joint spaces. It got its name from Sir James Paget who first described it in 1879.

The affected bones increase in width and hence become thicker. They lose their normal consistency, and have an increase in their blood supply, hence becoming spongy and weakened and leading to an increase in fractures (Crawford Adams & Hamblen 1990, Dandy 1993).

The disease can be localized to one bone for years before affecting others (skull, femur, pelvis, clavicle and spine). The patient complains of often quite severe pain, frequently worse at night, but is able to continue with life as before being diagnosed. The latter may be confirmed by:

1. a raised alkaline phosphase level in the plasma
2. raised hydroxyproline in the urine
3. 'hot spots' on the isotope (bone) scan.

On examination the painful bone is characteristically bent, thickened and hot to touch. As bone formation and resorption are increased, spaces are created by this absorption which are slowly filled by vascular tissues (Apley 1977). The body reacts to this by forming new osteoid tissue, on either side of the cortex, which does not get converted into mature bone tissue. The bone is therefore much thicker but also much weaker, easily giving way under loading and fracturing. Nerves can easily be compromised due to the decrease in available space caused by the increase in bone circumference.

The X-ray is characteristic (Figs 10.2–10.4).

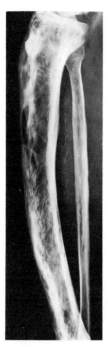

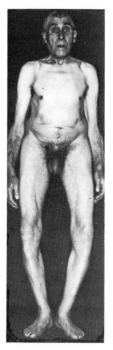

Figure 10.2 X-ray of tibia in patient with Paget's disease. (Reproduced with permission from Crawford Adams & Hamblen 1990.)

Figure 10.3 Typical appearance of a patient with widespread Paget's disease. (Reproduced with permission from Crawford Adams & Hamblen 1990.)

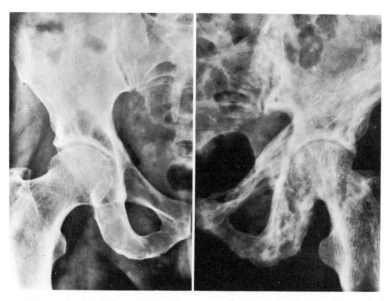

Figure 10.4 X-ray of half pelvis of a patient with Paget's disease, shown side by side with a normal one for comparison. (Reproduced with permission from Crawford Adams & Hamblen 1990.)

Management

Mr Jones' physician has already prescribed some painkillers and bisphosphonates. These latter drugs are a class of synthetic compounds used in the treatment of Paget's disease and various metabolic bone disease. Rosen & Kessenich (1996) have published an interesting review of the effect of these bisphosphonates. They identify several studies that have compared these drugs with placebo and have noted the paucity of research investigating the effect of these drugs compared with other pharmacological agents. The authors are nevertheless convinced that the effects of these drugs as documented so far, make them the treatment of choice for Paget's disease and for some other metabolic diseases at this time.

Problem-solving exercise 10.2

You have read about Mr Jones' referral and the detail of his disease history.

- **A.** What are your aims for assessment? Is there anything in particular that you might need to address or are there any special tests that you might need to make use of? How are you going to assess the impact of Mr Jones' problem on his present and future life?

- **B.** What are your aims for treatment/management? What is your problem list likely to look like? How are you and Mr Jones going to know if the treatment approach chosen is successful?

- **C.** What advice would you want to give Mr Jones with regard to the future?

If in doubt you will find all the answers in this chapter or the chapter on assessment (Ch. 3).

Osteosarcoma and other malignant tumours

Case history 10.3

Alan

Alan is 25-year-old man who describes himself as very fit and energetic. He is a motor

mechanic and loves motor bike racing. Eight weeks ago he jarred his knee by missing the last step on a staircase. He did not really give this incident any attention until he started to experience a dull ache in the upper end of his tibia near the knee, which did not react to any mechanical influences. It was the same whether he was sitting down or walking. He also started to notice a swelling near his knee which became tender to touch. Finally, as it started to interfere with his sport he decided to consult his doctor who gave him painkillers, and a cream. As his problems did not resolve but became more pronounced, his GP referred him to the local orthopaedic surgeon who after tests diagnosed an osteosarcoma.

Self-assessment question

- **SAQ 10.9.** What are the important aspects of this patient's history with regard to his diagnosis?

Osteosarcoma is a malignant tumour which is also known as osteogenic sarcoma. It predominantly occurs in younger people or even children but can also appear as a complication of Paget's disease in older adults. This malignant tumour occurs more often in males than females with a ratio of roughly 2:1 (Maxwell 1995). It arises from the bone-forming cells and most often appears at the lower end of the femur, the upper end of the tibia and the upper end of the humerus. Crawford Adams & Hamblen (1990) describe how osteosarcomas classically destroy the bone structure before bursting into the surrounding soft tissues. Any type of connective tissue may be represented, giving it a widely varying histological appearance. Always present though are areas of neoplastic new bone or osteoid tissue. Metastasis of this tumour occurs early via the bloodstream, particularly to the lungs. Dandy (1993) reported an average survival rate of about 30%.

Clinically there is pain and a local increasing swelling. On examination this swelling is usually found at the end of bones near to the joint (Figs 10.5, 10.6; Crawford Adams & Hamblen 1990).

The patient often indicates a minor injury disproportionate to the extent of the pain and the change of the affected region.

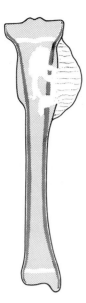

Figure 10.5 Osteosarcoma. (Reproduced with permission from Crawford Adams & Hamblen 1990.)

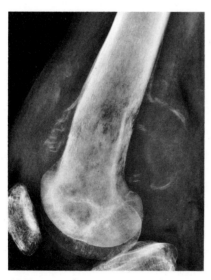

Figure 10.6 X-ray of osteosarcoma at lower end of femur. (Reproduced with permission from Crawford Adams & Hamblen 1990.)

The X-rays show the proliferation of bone and the destruction of the metaphysis. Often one can identify the Codman's triangle which is the appearance of new bone formation under the corners of the raised periosteum. Nuclear magnetic resonance (NMR) scanning is the best way of identifying spread into the surrounding soft tissues.

Management

The rest of the body, especially the lungs and the rest of the skeleton, must be scanned to identify possible metastases. Chemotherapy in conjunction with amputation has increased the survival rate greatly from the original 25–30% (Crawford Adams & Hamblen 1990). Chemotherapy is usually started before surgery and then continued for about a year afterwards. As the use of drug therapy has increased, radical resection has often taken over from amputation. Simon (1988) reported in excess of 70% disease-free survival after 5 years with this mixed approach.

Rehabilitation

Fulton (1994) discusses the different rehabilitation strategies as follows. She states that first of all care must be comprehensive, addressing the needs of the whole person, that is, psychological, social, vocational, economic and physical factors that shape a life. She continues by quoting Habeck et al (1984) on the need for an interdisciplinary approach which includes both the patient and his or her family. The members of the team also include the physician or surgeon, nurses, therapists and ancillary personnel. According to Habeck et al (1984) the remaining elements of the framework for the rehabilitation of cancer patients include:

1. Goals for rehabilitation that are derived from the effects of medical problems in accordance with prognostic expectations.
2. Intervention occurring as soon as the likelihood of disability is anticipated.
3. Reassessment, on a continuing basis, of rehabilitation needs and meeting of these needs throughout all phases of care.
4. Education, regarded as a major component of the rehabilitation process.

Concerning the goals of rehabilitation Dietz (1974, 1985) argues that these goals can be:

- preventive, when disability can be predicted
- restorative, when patients can be expected to have only minimal or residual handicap
- supportive, when patients have to cope with ongoing disease or permanent disability
- palliative, when patients are managing advanced disease and basic disability cannot

be corrected but where training can enhance performance.

Dietz (1985) states that these goals will be determined by an aggregate of factors relevant to the individual: age, type and stage of neoplastic disease, other concomitant disease, inherent physical ability, social background, basic education and job or work experience.

With regard to the timing of intervention, Fulton (1994) and Dietz (1985) argue that any rehabilitation programme for a cancer patient should be instituted as soon as possible. They comment further that preventive goals, such as breathing control, general muscle and joint range maintenance and fitness exercises, are crucial and the role of the physiotherapist is firmly established within this framework. Fulton (1994) refers to the work by Folkman & Lazarus (1980), stating that as a patient with a cancer diagnosis often initially feels out of control, exercises might help him to determine some control of his body and hence put him at a general psychological advantage.

Concerning the third point, that rehabilitation needs must be reassessed on a continuing basis, Fulton (1994) reiterates the point that these needs must be met throughout all phases of the disease, that is, diagnosis, primary treatment, adjuvant therapy, secondary recurrence and palliation. She emphasises that goals must be realistic for the current stage of the patient's disease process and the patient's abilities.

The fourth point states that education must be seen as a major element of rehabilitation. By concentrating on the rehabilitation process the multidisciplinary team is able to focus on the patient's abilities rather than the disease.

The aim of rehabilitation at this stage is therefore to concentrate on reducing the degree to which disabilities become permanent or interfere with everyday life, regardless of how long that life might be.

Fulton (1994) continues her review by stating that the main difficulties for effective rehabilitation for cancer patients seem to concern attitudinal problems and poor knowledge about the disease and the rehabilitation process. It is important to remember that part of the role of the physiotherapist is to identify problems with the rehabilitation process that are not purely physical, such as anxiety and depression, as the physiotherapist often spends more time than other team members with the patient. This might then result in a helpful referral to the psychologist on the team.

Fulton (1994) suggests that it is essential for the physiotherapist to address more specific issues in order to plan the most effective rehabilitation. The physiotherapist therefore must make it her business to fully understand all the aspects of the different stages of the disease, to be familiar with the medical tests and their implications and to have a realistic view of the process. This realistic outlook will have a direct influence on the physiotherapist's goals. If she is unrealistic or ignorant about the disease process, the short-term goals can result in inappropriate programmes, leading to trauma both physical as well as psychological for the patient and a feeling of helplessness for the physiotherapist. In the long term Fulton (1994) reminds us that the patient could lose out in rehabilitation achievement and the physiotherapist might feel deskilled and impotent.

Further issues in the physiotherapy management of patients with malignant bone disease

A physiotherapist's check list of medical tests and their implications prior to starting an assessment might look something like this (Fulton 1994):

1. What sort of cancer is it? Which organ and cell type are involved?
2. What is the stage of the patient's cancer? Is the patient dealing with an isolated growth or has metastasis already taken place? If so, have the metastases spread to the lung, other organs or another bony site?
3. What kind of medical treatment has been adopted? Is it surgery, chemotherapy and radiotherapy? Is it only one of these? Remember that some side-effects of cancer treatment may start only many years after the diagnosis.
4. What is the patient's prognosis? For the disease in general this is changing all the time and mostly for the better.
5. Which members of the multidisciplinary team are involved in the rehabilitation process?
6. Are there any obvious contraindications to certain modalities of physiotherapy?

With regard to the last point, Maxwell (1995) reviews the contradictory evidence regarding ultrasound therapy and tumour metastases. It has certainly always been thought that ultrasound therapy was contraindicated as it was felt that it could disturb tumours and hence increase the risk of metastases. This is thought to be due to the micro massage effect which could cause the separation of weakly bound tumour cells and the disruption of the very delicate tumour vessels. Once a tumour cell has been dislodged it can be disseminated by three different routes (Maxwell 1995):

1. Tumours growing in cavities may show a transcoelomic spread in which fragments attach themselves to and become implanted into the apposing serosal or mucosal surfaces to form secondary tumours.
2. The more predominant route for spread of carcinomas is via the lymphatic system. Hence the assessment of the lymph nodes is vital in this area.
3. Another route is via the bloodstream. It seems that the amount of tumour material escaping into the bloodstream is directly related to the size of the vessels in the tumour.

Maxwell (1995) reminds us that physiotherapists must be aware of the differential diagnosis of musculoskeletal tumours and the possibility that some of the latter might mimic conditions for which some physiotherapeutic modalities such as electrotherapy, might be helpful. A good and thorough assessment based upon a constant vigilance is required if these malignant tumours are not to be mismanaged.

Fallowfield (1990) notes that the mere knowledge of having a life-threatening disease is enough to seriously impair the quality of life. The psychosocial problems cancer patients might have to battle with are provoked by the actual knowledge of their diagnosis (Fallowfield 1990). They are concerned about the lack of information and the uncertainty of the prognosis, and there may be guilt about the causality and the fear of a painful and undignified death. On the other hand these patients also have to cope with radical treatments like surgery that might be mutilating and/or lead to loss of body image and/or rejection by the partner. Radiotherapy is linked to anxiety and depression, can cause nausea and vomiting, lethargy and skin problems. Chemotherapy again is linked to nausea and vomiting, and also to hair loss, mouth ulcers, hot flushes and other side-effects. All of these lead to economic, social and sexual disruption, resulting in depression and anxiety and hence a loss of quality of life (Fallowfield 1990). Some research has been done on this issue, using the Profile of Mood States (POMS) test with cancer patients (Silberfarb et al 1983).

Problem-solving exercise 10.3

Alan is facing rigorous chemotherapy, perhaps radiotherapy and either an above-knee amputation or a radical resection of his tumour involving the upper end of his tibia, his knee and the lower end of his femur, resulting in a massive total knee replacement.

- **A.** What are the general strategies going to be?
- **B.** Regardless of Alan's prognosis, what are realistic goals for him?
- **C.** Which members of the multidisciplinary team will the physiotherapist have to work with?

Refer to the assessment chapter and the chapter on joint replacement (Chapters 3 and 8) if you are stuck.

Summary

In this chapter an attempt has been made to give you a framework to assess and then manage patients with bone diseases. In contrast to soft tissue injuries or fractures you need to be able to form an assessment strategy that will include not just the search for a mechanical cause but that will help you to identify non-mechanical disease states. It is not necessary to know all the details of the medical diagnosis but rather to arrive at a reasoned and well thought out treatment plan.

ANSWERS TO QUESTIONS AND EXERCISES

Self-assessment question 10.2 (page 270)

■ **SAQ 10.2.** How will you be able to detect whether your communication skills are effective and appropriate?

Answer: The patient will be relaxed and cooperative. He or she will be able to be specific and precise during the subjective and objective assessments, and will be able to adhere to advice or to treatment approaches that have been planned collaboratively.

Self-assessment question 10.4 (page 275)

Refer to Chapter 9 for information.

Self-assessment questions 10.5, 10.6 (page 275)

See information in text.

Self-assessment question 10.7 (page 279)

■ **SAQ 10.7.** What sort of pointers might you come across in your assessment that would alert the physiotherapist to the fact that disability is a bigger problem than the measured impairment?

Answer: For example, the patient may be off work, may be avoiding daily tasks such as domestic chores and may be withdrawing from social interactions.

Problem-solving exercise 10.1 (page 280)

See information in text.

Self-assessment question 10.8 (page 280)

■ **SAQ 10.8.** Listening to Mr Jones' story, what characteristic features of Paget's disease have you identified so far?

Answer:
1. *Mr Jones' age.*
2. *The main site of his problem (his (R) thigh), and the fact that pain and deformity are appearing together.*
3. *The possibility of associated symptoms (headaches, increased kyphosis).*

Problem-solving exercise 10.2 (page 282)

See information in this chapter and in Chapter 3.

Self-assessment question 10.9 (page 282)

■ **SAQ 10.9.** What are the important aspects of this patient's history with regard to his diagnosis?

Answer:
1. *The problem began with a seemingly insignificant injury.*
2. *The patient noticed a non-mechanical behaviour of his pain.*
3. *The patient noticed swelling.*

Problem-solving exercise 10.3 (page 285)

See information in Chapters 3 and 8.

REFERENCES

Adami M 1994 Optimising peak bone mass – what are the therapeutic possibilities? Osteoporosis International Suppl 1:S27–30

Apley A G 1977 System of orthopaedics and fractures, 5th edn. Butterworths, London

Barlow W 1952 Postural homeostasis. Annals of Physical Medicine 1:77

Chappard D, Minaire P, Privat C et al 1995 Effects of tiludronate in bone loss in paraplegic patients. Journal of Bone and Mineral Research 10(1):112–118

Crawford Adams J, Hamblen D L 1990 Outline of orthopaedics, 11th edn. Churchill Livingstone, Edinburgh

Dandy D 1993 Essential orthopaedics and trauma, 2nd edn. Churchill Livingstone, Edinburgh

Delmas P D 1993 Biochemical markers of bone turnover. Journal of Bone and Mineral Research 8(S2):S549–S555

Dietz J H Jr 1974 Rehabilitation of the cancer patient. Its role in the scheme of comprehensive care. Clinical Bulletin 4(4):104–107

Dietz J H Jr 1985 Rehabilitation of the patient with cancer. In: Cabresi P, Schein P S, Rosenberg S A (eds) Medical oncology: basic principles and clinical management of cancer. Macmillan, New York

Dinan S, Rutherford O 1994 Osteoporosis. Asset: Magazine of the association of exercise teachers 2:14–21

Fallowfield L 1990 The quality of life. The missing measurement in health care. Human horizons series. Souvenir Press, London

Folkman S, Lazarus R S 1980 An analysis of coping in a middle aged community sample. Journal of Health and Social Behaviour 2:219–239

Fulton C 1994 Physiotherapists in cancer care. A framework for rehabilitation of patients. Physiotherapy 80(12):830–834

Grieve G P 1981 Common vertebral joint problems. Churchill Livingstone, Edinburgh

Habeck R V, Romsaas E P, Olson S J 1984 Cancer rehabilitation and continuing care: a case study. Cancer Nursing 7:315–319

Hall S J 1991 Basic biomechanics. Mosby Yearbook, St Louis

Helmes E, Hodsman A, Lazowski D et al 1995 A questionnaire to evaluate disability in osteoporotic patients with vertebral compression fractures. Journals of Gerontology Series A – Biological Sciences and Medical Sciences 50(2):M91–M98

Lloyd C, Maas F 1992 Interpersonal skills and occupational therapy. British Journal of Occupational Therapy 55(10):379–382

Maxwell L 1995 Therapeutic ultrasound and tumour metastasis. Physiotherapy 81(5):272–275

Payton O, Nelson C 1996 A preliminary study of patients' perceptions of certain aspects of their physical therapy experience. Physiotherapy Theory and Practice 12:27–38

Pettifor J 1981 Calcium in the young and the old. Transactions of the College of Medicine, South Africa, 3rd interdisciplinary symposium – rehabilitation 25:120–123

Ramsden E 1975 The patient's right to know: implications for interpersonal communication processes. Physical Therapy 55:133–138

Revel M, Mayoux-Behamon M A, Rabourdin J P, Baghen F, Roux C 1993 One year psoas training can prevent lumbar bone loss in post-menopausal women: a randomised controlled trial. Calcium Tissue International 53:307–311

Ritson F, Scott S 1996 Physiotherapy for osteoporosis. A pilot study comparing practice and knowledge in Scotland and Sweden. Physiotherapy 82(7):390–394

Roaf L 1978 Posture. Academic Press, London

Rosen C J, Kessenich C R 1996 Comparative clinical pharmacology and therapeutic use of bisphosphonates in metabolic bone diseases. Drugs 51(4):537–551

Schnitzler C M 1987 Osteoporosis. Sandoz Booklet Publications, Sandoz Ltd, South Africa

Sherwood L 1995 Fundamentals of physiology. A human perspective, 2nd edn. West Publishing, Minneapolis

Silberfarb P M, Holland J, Anbar D et al 1983 Psychological response of patients receiving two drug regimens for lung carcinoma. American Journal of Psychiatry 140:110–111

Simon M A 1988 Limb salvage for osteosarcoma. Journal of Bone and Joint Surgery 70A:307

Sinaki M, Mikkelson M 1984 Post-menopausal spinal osteoporosis. Flexion versus extension exercises. Archives of Physical Medicine and Rehabilitation 65:593–596

Spector T D 1990 Trends for admissions of hip fractures in England and Wales 1968–1985. British Medical Journal 300:1173–1174

Thomson D J, Hassenkamp A M, Mansbridge C 1997 The measurement of empathy in a clinical and a non-clinical setting. Does empathy increase with clinical experience? Physiotherapy 83(4):173–180

Turner P 1991 Osteoporotic back pain – its prevention and treatment. Physiotherapy 77:642–646

Vogelsang H, Ferenci P, Resch H, Kiss A, Gangl A 1995 Prevention of bone mineral loss in patients with Crohn's disease by long-term oral vitamin D supplementation. European Journal of Gastroenterology and Hepatology 7(7):609–614

Worthington J 1994 Team approach to multidisciplinary care. British Journal of Therapy and Rehabilitation 1(3):119–120

Wynne-Davies R, Fairbank T J 1976 Fairbank's atlas of general afflictions of the skeleton. Churchill Livingstone, Edinburgh

Index